T0205948

Cases in Pediatric Occupational Therapy

Assessment and Intervention

Cases in Pediatric Occupational Therapy

Assessment and Intervention

Editors

Susan M. Cahill, PhD, OTR/L
Assistant Professor
Occupational Therapy Program
Associate Director
Doctorate of Health Sciences Program
College of Health Sciences
Midwestern University
Downers Grove, Illinois

Patricia Bowyer, EdD, MS, OTR, FAOTA
Associate Director and Professor
School of Occupational Therapy-Houston
College of Health Sciences
Texas Woman's University
Texas Medical Center
Houston, Texas

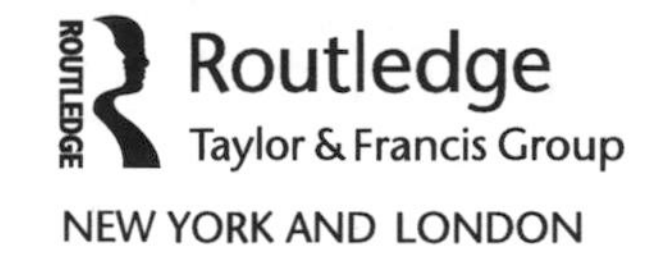

NEW YORK AND LONDON

Cases in Pediatric Occupational Therapy: Assessment and Intervention Instructor's Manual is also available. Don't miss this important companion to *Cases in Pediatric Occupational Therapy: Assessment and Intervention.* To obtain the Instructor's Manual, please visit www.routledge.com/9781617115974

First published 2015 by SLACK Incorporated

Published 2024 by Routledge
605 Third Avenue, New York, NY 10158

and by Routledge
4 Park Square, Milton Park, Abingdon, Oxon, OX14 4RN

Routledge is an imprint of the Taylor & Francis Group, an informa business

Library of Congress Cataloging-in-Publication Data

Cases in pediatric occupational therapy : assessment and intervention / editors, Susan M. Cahill, Patricia Bowye.
p. ; cm.
Includes bibliographical references and index.
ISBN 978-1-61711-597-4 (alk. paper)
I. Cahill, Susan M., editor. II. Bowyer, Patricia, editor.
[DNLM: 1. Child--Case Reports. 2. Occupational Therapy--Case Reports. 3. Disabled Children--rehabilitation--Case Reports. 4. Early Intervention (Education)--Case Reports. 5. Mentally Disabled Persons--rehabilitation--Case Reports. WS 368]
RJ53.O25
615.8'515083--dc23

2014032731

ISBN: 9781617115974 (pbk)
ISBN: 9781003522867 (ebk)

DOI: 10.4324/9781003522867

Dedication

To Charlotte and Alex; you are my joy and my best teachers.
—Susan M. Cahill, PhD, OTR/L

To Bobby, for being an extraordinary man in an ordinary world; you make the seemingly impossible possible. And for Jim and Barbara, who believed, hoped, and stood the test of time. What an inspiration!
—Patricia Bowyer, EdD, MS, OTR, FAOTA

Contents

Dedication . . . *v*
Acknowledgments . . . *xi*
About the Editors . . . *xiii*
Contributing Authors . . . *xv*
Introduction . . . *xix*

Chapter 1 The Neonatal Intensive Care Unit . . . 1
Jaylene: Prematurity/Neonatal Intensive Care Unit . . . 2
Jennifer J. Hofherr, MS, OTR/L, C/NDT
Maya: Premature Infant/Neonatal Intensive Care Unit . . . 9
Maureen Connors Lenke, OTR/L
Sam: Premature Infant/Neonatal Intensive Care Unit . . . 13
Maureen Connors Lenke, OTR/L
Marco: Premature Infant/Neonatal Intensive Care Unit . . . 16
Mary J. Greer, MOT
Pablo: Premature Infant/Neonatal Intensive Care Unit . . . 21
Sonia F. Kay, PhD, OTR/L and Marvieann Garcia-Rodriguez, MHS, BHS, OTR

Chapter 2 Introduction to Early Intervention . . . 25
Royce: Developmental Delay/Early Intervention . . . 26
Ashley Stoffel, OTD, OTR/L and M. Veronica Llerena, MS, OTR/L
Catherine: Agenesis of the Corpus Callosum/Early Intervention Transition . . . 31
Deborah K. Anderson, PT, MS, PCS
Tommy: Sensory Dysmodulation and Dyspraxia/Early Intervention . . . 33
Kimberly Bryze, PhD, OTR/L and Roberta K. O'Shea, PT, DPT, PhD
Cooper: Developmental Delay/Early Intervention . . . 38
Susan M. Cahill, PhD, OTR/L
Ricky: Developmental Delay and Sensory Processing Disorder/Early Intervention . . . 40
Robin Elaine Fogerty, OTD, OTR/L; Thelma Haydee Montemayor, MOTS; and Patricia Bowyer, EdD, MS, OTR, FAOTA

Chapter 3 Introduction to School Systems . . . 47
Denny: Autism and Attention Deficit Hyperactivity Disorder/School Systems . . . 48
Meghan Suman, MS, OTR/L, BCP
Donovan: Emotional Disturbance/Middle School . . . 54
Heather Roberts, MHA, OTR/L
Serena: At Risk for Learning and Social Emotional Disabilities/School Systems . . . 56
Susan M. Cahill, PhD, OTR/L
Kendra: Cerebral Palsy . . . 59
Robin Elaine Fogerty, OTD, OTR/L; Meagan E. Wisniewski, BS; and Patricia Bowyer, EdD, MS, OTR, FAOTA
Wilson: Learning Disability/School Systems . . . 67
Susan M. Cahill, PhD, OTR/L
Johanna: Cerebral Palsy/School Systems . . . 69
Susan M. Cahill, PhD, OTR/L
April: Autism/Private Separate Day School . . . 73
Wanda Mahoney, PhD, OTR/L
Abby: Down Syndrome/School Systems . . . 76
Mickenzie Wilson, OTS; Jennifer Clone, OTS; and Agnieszka Moroni, OTS
Gina: Cerebral Palsy/School Systems . . . 79
Minetta Wallingford, DrOT, OTR/L
Jefferson Union High School District: Sexuality and Dating Skills Training/School Systems . . . 82
Joanna Swanton, MS, OTR/L
Ozzy: Childhood Trauma With Neuromotor Sequelae . . . 84
Kimberly Bryze, PhD, OTR/L

Chapter 4 Introduction to Outpatient Services 89
Conrad: Sensory Processing Disorder, Fine- and Gross-Motor Delay/Outpatient Clinic 89
Erin Anderson, OTR/L; Michelle Bednarek, MS, OTR/L; and Melissa Williamson, OTR/L
Jacob: Sensory Processing Disorder/Outpatient Clinic 93
Dana Pais, OTD, OTR/L
Brad: Brain Tumor/Outpatient 98
Kendall Carithers, OTR and Lauro A. Munoz, OTR, MOT, CHC
Nadir: Motor Disorder/Outpatient Rehabilitation 101
Carly Thom, MA, OTR/L
Renee: CHARGE Syndrome/Outpatient. 103
Leon Washington, OTR, PhD, LMSW, C/NDT
Finn: Autism Spectrum Disorder and Feeding Concerns 106
Kristin Winston, PhD, OTR/L

Chapter 5 Introduction to Hospital-Based Settings. 109
Alexa: Pediatric Traumatic Brain Injury/Inpatient Rehabilitation 110
Sara Clark, MS, OTR/L and Jennifer Schmidt, OTR/L
Jenna: Complex Regional Pain Syndrome/Hand Therapy 114
Susanne Higgins, MHS, OTR/L, CHT and Jennifer Bobo, MOT, OTR/L, CHT
Jonathon: Pediatric Spinal Cord Injury/Rehabilitation 117
Gail A. Poskey, PhD, OTR
Martha: Spina Bifida/Hospital Clinic 120
Rachel Galant, MS, OTR/L
Liam: Acute Myeloid Leukemia, Septic Shock, Cardiac Myopathy/Oncology 123
Lisa Robken, OTR
Robby: Feeding Disorder/Hospital-Based Feeding Clinic 127
Patricia W. Ideran, OTR/L, CEIM and Jennifer L. Zieman, MOTR/L, CEIM
Lyrik: Amyoplasia Multiplex Congenita/Outpatient. 128
Angela R. Shierk, PhD, OTR
Jane: Pediatric Spinal Cord Injury/Inpatient Rehabilitation 131
Elizabeth Kohler-Rausch, OTR/L

Chapter 6 Introduction to Mental Health Settings 135
Abigail: Aggression/Inpatient Psychiatric Unit. 136
Lisa Mahaffey, MS, OTR/L, FAOTA
Tiffany: Pediatric Depression/Community-Based Mental Health 138
Brad E. Egan, OTD, MA, OTR/L and Eric Howard, COTA/L
Sophia: Early Intervention/Infant Mental Health 144
Kris Pizur-Barnekow, PhD, OTR/L; Jennifer Nash, PhD, OTR/L; Susan Wendel, MS, OTR/L; and Molly Chopper
William: Bipolar Disorder/School 148
Sally W. Schultz, PhD, OTR, LPC
James: Posttraumatic Stress Disorder/Inpatient Psychiatry. 150
Ann Aviles de Bradley, PhD, OTR/L
Emma: Anxiety Disorder/Inpatient. 153
Kristin Winston, PhD, OTR/L and Jamie Harmon, MS, OTR/L

Chapter 7 Introduction to Community Settings 155
Michael: Anoxic Brain Injury/Hippotherapy 155
Monica Griffin, OTD, OTR/L, C/NDT
Opening Doors/Community Organization. 158
Brittany Diasio, MOT, OTR/L; Brooke Nicole Dudley, MOT, OTR/L; Brianne N. Heiland, MOT, OTR/L; Elizabeth Kohler-Rausch, OTR/L; and Kiley Rich, MOT, OTR/L

Ivan: Status Post Burns and Left Lower Extremity Amputation/Village in Ecuador 163
Mark Kovic, OTD, OTR/L
La Fuente: Community-Based Parent Education and Advocacy Training in Special Education 166
Cindy DeRuiter, OTD, OTR/L
Carlos: Duchenne Muscular Dystrophy/Hospice 170
Wanda Mahoney, PhD, OTR/L

Financial Disclosures 175
Index 179

Acknowledgments

Thank you to all of the practitioners who contributed their time and expertise to the development of the cases in this book. Your passion for pediatric occupational therapy will inspire students to think critically and provide quality intervention to children. Thank you to the Midwestern University Occupational Therapy class of 2014 for your thoughtful commentary on the case materials. Finally, thank you to Brian Cahill for prioritizing this project and my work as if it were his own.

—Susan M. Cahill, PhD, OTR/L

To the children featured in the cases and their families, thank you for opening up your lives to teach others. In learning, we will all be better prepared to serve.

This book was helped along by the organizational skills of Jackson Parker and Haydee Montemayor. Thank you both for your assistance in bringing this book to fruition.

—Patricia Bowyer, EdD, MS, OTR, FAOTA

The Editors would like to acknowledge the contributions of Ashley Stoffel, M. Veronica Llerena, and Meghan Suman for their contributions to the chapter introductions for Chapters 2 and 3.

About the Editors

Susan M. Cahill, PhD, OTR/L completed her entry-level occupational therapy education at the University of Illinois at Chicago. She received a Master's Degree in Educational Leadership from Dominican University in River Forest, Illinois, and a PhD in Special Education from the University of Illinois at Chicago. Dr. Cahill has 17 years of experience as an occupational therapist, working primarily in pediatrics and the school systems. Her professional roles have included school administration, leadership of faculty, and implementation and evaluation of school-wide programs. Her research interests include supporting the occupational performance of children who are at-risk for learning and social emotional disabilities at school. Dr. Cahill is the author of many journal articles and chapters focused on pediatric occupational therapy practice and the co-author of another pediatric text. She has presented at local and national conferences and consults with many school districts.

Patricia Bowyer, EdD, MS, OTR, FAOTA is Associate Director and Professor in the School of Occupational Therapy-Houston, Institute of Health Sciences, Texas Woman's University, the Texas Medical Center. Dr. Bowyer's interests focus on increasing levels of life participation for children and youth with disabilities through the development of theory-based assessments and interventions. Dr. Bowyer is the primary developer of the Short Child Occupational Profile (SCOPE). Dr. Bowyer's research applies qualitative, quantitative, and mixed methods. Dr. Bowyer has 13 years of experience working with children and youth with disabilities. She has worked in school settings, home health, community based centers, and private practice. She received a certificate and Masters in Occupational Therapy from Eastern Kentucky University and a doctorate from East Tennessee State University. Dr. Bowyer was a postdoctoral research associate at Johns Hopkins University and a postdoctoral research assistant at the University of Illinois at Chicago in the Department of Occupational Therapy (NIDRR ARRT Grant, PI Dr. Gary Kielhofner).

Contributing Authors

Deborah K. Anderson, PT, MS, PCS (Chapter 2)
Associate Professor
Codirector of Clinical Education
Physical Therapy Program
Midwestern University College of Health Sciences
Downers Grove, Illinois

Erin Anderson, OTR/L (Chapter 4)
Owner
Erin Anderson Associates
Chicago, Illinois

Ann Aviles de Bradley, PhD, OTR/L (Chapter 6)
Assistant Professor
Department of Educational Inquiry & Curriculum Studies
Northeastern Illinois University
Chicago, Illinois

Michelle Bednarek, MS, OTR/L (Chapter 4)
Lurie Children's Hospital
Erin Anderson Associates
Chicago, Illinois

Jennifer Bobo, MOT, OTR/L, CHT (Chapter 5)
Occupational Therapist, Certified Hand Therapist
Dupage Medical Group
Naperville, Illinois

Kimberly Bryze, PhD, OTR/L (Chapters 2, 3)
Director and Associate Professor
Occupational Therapy Program
Midwestern University
Downers Grove, Illinois

Kendall Carithers, OTR (Chapter 4)
Occupational Therapist
The University of Texas M.D. Anderson Cancer Center
The Texas Medical Center
Houston, Texas

Molly Chopper (Chapter 6)
Seattle, Washington

Sara Clark, MS, OTR/L (Chapter 5)
Academic Fieldwork Coordinator
Faculty Clinical Specialist
Department of Occupational Therapy
College of Health and Human Services
Western Michigan University
Kalamazoo, Michigan

Jennifer Clone, OTS (Chapter 3)
Master of Occupational Therapy Student
Occupational Therapy Program
Midwestern University
Downers Grove, Illinois

Cindy DeRuiter, OTD, OTR/L (Chapter 7)
Easter Seals Therapeutic Day School
Chicago, Illinois

Brittany Diasio, MOT, OTR/L (Chapter 7)
Midwestern University
Downers Grove, Illinois

Brooke Nicole Dudley, MOT, OTR/L (Chapter 7)
Midwestern University
Downers Grove, Illinois

Brad E. Egan, OTD, MA, OTR/L (Chapter 6)
Assistant Professor
Occupational Therapy Program
Midwestern University
Downers Grove, Illinois

Robin Elaine Fogerty, OTD, OTR/L (Chapters 2, 3)
Doctoral Student
Texas Woman's University–Houston
Owner
New Horizons Therapy Services
Hobbs, New Mexico

Rachel Galant, MS, OTR/L (Chapter 5)
Director of Rehabilitation Services
Shriners Hospitals for Children – Chicago
Chicago, Illinois

Marvieann Garcia-Rodriguez, MHS, BHS, OTR (Chapter 1)
Clinical Specialist
Student Program Coordinator
NICU
Miami Children's Hospital
Miami, Florida

Mary J. Greer, MOT (Chapter 1)
Doctoral Student
Occupational Therapy Program
Texas Woman's University
Dallas, Texas

Monica Griffin, OTD, OTR/L, C/NDT (Chapter 7)
Occupational Therapist
BraveHearts Therapeutic Riding & Educational Center
Poplar Grove, Illinois
Arlington Pediatric Therapy Management Services, Ltd
Arlington Heights, Illinois

Jamie Harmon, MS, OTR/L (Chapter 6)
Spring Harbor Hospital
Westbrook, Maine

Brianne N. Heiland, MOT, OTR/L (Chapter 7)
Midwestern University
Downers Grove, Illinois

Susanne Higgins, MHS, OTR/L, CHT (Chapter 5)
Assistant Professor
Occupational Therapy Program
Midwestern University
Downers Grove, Illinois

Jennifer J. Hofherr, MS, OTR/L, C/NDT (Chapter 1)
PT/OT Clinical Leader–NICU
Nationwide Children's Hospital
Columbus, Ohio
NIDCAP Trainer, Children's Hospital
University of Illinois
Chicago, Illinois
Fussy Baby Network Trainer
Erikson Institute
Chicago, Illinois

Eric Howard, COTA/L (Chapter 6)
Select Rehab
Niles, Illinois

Patricia W. Ideran, OTR/L, CEIM (Chapter 5)
Pediatric Occupational Therapy
Cadence Health-Central DuPage Hospital
Winfield, Illinois

Sonia F. Kay, PhD, OTR/L (Chapter 1)
Assistant Professor
Occupational Therapy Program
Nova Southeastern University
Fort Lauderdale, Florida

Elizabeth Kohler-Rausch, OTR/L (Chapters 5, 7)
Master of Occupational Therapy
Occupational Therapy Program
Midwestern University
Downers Grove, Illinois

Mark Kovic, OTD, OTR/L (Chapter 7)
Assistant Program Director & Associate Professor
Occupational Therapy Program
Midwestern University
Downers Grove, Illinois

Maureen Connors Lenke, OTR/L (Chapter 1)
Pediatric Therapy Coordinator
Developmental and Behavioral Pediatrics
Alexian Brothers Women's and Children's Hospital
Hoffman Estates, Illinois
Co-owner, Infant Motor Performance Scales
Contract Pediatric OT
Advocate Lutheran General Children's Hospital
Park Ridge, Illinois

M. Veronica Llerena, MS, OTR/L (Chapter 2)
Occupational Therapist–Early Intervention
Adjunct Clinical Instructor
Department of Occupational Therapy
University of Illinois at Chicago
Chicago, Illinois

Lisa Mahaffey, MS, OTR/L, FAOTA (Chapter 6)
Associate Professor
Occupational Therapy Program
Midwestern University
Downers Grove, Illinois

Wanda Mahoney, PhD, OTR/L (Chapters 3, 7)
Assistant Professor
Occupational Therapy Program
Midwestern University
Downers Grove, Illinois

Thelma Haydee Montemayor, MOTS (Chapter 2)
Master of Occupational Therapy Student
Occupational Therapy Program
School of Occupational Therapy–Houston
Texas Woman's University
Houston, Texas

Agnieszka Moroni, OTS (Chapter 3)
Master of Occupational Therapy Student
Occupational Therapy Program
Midwestern University
Downers Grove, Illinois

Lauro A. Munoz, OTR, MOT, CHC (Chapter 4)
Rehabilitation Regulatory Specialist
The University of Texas M.D. Anderson Cancer Center
Texas Medical Center
Houston, Texas

Jennifer Nash, PhD, OTR/L (Chapter 6)
University of Washington
Seattle, Washington

Roberta K. O'Shea, PT, DPT, PhD (Chapter 2)
Professor
Department of Physical Therapy
Governors State University
University Park, Illinois

Dana Pais, OTD, OTR/L (Chapter 4)
North Shore Pediatric Therapy
Chicago, Illinois

Kris Pizur-Barnekow, PhD, OTR/L (Chapter 6)
Associate Professor
Department of Occupational Science and Technology
University of Wisconsin–Milwaukee
Milwaukee, Wisconsin

Gail A. Poskey, PhD, OTR (Chapter 5)
Assistant Professor
School of Occupational Therapy
Texas Woman's University
Denton, Texas

Kiley Rich, MOT, OTR/L (Chapter 7)
Midwestern University
Downers Grove, Illinois

Heather Roberts, MHA, OTR/L (Chapter 3)
Occupational Therapist
Denton, Texas

Lisa Robken, OTR (Chapter 5)
Occupational Therapist
Shriner's Hospital for Children
Houston, Texas

Jennifer Schmidt, OTR/L (Chapter 5)
Allied Health Manager–Pediatrics
Rehabilitation Institute of Chicago
Chicago, Illinois

Sally W. Schultz, PhD, OTR, LPC (Chapter 6)
Professor and Coordinator, PhD in OT Program
School of Occupational Therapy
Texas Woman's University
Dallas, Texas

Angela R. Shierk, PhD, OTR (Chapter 5)
Occupational Therapist
Texas Scottish Rite Hospital for Children
Dallas, Texas

Ashley Stoffel, OTD, OTR/L (Chapter 2)
Clinical Assistant Professor
Department of Occupational Therapy
University of Illinois at Chicago
Chicago, Illinois

Meghan Suman, MS, OTR/L, BCP (Chapter 3)
Occupational Therapy Coordinator
AOTA Board Certified Pediatric Specialist
Indian Prairie School District
Aurora, Illinois

Joanna Swanton, MS, OTR/L (Chapter 3)
Jefferson Union High School District
Daly City, California

Carly Thom, MA, OTR/L (Chapter 4)
Occupational Therapist III
TIRR Memorial Hermann Adult and Pediatric Rehabilitation
Houston, Texas

Minetta Wallingford, DrOT, OTR/L (Chapter 3)
Assistant Professor and Academic Fieldwork Coordinator
Midwestern Occupational Therapy Program
Downers Grove, Illinois

Leon Washington, OTR, PhD, LMSW, C/NDT (Chapter 4)
Owner, Kidz and Caregivers at Heart, PC
Humble, Texas

Susan Wendel, MS, OTR/L (Chapter 6)
Center on Human Development and Disability
University of Washington
Seattle, Washington

Melissa Williamson, OTR/L (Chapter 4)
Early Intervention Provider
Erin Anderson Associates
Chicago, Illinois

Mickenzie Wilson, OTS (Chapter 3)
Master of Occupational Therapy Student
Occupational Therapy Program
Midwestern University
Downers Grove, Illinois

Kristin Winston, PhD, OTR/L (Chapters 4, 6)
Director, PhD Program
Assistant Professor
Occupational Therapy Program
Nova Southeastern University
Fort Lauderdale, Florida

Meagan E. Wisniewski, BS (Chapter 3)
Master of Occupational Therapy Student
Occupational Therapy Program
School of Occupational Therapy–Houston
Texas Woman's University
Houston, Texas

Jennifer L. Ziemann, MOTR/L, CEIM (Chapter 5)
Pediatric Occupational Therapy
Cadence Health–Central Dupage Hospital
Winfield, Illinois

Introduction

Cases in Pediatric Occupational Therapy: Assessment and Intervention is designed to provide occupational therapy instructors and students with a comprehensive collection of case studies that reflect the scope of current pediatric occupational therapy practice. Currently, instructors are forced to enter into the time-consuming and lengthy process of referring to multiple resources to learn about different practice settings, develop their own case studies, and identify and collect relevant resources to support their cases. *Cases in Pediatric Occupational Therapy: Assessment and Intervention* eliminates this need by providing real-world examples of scenarios written by clinicians with experience in their practice settings. In addition, supplemental information, photographs, and video clips help to bring the cases to life.

This text is organized by practice setting. Each section begins with an introduction to the practice setting and directs instructors and students to additional resources for more information. Each case includes an overview of the client, relevant history and background information, information regarding the analysis of occupational performance, information about progress in treatment, as well as questions to guide clinical reasoning about the case. Supplemental information for each chapter is located on efacultylounge.com and can be downloaded for the instructor's use.

CHAPTER 1

The Neonatal Intensive Care Unit

The neonatal intensive care unit (NICU) is a highly specialized area of occupational therapy practice that requires advanced knowledge, skills, and expertise. The primary function of the NICU is to provide the necessary medical support for physiologically compromised infants. Occupational therapists (OTs) who work in the NICU provide developmentally supportive care to infants once they are medically stable (Hunter, 2010). OTs coach other medical professionals and the infant's parents on issues related to therapeutic positioning and feeding. In addition, OTs in the NICU may perform range of motion and infant massage and fabricate orthotics.

As in other areas of pediatric practice, OTs in the NICU are concerned with providing child-focused and family-centered care. OTs understand how the NICU experience influences attachment, family relationships, and the development of co-occupations. OTs working in this practice setting must be versed in theory related to infant mental health, early social emotional development, coping, and families.

It is recommended that clinicians interested in working in the NICU have previous pediatric experience. An extensive knowledge of development, both pre- and postnatal, as well as neurobehavioral organization is critical. Previous hospital experience is also beneficial because OTs with this experience will have prior knowledge of different medical procedures and equipment.

Role of Occupational Therapy in the Neonatal Intensive Care Unit

OTs work with the medical team to support and build the family's capacity to care for their infant while he or she is in the hospital and in preparation for his or her discharge to home. The Occupational Therapy Process can be used to guide practice in the NICU. Close collaboration with the family and medical team is crucial throughout this process. According to the American Occupational Therapy Association (2006), some of the specific skills that OTs perform in the NICU include the following:

- Educating parents and medical team members
- Performing assessments (e.g., motor function, pain, neurobehavioral organization)
- Evaluating factors of the physical environment and how these factors influence the infant's ability to maintain homeostasis
- Developing individual plans of care that support development and optimize opportunities for caregiver interaction
- Observing the infant's reaction to care routines and recommending adjustments
- Incorporating occupational therapy services into existing care routines
- Making recommendations for discharge

The need to provide specialized care to a medically fragile infant is in constant conflict with the infant's need to grow and develop in a safe and stress-free environment. One of the critical roles of the OT is preventing and addressing mismatches between the infant and the complex NICU environment (AOTA, 2006; Hunter, 2010). The OT engages in a systematic analysis of the multitude of environmental factors and attends to how the infant responds to each factor. The therapist then recommends how environmental factors can be adapted or modified to reduce the infant's stress. For example, an OT might consider the timing of nursing procedures as well as the frequency and intensity of the handling used by the staff to perform such procedures. The OT might also make

Cahill SM, Bowyer P, eds. *Cases in Pediatric Occupational Therapy: Assessment and Intervention (pp 1-24).*

recommendations associated with visual and auditory properties of the environment.

The NICU is an advanced area of practice for OTs. Specialized knowledge and skills are essential to working in this context. OTs who are interested in working in this area of practice should have experience in pediatrics as well as in medical settings. In addition, it is highly recommended that they receive additional specialized training.

Questions to Consider

1. Why is the NICU considered an advanced area of practice?
2. What types of knowledge and skills are needed to work in the NICU?
3. Review the AOTA (2006) paper on specialized knowledge and skills for work in the NICU. Reflect on what knowledge and skills you feel are unique to practice in the NICU compared with other areas of pediatric practice.

References

American Occupational Therapy Association. (2006). Specialized knowledge and skills for practice in the neonatal intensive care unit. *American Journal of Occupational Therapy, 60*(6), 659-668.

Hunter, J. (2010). Neonatal intensive care unit. In J. Case-Smith & J. O'Brien (Eds.), *Occupational therapy for children* (pp. 649-677). Maryland Heights, MI: Mosby.

Jaylene: Prematurity/ Neonatal Intensive Care Unit

Jennifer J. Hofherr, MS, OTR/L, C/NDT

History and Background Information

Jaylene was born on February 7, 29 weeks and 3 days into her mother's pregnancy. Her mother, Irene, was 19 years old and attended community college, and her father, Paul, also 19 years old, was going to school for his high school diploma. Irene was due to deliver on April 22, but on January 29 she developed high blood pressure and was admitted to the hospital for treatment. Irene was readmitted to the hospital on February 5, again with increased blood pressure. Ultrasound pictures of the baby showed that Jaylene was very small for her age. Jaylene's heart rate began to slow and a decision was made to deliver her by cesarean section. At birth, Jaylene's score of well-being (Apgar score) was 7 out of 10 at 1 minute and 9 out of 10 at 5 minutes. Jaylene weighed just 1 pound, 10 ounces (753 g), which is at the 4th percentile for infants at Jaylene's gestational age. She measured 12.5 inches (32 cm; < 3rd percentile) and had a head size of 9.5 inches (25 cm; 9th percentile).

Jaylene had some difficulty breathing right after she was born. She was placed on a ventilator via an endotracheal tube placed down her mouth and throat to assist her breathing and was given Survanta (beractant) to lubricate the tissue in her lungs because this is typically underdeveloped in premature infants. Jaylene was admitted to the NICU, which was on the same floor as the labor and delivery suite and also was adjacent to the postpartum care unit for mothers and babies.

The NICU at University Hospital has two large, rectangular care rooms. Between the two care rooms is the main entrance, where families ring a buzzer to be let into the locked unit. A reception desk stands a few steps past the entry, along with a bathroom and a small white sink for families to wash their hands and put on blue paper gowns to cover their clothing. A 6-foot-high wall divides each care room in half lengthwise. Up to 12 babies are cared for in each room. A long counter with phones, computers, and binders stands at the front of the room, where NICU staff document and discuss patient care. There are also two white sinks and a counter with a small refrigerator at the front of each room where breast milk is kept. A row of uncovered windows along the top of the south wall in each room opens onto a corridor, from which sunshine streams through outer windows and into the care rooms. At each bed space, incubators stand perpendicular to the outer and inner dividing walls of the room. Above the beds, monitors stand on shelves and various pieces of medical equipment stand near the beds. Rocking chairs and recliners are scattered throughout the room. On a typical day, the room is quite busy with doctors doing rounds, specialists conducting assessments, and nurses providing care using normal speaking voices. At times, the nurses raise their voices to request assistance or to relay information to one another across the room. The sounds of monitors beeping, medication pumps alarming, breathing machines humming, oxygen and heating/cooling systems hissing, infants crying, and phones ringing are constant.

Paul came into the NICU to see Jaylene for a few moments after her birth and Irene saw Jaylene on the second day, when her nurse helped her walk down to the NICU. After 2 days on the ventilator, Jaylene was strong enough to breathe on her own without any assistance. By the fourth day, she no longer required any additional oxygen but still received some extra flow of room air through a small set of plastic nasal prongs. Irene was able to pump and provide some milk for Jaylene before being discharged home to her mother's house on the fourth day. On the fifth day, Jaylene's phototherapy treatment for jaundice, a common condition in premature infants due to the immaturity of the liver, was stopped and she was started on small amounts of her mother's breast milk—in addition to the intravenous fluid and nutrition she had been receiving—through a nasogastric (NG) feeding tube, which is a very narrow tube that goes into one of the nostrils, down the esophagus, and into the stomach. Occupational therapy received a referral to evaluate and treat Jaylene on the sixth day of life. On that day, Jaylene was 30 weeks and 2 days old postconception. Jaylene was one of 11 babies in the west care room; her bed was on the left side of the room from the doorway under the windows with the sunshine streaming through.

Evaluation Information

Jaylene's OT reviewed the medical record and queried the nurse on duty about what it was like for her to take care of Jaylene. The nurse, Cathy, noted that Jaylene had been stable and doing well. Cathy shared that Irene planned to stay at home for several days before coming in again because she wanted to rest after the c-section. Jaylene's father, Paul, had been stopping by for just a few minutes each day to bring the small amounts of breast milk that Irene was pumping at home. The OT and Cathy planned on a time later that day when she could observe Jaylene before, during, and after a planned care time using the Newborn Individualized Developmental Care and Assessment Program (NIDCAP) naturalistic observation method.

The OT returned at the planned time and began to observe Jaylene and her environment. A pink plaid blanket covered the top of Jaylene's incubator to help protect her from the overhead lights. Inside the incubator, Jaylene lay on a soft foam mattress covered with a flowered flannel blanket and surrounded by a white blanket rolled into a "U" shape. Jaylene lay slightly turned to the right side with her arms folded across her chest. She wore a small fitted diaper and her legs were crossed and tucked up to her belly. The blanket roll provided a boundary below her bottom that supported her in this position. A pole with three machines used to deliver medications, fluids, and nutrition stood next to her incubator. Small, flexible plastic tubes led from the machines to a small opening at the head of Jaylene's incubator. IV tubes entered her left arm and were taped carefully into place. The NG tube entered her left nostril to provide breast milk directly into her stomach. The end of this short tube was attached to a small, empty syringe that hung from the top of the roof of the incubator. Three small patches with wires placed on her chest and abdomen connected Jaylene to a monitor that kept track of her breathing and heart rate. A special glowing piece of tape wrapped around her right foot measured the amount of oxygen in her blood. A pink pacifier lay at the foot of her incubator and a pillow with the words "angel sleeping" lay at the head of her bed. A pink name card with stenciled pictures was taped onto the front of her incubator. Several alarms sounded throughout the room, staff busily moved around, and the sunlight brightened the room, creating a pink glow inside Jaylene's incubator through the lightweight blanket that lay on top.

Jaylene was observed for 30 minutes before her nursing care interaction. She appeared to be sleeping lightly and comfortably, yet her face looked pale and her breathing sped up and slowed down frequently. Her heartbeat was steady at 129 beats per minute. The level of oxygen in her blood also was steady at a saturation of 99%. For the first 10 minutes, Jaylene maintained her curled up position and moved only to squirm briefly and kick her right leg over the blanket roll. At times, sound in the room peaked sharply and Jaylene responded by twitching, sighing, and squirming more. After each squirm, Jaylene tucked herself back into a little ball and put her hands near or on her mouth. The level of sound in the room was steady, with frequent bursts from alarms ringing, doors closing, and staff members directing questions across the room. Jaylene breathed rapidly and her face paled with each burst of sound. When she squirmed, her face turned red and she stuck out her tongue, yawned, and frowned. Her legs stretched upward as she straightened her knees. She tried to kick her left leg but the blanket roll prevented her from stretching out her hips, so she kept stretching her feet up into her face. Jaylene grasped at her feeding tube and made sucking movements with her tongue. She covered her eyes with her right arm and was able to lie quietly for a moment. She then breathed quickly and turned her body by stretching her head to the left. Each time she squirmed and stretched her feet into her face, she grimaced and struggled to reposition herself. She alerted a bit toward the end of the 30 minutes, just before Cathy arrived at her bedside.

Cathy and one of the doctors approached Jaylene's incubator while discussing her care. Cathy was briefly distracted as she opened the little doors to Jaylene's incubator. Cathy placed a small plastic thermometer under Jaylene's left arm and put one hand on Jaylene's head and then the other on her left arm. Jaylene lay quietly but appeared tense, with her hands fisted, her left leg cramped into the blanket roll, her face dark, and hiccupping. When Cathy lifted her hands to get the stethoscope, Jaylene arched her back and breathed rapidly at 197 beats per minute. Cathy quickly lifted Jaylene up the mattress about 4 inches by grasping her by her hips and shoulders and tucking her body further into a ball as she lifted. Jaylene did not move but continued to hiccup, and her face alternated between pale and dark. Cathy used the stethoscope to listen to Jaylene's stomach as she pushed some air into the feeding tube and checked its placement in her stomach. Cathy then turned Jaylene so that she now lay on her back for a diaper change. Jaylene continued to hiccup and was pale. Her legs could now extend and she thrust them into the air for a moment then tucked them back close to her body. Cathy gently but quickly replaced the diaper by lifting Jaylene's hips slightly. Cathy moved the glowing oxygen monitor strip from Jaylene's right foot to the left. Cathy again scooted Jaylene up the bed a few inches and turned her to her left side. Jaylene's face turned dark after being moved; she arched her back and struggled to catch her breath. Cathy wiped Jaylene's mouth and then offered her the pink pacifier. Jaylene still had the hiccups and did not suck on the pacifier. Her squirms a few moments earlier had dislodged the glowing oxygen strip and Cathy rewrapped it onto her foot. Cathy again offered the pacifier, but now Jaylene turned her head away and extended her neck. Cathy scooted her up the bed once again and then held her by the head, shoulders, and upper back with her left hand as she repositioned the blanket under her with her right hand. Jaylene's face paled, her body became limp, and she continued to hiccup. Cathy laid her down on her left side and walked away for 2 minutes. Jaylene appeared tired; her arms remained limp and her face paled even more. After resting for a minute, Jaylene twitched, squirmed, and used her right hand to grab onto her face. She breathed rapidly, then held her breathing as she tried to turn her head back to the right. Cathy returned to her incubator with a small syringe of breast milk that she attached to Jaylene's feeding tube without touching Jaylene. As soon as the milk began to drip into her stomach, Jaylene mouthed her lips and tongue and her face was pink for a moment. The tube brushed her arm as Cathy attached the syringe back to the rubber band hanging from the roof of the incubator. Jaylene responded by squirming slightly, frowning, and then smiling briefly. Cathy then closed the doors to her incubator and turned away.

Jaylene squirmed and tucked her body into the roll of blankets. She stuck out her tongue, yawned, and then frowned as she struggled to stretch out her legs. She breathed quickly and her face looked dark. She sighed and relaxed with her hands on her face. She twitched once, then covered her eyes with her right arm and remained still. Her breathing paused and then quickened. Jaylene's room quieted and she appeared to be steadying her breathing pattern. Twice an alarm beeped suddenly; Jaylene twitched and breathed quickly in response. She lay on her left side with her right shoulder extended behind her body and with her arms folded across her chest and her legs tucked into her body. As the observation ended, Jaylene appeared to be tired, her posture was somewhat tense and limp, and she remained in a light sleep.

The OT thanked Cathy for allowing her to observe Jaylene and her care and asked Cathy what it was like to take care of Jaylene this time. Cathy replied that she had felt more hurried than she would have liked because she knew that a new admission was coming soon that would be on her caseload. "That baby doesn't like to be touched so I wasn't sure if going faster would be better for her anyway but I guess not, she seemed pretty worn out at the end." Cathy also commented that she was surprised that Jaylene didn't take the pacifier because she'd been able to soothe her easily before with the pacifier. The OT shared her observations that Jaylene had many strengths, such as an ability to keep her body tucked in tightly as if she was still in the womb, as well as some nice mouthing movements. These skills seemed to help her remain relaxed; however, she was very sensitive to bursts of sound in the room and perhaps the overhead lights. The OT shared that Jaylene's bedding helped her keep this tucked position, but it may have been too restrictive when she wanted to stretch. The OT confirmed Cathy's assessment that Jaylene was sensitive to touch and movement. She also shared what she had seen in terms of how the activity and handling appeared to upset her breathing pattern, from which it took her a long time to recover. Cathy and the OT also noted that Jaylene seemed aware of the breast milk stimulating her stomach, and she responded with mouthing movements to this input. Because of the impending admission, the OT and Cathy agreed to meet toward the end of the day to discuss goals and recommendations.

The OT documented the assessment in a narrative format according to the NIDCAP approach and created a bedside summary to review with the staff (Figure 1-1). Copies of both the NIDCAP assessment report and the bedside summary were placed in the parent binder at the bedside so that the parents could take them home and share with other family members.

Occupational Therapy Intervention and Recommendations

Later in the afternoon, the OT met with Cathy to collaborate on the goals and recommendations for Jaylene's care. The OT and Cathy agreed that Jaylene appeared to be working toward the following:

1. Breathing more steadily when on her own and particularly when she was cared for
2. Stretching and practicing smoother movements when uncomfortable
3. Keeping her energy level up when cared for
4. Using tucking and sucking movements as strategies to achieve and maintain regulation

Together, they thought through recommendations that might help Jaylene be more successful in staying regulated, both between and during care sessions. They also thought and wondered together about Irene and Paul's experience and how the care team might support both their participation and the important parent-infant bond.

The OT again thanked Cathy for her time and input, then wrote up the following recommendations to add to the care plan:

Neurodevelopmental and Behavioral Assessment (Infants less than 32 weeks)

Name: Jaylene **GA at Birth**: 29 weeks, 3 days	**DOB**: February 7 **Birth Weight**: 756 grams (1 pound, 10 oz)
Date of Assessment: February 13 **Current Post-Menstrual Age**: 30 weeks	**Current Weight**: 756 grams **Developmental Specialist**: Jennifer Hofherr, OTR/L

Infant's Current Medical Status:

Respiratory support: none **Meds: caffeine** **Head U/S: WNL** **Phototherapy: d/c**

Bed type: incubator **Nutrition by: IV/NG** **Other:**

Vital Signs:	**HR: 150**	**RR: 60-70**	**Oxygen Sat: 95%**	**Comments:**

Attempts to Self-Calm/Regulate by:

☒ **Sucking/suck searching** ☒ **Body tucking** ☐ Grasping ☒ **Hands to face/mouth** ☐ Bracing one leg against the other

Baby shows stress in the following ways:

☐ Low-keyed responses
- ☐ Minimal arousal
- ☒ **Periods of lower tone**
- ☒ **Breathing pauses/shallow breathing**
- ☐ Subtle color changes
- ☒ **Twitches/tremors**

☐ Energetic responses
- ☐ Frequent state changes, irritability
- ☒ **Muscle tension: finger splays, leg/arm extensions**
- ☒ **Grunting, hiccups**
- ☒ **High fluctuations in RR, HR, and/or color**
- ☐ Yawns, sneezes

When does baby become moderately upset (can no longer calm himself or herself)?

____|______X____________|____________________|____________________|____________________

Environmental disturbances (light, sounds)	Light touch (unwrapping, temperature taking, changing sat probe)	Moderate touch (diaper or position change, feeding)	Painful/abrupt touch (heelstick, NG insertion, suctioning)

Minimal amount of support needed to regain or maintain relative regulation:

____|________________X__|____________________|____________________|____________________

Care needs to be very slow with two people and long delays between care tasks or with prolonged skin to skin care	Care should be done with two people, some pacing, and delay of tasks; Good support of posture	One person can care for infant with frequent short breaks and good postural support, or two people can care for infant with fewer breaks	One person can care for infant with containment; some pacing boundaries at rest	Infant self-soothes, uses pacifier, and can hold a flexed midline position; able to go back to sleep

Functional Goals for infants less than 32 weeks gestation currently:

1. On current medical support, infant can maintain heart rate, breathing, skin color, and oxygen level while sleeping:

   ______|____________|____________|X______________|______________
   Does easily — at times — beginning to show ability — not yet — not assessed

2. Infant can maintain muscle tone while relaxed, and when awake or being handled, keeps tone within moderately hypertonic and hypotonic ranges.

   ______|____________|____________|________X________|______________
   Does easily — at times — beginning to show ability — not yet — not assessed

3. Infant can make use of calming strategies offered to him/her, such as a pacifier, grasping, boundaries, etc and can calm self from a moderately disorganized state.

   ______|____________|____________|__________X______|______________
   Does easily — at times — beginning to show ability — not yet — not assessed

4. The infant shows some interest in social interaction.

   ______|____________|____________|________________|______X________
   Does easily — at times — beginning to show ability — not yet — not assessed

5. The infant can change state (from sleep to wake and back to sleep) without significantly compromising his or her heart rate, breathing pattern, color, muscle tone, or other parameters.

   ______|____________|____________|________X________|______________
   Does easily — at times — beginning to show ability — not yet — not assessed

Figure 1-1. NIDCAP Approach Summary. *(continued)*

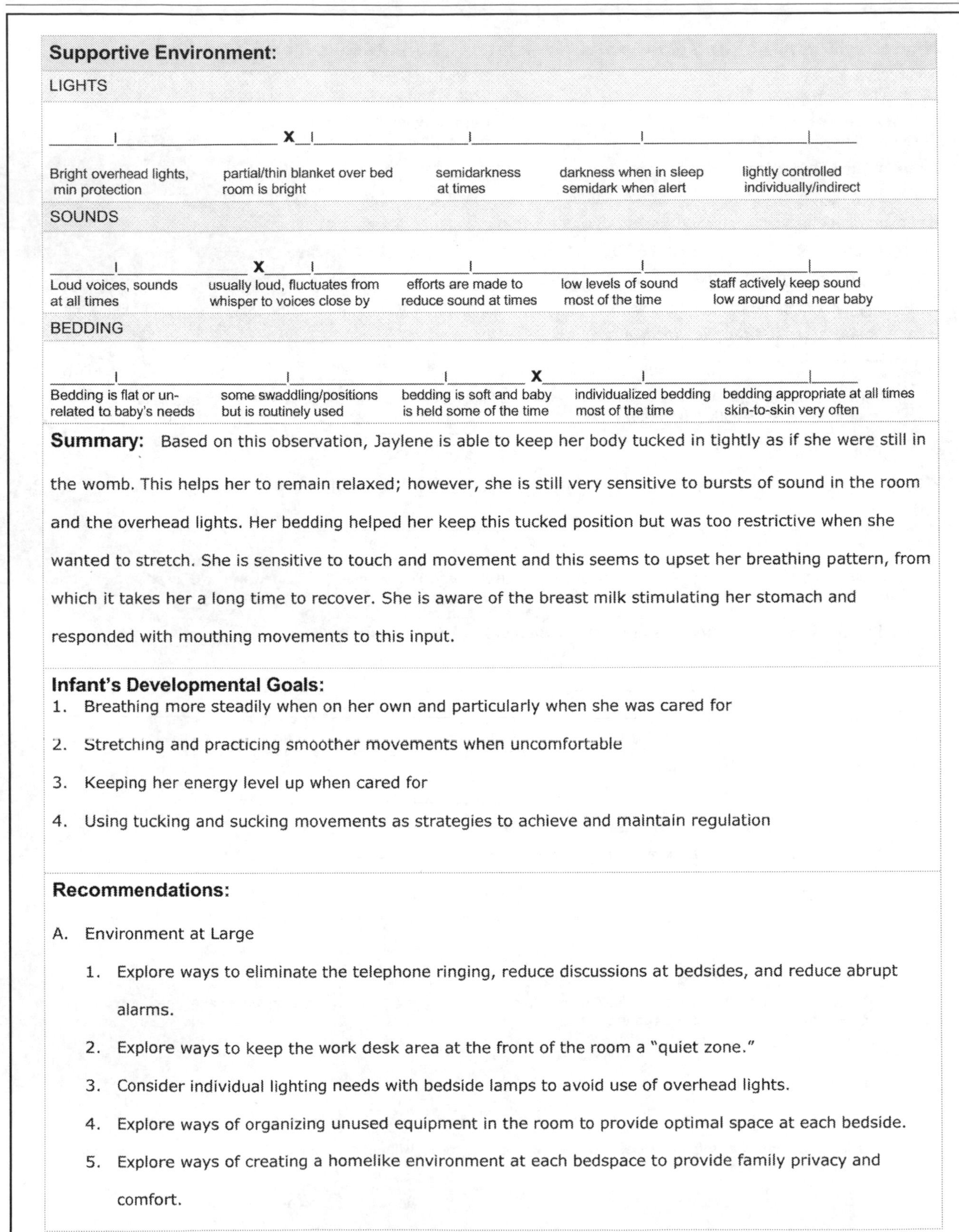

Supportive Environment:

LIGHTS

________|____________________X__|____________________|____________________|____________________|_____

Bright overhead lights, min protection	partial/thin blanket over bed room is bright	semidarkness at times	darkness when in sleep semidark when alert	lightly controlled individually/indirect

SOUNDS

________|________________X_____|____________________|____________________|____________________|_____

Loud voices, sounds at all times	usually loud, fluctuates from whisper to voices close by	efforts are made to reduce sound at times	low levels of sound most of the time	staff actively keep sound low around and near baby

BEDDING

________|____________________|____________________|_________X__________|____________________|_____

Bedding is flat or unrelated to baby's needs	some swaddling/positions but is routinely used	bedding is soft and baby is held some of the time	individualized bedding most of the time	bedding appropriate at all times skin-to-skin very often

Summary: Based on this observation, Jaylene is able to keep her body tucked in tightly as if she were still in the womb. This helps her to remain relaxed; however, she is still very sensitive to bursts of sound in the room and the overhead lights. Her bedding helped her keep this tucked position but was too restrictive when she wanted to stretch. She is sensitive to touch and movement and this seems to upset her breathing pattern, from which it takes her a long time to recover. She is aware of the breast milk stimulating her stomach and responded with mouthing movements to this input.

Infant's Developmental Goals:

1. Breathing more steadily when on her own and particularly when she was cared for
2. Stretching and practicing smoother movements when uncomfortable
3. Keeping her energy level up when cared for
4. Using tucking and sucking movements as strategies to achieve and maintain regulation

Recommendations:

A. Environment at Large
   1. Explore ways to eliminate the telephone ringing, reduce discussions at bedsides, and reduce abrupt alarms.
   2. Explore ways to keep the work desk area at the front of the room a "quiet zone."
   3. Consider individual lighting needs with bedside lamps to avoid use of overhead lights.
   4. Explore ways of organizing unused equipment in the room to provide optimal space at each bedside.
   5. Explore ways of creating a homelike environment at each bedspace to provide family privacy and comfort.

Figure 1-1 (continued). NIDCAP Approach Summary. *(continued)*

B. Bedspace and Bedding

1. Consider using a heavier, fitted incubator cover to block out light inside Jaylene's bed.
2. Consider asking Jaylene's parents to bring in a small soft cloth with their scent on it to give Jaylene a calming, familiar smell to rely on when they are not present.
3. Consider creating a bedding nest that supports Jaylene's ability to keep her body nicely tucked while still allowing her some freedom of movement.
4. Consider covering Jaylene in a light blanket to help her feel relaxed and supported from all sides while helping her maintain good trunk, head, and limb alignment.

C. Caregiving Interaction

1. Consider observing Jaylene between and before care interactions as an opportunity to let Jaylene communicate how sensitive or relaxed she may be at the moment.
2. Consider gathering all materials and supplies you plan to use for your caregiving before opening the incubator.
3. Consider using supportive measures such as containment and sucking as a response to Jaylene's own communications instead of routinely.
4. Consider that Jaylene uses tucking and sucking as signs that she is feeling regulated and use these strategies to guide the pace of care.
5. Consider holding Jaylene or staying with her as her feeding goes into her stomach so you can observe her response to this stimulation and offer the pacifier if she is ready.
6. Consider Jaylene's response to changes in position and explore ways of bedding her that will require less movement during the care interaction. For example, the bedding roll required lifting Jaylene's hips up higher in order to place the diaper under her bottom.
7. Consider inviting Paul, when he comes to drop off milk, to support Jaylene when it is time for her care. Offer him a simple task such as holding her hand to help him gain confidence that his touch will be healing for Jaylene.
8. Encourage both parents to provide skin-to-skin holding ("Kangaroo care") and explain the benefits of this care for baby's weight gain, steadying of vital signs, Irene's milk supply, and as a chance for the family to experience relaxation and closeness despite the hectic and stressful NICU environment.

Plan: OT will provide direct intervention, consultation, collaboration, and parent education two to three times per week to address functional goals and provide support to Jaylene's care team.

Figure 1-1 (continued). NIDCAP Approach Summary.

After documenting in the electronic medical record and leaving the assessment and care plan at Jaylene's bedside, the OT called Irene to introduce herself and shared with her the observations that were made about Jaylene's strengths and challenges. Irene was quiet and did not offer much information or response to the OT's comments and questions. The OT asked, "How has this experience been for you?" Irene seemed to choke back tears and replied, "Really hard, I just want her to be home with me." The OT empathized with her feeling and acknowledged that dealing with her own C-section recovery must be additionally very challenging. "Yes, it is, but I'm just afraid to see Jaylene with all of those wires and tubes." Again, the OT acknowledged Irene's feelings and asked, "What would be helpful for you when you come to be with Jaylene here?" Irene was silent for a moment and then sighed, "I don't know, I just need to be there for her. It's going to be hard, but I need to just do it. That's what my mom has been telling me all week! I know she's right." The OT concluded the conversation with an invitation to meet her the following day in the NICU. Irene accepted the invitation and thanked the OT for the call.

On the following day, the OT met again with Cathy, the nurse, who had asked to be a primary nurse for Jaylene. The OT shared that Irene was planning to come in after noon. Cathy had swapped the light incubator cover for a thicker one that more fully covered the hood and sides of Jaylene's incubator. The OT and Cathy moved a recliner into place next to Jaylene's bed. The OT peeked in at Jaylene, who she saw was resting quietly in a soft nest of blankets, a pacifier resting in her mouth. Cathy shared that she had paid attention to Jaylene's sensitivities during the care time and made sure that she paced the care more slowly. "What was that like for you?" the OT asked. Cathy replied that she felt good about going a bit slower and focusing on keeping Jaylene calm during the care without tiring her. "It was kind of like a little challenge for myself. But I know that there are times when I will feel rushed, so I don't know about doing that all the time." The OT empathized with Cathy that she had many tasks and responsibilities that are common barriers to providing the ideal environment for Jaylene and other babies in the NICU. The OT reminded her that whenever possible those regulating experiences that she and Jaylene had shared earlier still had a positive impact on the development of the brain. Cathy sighed and said, "I should try and remember that more often."

Later in the day, Cathy paged the OT to let her know that Irene and Paul had arrived. The OT met both parents at the bedside. Irene sat stiffly in the recliner, holding a swaddled Jaylene in her arms. Paul stood at the foot of the incubator, some distance from the pair. The OT greeted the new parents warmly and noticed their discomfort. "How does it feel for you to hold her like that?" she asked. Irene said that she felt nervous but that she felt really happy because Jaylene had peeked at her, then fell asleep. "Maybe she knows that I'm here and she can relax." The OT smiled and concurred. The OT then turned to Paul and asked him what it was like to be there. Paul shrugged and looked away. "Some parents tell me what mixed feelings they have when their baby is in the NICU," the OT said gently. Paul nodded, looking down at his feet. The OT then showed them the bedside baby journal and where to find the assessment and care plan, a diary, growth chart, and other resources to use while in the NICU with Jaylene. The OT highlighted a few of the recommendations, including skin-to-skin holding. Irene appeared interested in this but declined trying it that day. The OT gave the parents her contact information, congratulated them on the birth of their beautiful baby, and left them to enjoy some time alone with her. As the OT left, Paul stepped closer to Irene and leaned down to lightly touch Jaylene's head.

Questions to Consider

1. What are some examples of cues that Jaylene gave when she was anxious or overwhelmed?
2. What are some examples of cues that Jaylene gave when she was content?
3. What aspects of the care routine were particularly stressful for Jaylene?
4. Compare and contrast the care Cathy provided before and after the OT evaluation.
5. Describe reasons why it might be difficult for Cathy to implement the OT's suggestions.
6. Which other professionals would benefit from learning about the OT's recommendations?
7. What strategies and techniques could the OT use to convey the recommendations to Jaylene's parents?
8. If the OT had only had 30 minutes to spend with Jaylene's parents, which recommendations should be prioritized and why?
9. Search the Internet for examples of positioning equipment that could be used to facilitate an optimal resting position for Jaylene.
10. Describe how a homelike environment at each infant's bedspace would look.
11. Describe additional ways that the OT could support Jaylene's parents.

Resources

Als, H. (1998). Developmental care in the newborn intensive care unit. *Current Opinion in Pediatrics, 10*(2), 138-142.

American Occupational Therapy Association. (2006). Specialized knowledge and skills for practice in the neonatal intensive care unit. *American Journal of Occupational Therapy, 60*(6), 659-668.

Gilkerson, L., Hofherr, J., Steir, A., Cook, A., Arbel, A., Heffron, M., ... Paul, J. (2012). Implementing the fussy baby network approach. *Zero to Three, 33*(2), 59-65.

Hunter, J. (2010). Neonatal intensive care unit. In J. Case-Smith & J. O'Brien (Eds.), *Occupational therapy for children* (6th ed.). (pp. 649-680). St. Louis: Elsevier. www.nidcap.org

McAnulty, G. B., Butler, S. C., Bernstein, J. H., Als, H., Duffy, F. H., & Zurakowski, D. (2010). Effects of the newborn individualized developmental care and assessment program (NIDCAP) at age 8 years: Preliminary data. *Clinical Pediatrics, 49*(3), 258-270.

Maya: Premature Infant/ Neonatal Intensive Care Unit

Maureen Connors Lenke, OTR/L

History and Background Information

Maya was born at 24 and 6/7 weeks gestation to a 32-year-old mother via cesarean section with a birth weight of 1 pound, 7 ounces (639 g). Her mother had premature rupture of membranes on December 7 and was given antibiotics and steroids to delay the onset of labor. She was hospitalized and put on bed rest. Complications during pregnancy included gestational diabetes and insulin-dependent diabetes. Maya was born on January 3 and spent 41 days in a Level III NICU. The Level III NICU is an environment that provides highly specialized care to infants requiring complex medical care, mechanical ventilator support, specialized nursing, advanced diagnostic services, or surgical care. Maya was discharged on April 27 at 41 weeks gestation, day of life 114, with a weight of 7 pounds, 2 ounces (3270 g).

Medical problems/presenting concerns during Maya's NICU hospitalization included the following:

- Nutrition: Maya initially required an umbilical venous catheter and peripherally inserted catheter for parenteral nutrition. NG feeds were begun January 26; she then advanced to bottle and breastfeeding. Maya went home on ad lib demand feeds with consistent weight gain.
- Bronchopulmonary dysplasia: Maya was intubated in the delivery room, given surfactant one time, and was on a ventilator for 1 month. She received albuterol, Pulmicort (budesonide), and a 5-day course of Decadron (dexamethasone) to promote lung maturity. She was extubated to high-flow nasal cannula (HFNC) on February 8 and tolerated weaning to a nasal cannula on March 23. She was placed on room air on April 19. She was treated with Pulmicort, Aldactone (spironolactone), and Diuril (chlorothiazide), which were discontinued on April 11. She required continued evaluation by a pulmonologist.
- Sepsis: Maya was initially treated with 7 days of vancomycin and cefotaxime for clinical deterioration, which were discontinued following negative blood cultures.
- Maya developed late-onset group B streptococcus as she was preparing for discharge home. She was treated with 14 days of ampicillin and 7 days of gentamicin with a consult from pediatric infectious disease.
- Hyperbilirubinemia: Maya was treated with phototherapy for 1 week, with a peak bilirubin of 7.4.
- Neurologic: Head ultrasounds on January 7, January 17, and February 7 revealed no intracranial hemorrhage.
- Patent ductus arteriosus (PDA): Maya received two courses of Indocin (indomethacin) and underwent a PDA ligation on January 19.
- Apnea: Maya was treated with caffeine, which was discontinued on March 18.
- Hyperglycemia: Maya was hyperglycemic while on Decadron and needed to be treated with insulin.
- Anemia of prematurity: Maya required blood transfusions due to anemia.
- Retinopathy of prematurity: Maya had repeated eye exams because she was at high risk due to her low gestational age, low birth weight, and exposure to high levels of oxygen.
- Congenital heart anomaly: Maya had a small patent foramen ovale/atrial septal defect noted on an echocardiogram, requiring follow-up with cardiology.
- Hearing screen: Maya had an auditory brainstem response on January 5 and passed for both ears.
- Gastroesophageal reflux: Maya experienced multiple oxygen desaturations occurring after oral feedings and/or toward the end of NG tube feedings; Zantac (ranitidine) was begun on March 7. Episodes of oxygen desaturations were still occurring at the middle and end of feedings 2 weeks later. On March 28, Zantac was discontinued.

Evaluation Information

The objectives and goals of OT assessment and intervention in the NICU are based on a strong knowledge of the NICU environment (including equipment and terminology), an understanding of normal infant development, a knowledge of the differences between preterm and full-term infants, and an understanding of the capacities of the preterm infant in relation to state, behavioral organization, and sensory systems. A thorough review of Maya's medical records provided important information regarding prenatal factors, delivery, medical status, and complications she had encountered since birth that may have an impact on her development. A discussion with the primary nurse prior to the evaluation provided important information regarding Maya's immediate status, including IV placement, oxygen support, and any positioning restrictions as well as information regarding her family.

Maya was referred for an OT evaluation at 31 weeks, when her medical stability had improved, although she remained in the isolette for temperature regulation, was fed via NG tube, and required respiratory support with an HFNC.

The initial contact with Maya and her parents following the referral for OT occurred while her mother was providing kangaroo care, or holding Maya with skin-to-skin contact on her chest. Kangaroo care is promoted in the NICU to assist with parent-infant bonding and provide positive tactile input. Maya's mother was encouraged that Maya was stable enough for an initial developmental assessment and requested that OT come to the bedside during her skin-to-skin holding with Maya. The role of OT in the NICU was explained to her mother, with reassurance that OT consults were performed on many infants in the NICU and that this did not necessarily indicate that Maya would have deficits in her development. The initial observation provided an opportunity to point out many positive behaviors that Maya was demonstrating while her mother was holding her.

During the initial observation, Maya maintained physiological stability because she had a stable heart rate, respiratory rate, and oxygen saturation. She demonstrated attempts to grasp at her blanket, and her mother was shown how to facilitate Maya's grasp of her finger and to bring her hand toward her mouth with support. Maya made attempts to clear her airway before her head went to either side while held in prone on her mother's chest. An explanation of the neuromotor differences between full-term and preterm infants, states of alertness, containment with handling and holding, and swaddling to support flexor tone was introduced to Maya's mother. A complete assessment was deferred to support the parent-infant bonding that was occurring as Maya was held supportively by her mother.

Prior to the gentle and graded hands-on assessment, Maya was observed at rest to note positioning and spontaneous activity. Clinical observations of Maya's muscle tone, state control, neurobehavioral organization, and spontaneous movements were made. She was assessed in her isolette to promote continued physiological stability and temperature control. Maya demonstrated appropriate muscle tone, reflexes, spontaneous activity, and behavior for her gestational age and current medical status. The following goal areas were selected to support Maya's development in collaboration with her NICU team:

1. Support behavioral organization to provide systematic touch, visual, and auditory input and facilitate Maya's adjustment to the extrauterine environment.
2. Promote co-regulation of parent and infant to enhance parent-infant interaction and support positive caretaking experiences.
3. Optimize neuromotor development by normalizing and promoting appropriate muscle tone through proper positioning and handling; prepare for functional movement, such as hands to face and to midline, to assist in calming and behavioral organization.

Maya's treatment was always coordinated with nursing to ensure that there was no interruption to her sleep, as her schedule might change due to medical interventions. Communication with nursing following each treatment session provided OT input into Maya's care plan and included strategies that improved Maya's movement and behavioral organization. The OT also shared Maya's progress with her parents via phone conversations if they were not present during treatment.

Progress Information

At 34 to 35 weeks gestation, Maya was initially evaluated with the Test of Infant Motor Performance Screening Items (TIMPSI). The Test of Infant Motor Performance (TIMP) and TIMPSI screening version assess the functional and postural control needed for functional movement in infants from 34 weeks gestation to 5 months of age. The TIMPSI is a shorter screening version of the TIMP and is used with medically fragile infants who may not yet tolerate the full TIMP assessment. During the TIMPSI, Maya demonstrated improved muscle tone appropriate for her gestational age. She maintained physiological stability during graded movement and handling. She demonstrated improved movement against gravity in attempts to flex her hips and knees or bring her hands to her face. Maya tolerated position changes well. She was able to maintain stable oxygen saturation levels when held in a semi-upright supported sitting position. Her mother was frequently present during treatment sessions and asked appropriate questions regarding Maya's continued development as well as strategies that could be incorporated during her visits to promote this.

Maya was evaluated using the full version of the TIMP prior to discharge. She scored within the average range for her gestational age at 38 to 39 weeks gestation on the TIMP. Maya's muscle tone continued to progress with supportive positioning and handling. These strategies allowed Maya to maintain her head in midline while supine and to actively turn her head to either side. In prone, Maya was able to lift her head from the surface momentarily and turn to either side. She was able to visually fixate on a face but was not yet visually tracking a face or object. She grasped a small lightweight ring placed in her hand for a few seconds.

Maya brightened to auditory stimuli presented to either side and began to orient to her mother's voice with active head turning. She demonstrated good state control with smooth transitions from light sleep to an alert state with handling. She brought her hands to her mouth for self-calming and was calmed easily with a pacifier. She tolerated being in a supported upright position and made attempts to right her head with support at her trunk.

Neonatal Intensive Care Unit Discharge Conference

An interdisciplinary conference was held with the neonatologist, Maya's parents, the nutritionist, the social worker, the discharge planner, and the OT prior to discharge. The role and importance of ongoing visits at the NICU follow-up clinic were discussed and an initial follow-up appointment was scheduled with written information describing the visit. Anticipatory guidance regarding Maya's continued development and skills that might be expected at the first follow-up visit were discussed. A handout regarding the importance of tummy time during wakeful periods was given.

Maya was discharged with home health nursing visits scheduled three times per week for 10 visits. She was referred to the state's early intervention program due to her extreme prematurity and low birth weight.

Neonatal Intensive Care Unit Follow-Up, First Visit

With her mother present, Maya was seen at the outpatient clinic setting at an adjusted age of 1 month 23 days and chronological age of 5 months 6 days. Her mother did not have specific concerns regarding Maya and described her as "a good baby." Maya lives with both of her parents and her mother is on family leave from her job as a teacher until August.

Since discharge from the NICU, Maya had one inpatient hospitalization for 4 days on the pediatric unit with an upper respiratory infection and fever. She underwent laser eye surgery for retinopathy of prematurity by the pediatric ophthalmologist. She continued use of an apnea monitor at night. She had been weaned off her nasal cannula by the pulmonologist a few days prior to clinic and was doing well. Maya had been evaluated at home by the state Early Intervention Program following discharge from the NICU but did not qualify for ongoing therapy services. The early intervention evaluation team will continue to monitor her development with periodic reassessments in the home.

Maya's physical exam revealed that she weighed 9.7 pounds (4.4 kg), was 25 inches (54 cm) in length, and had a head circumference of 36 cm. When plotted on the growth chart for her adjusted age, her weight was at the 10th to 25th percentile, height was at the 10th percentile, and head circumference was at the 3rd percentile.

During her first follow-up clinic visit, Maya was reassessed with the TIMP and scored within the average range for her adjusted age. She had made significant progress since her discharge from the NICU. She was very alert and responsive and was able to visually track from midline to either side. She was beginning to smile occasionally. In prone, she was able to lift her head to 45 degrees with forearm support. She was able to maintain head control in supported sitting with head-righting reactions. She was able to bear weight briefly through both lower extremities in a supported standing position. She was not yet rolling independently but could roll with facilitation at her arms or legs from supine to prone. Maya demonstrated mild flattening on the posterior right side of her skull but was able to actively rotate her head to the left. She had a preference for head turning to the right, as noted in the NICU. Maya was able to grasp a small lightweight ring placed in either hand, and recommendations to provide opportunities for active grasp with either hand were given.

Neonatal Intensive Care Unit Follow-up, Second Visit

Maya (Figure 1-2) was seen for her second follow-up clinic visit at the chronological age of 8 months and 22 days and adjusted age of 4 months 22 days. She had no hospitalizations, illnesses, or surgeries since her last visit. She does qualify for Synagis (palivizumab) during the respiratory syncytial virus season to reduce illnesses. Maya's physical exam revealed that she weighed 12.6 pounds (5.75 kg) and her height was 23 inches (59 cm). Her weight was at the 10th percentile, height at the 5th percentile, and head circumference at the 5th to 10th percentile. Her parents had no specific concerns regarding Maya's development. Her mother has returned to her job as a teacher and Maya is cared for by a family friend during the parents' work hours.

Maya was assessed with the Alberta Infant Motor Scale (AIMS). She scored at the 25th to 50th percentile with skills appropriate for her corrected age. She had made significant progress since her last follow-up visit. Maya was a happy, social baby who was very attentive to her surroundings. She was able to visually track a face or object in vertical and horizontal planes. She smiled and vocalized to the examiner and her mother. She was able to grasp a rattle with both hands and bat at toys. She was briefly able to grasp a cube with an ulnar palmar grasp. Maya was able to roll prone to supine independently and supine to prone with minimal facilitation. She was able to briefly sit independently with forward propping. She was able to bear weight through both lower extremities in supported standing with active trunk extension. Maya was able to easily rotate her head to either side. Her mother was very pleased with her progress.

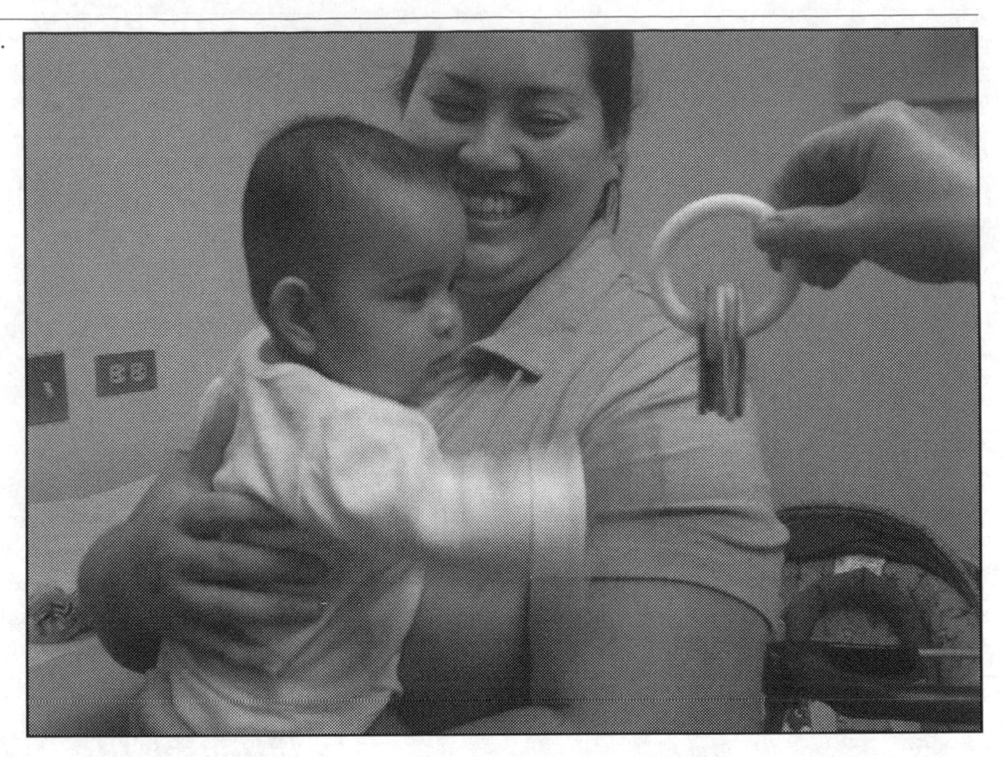

Figure 1-2. Maya batting at toys.

Questions to Consider

1. Construct a time line that includes Maya's medical care and development. Include important events like being discharged from the NICU and attending visits at the NICU follow-up clinic.
2. How would you conduct an occupational profile for Maya? What methods would you use to collect information? Describe some specific information that you would like to include.
3. What are some examples of the neuromotor differences found between full-term and preterm infants?
4. What are the different states of alertness? What does each state look like?
5. What are some examples of positioning devices that are used to contain preterm infants in the NICU?
6. Why is swaddling to support flexor tone introduced to Maya's mother in the NICU? How will spending time in this position support Maya's development?
7. What are the key characteristics of the TIMP and AIMS? What are the age ranges associated with these assessments? What are some examples of different items? Why would an OT choose one assessment tool over another?
8. Develop a tummy time information sheet that could be presented to Maya's parents at the NICU discharge conference.
9. After Maya's first visit to the NICU follow-up clinic, her mother was given written instructions and provided with a demonstration to increase head turning to the left, as well as suggestions for crib placement and toy placement to encourage head turning to the left. What do you think was included in the instructions? Describe what you think took place in the demonstration.
10. After Maya's second visit to the NICU follow-up clinic, instructions were given to her mother to promote Maya's ability to actively reach her hands to her knees and feet as well as to promote prop sitting. What do you think was included in the instructions?
11. During Maya's second visit to the NICU follow-up clinic, Maya's mother asked if she could begin placing Maya in an infant walker or exersaucer. Discuss the pros and cons of using this type of equipment with Maya and decide whether you would recommend its use.

Resources

American Occupational Therapy Association. (2006). Specialized knowledge and skills for practice in the neonatal intensive care unit. *American Journal of Occupational Therapy, 60*(6), 659-668.

Campbell, S. (2004). *Test of infant motor performance.* Chicago: Infant Motor Performance Scales, LLC.

Feldman, R. (2004). Mother-infant skin-to-skin contact (kangaroo care): Theoretical, clinical, and empirical aspects. *Infants & Young Children, 17*(2), 145-161.

Hunter, J. (2010). Neonatal intensive care unit. In J. Case-Smith & J. O'Brien (Eds.), *Occupational therapy for children* (6th ed.). (pp. 649-680). St. Louis: Elsevier.

Piper, M., & Darragh, J. (1994). *Alberta infant motor scales.* Alberta: Saunders.

Sam: Premature Infant/ Neonatal Intensive Care Unit

Maureen Connors Lenke, OTR/L

History and Background Information

Sam, the first of twins, was born at 24 6/7 weeks to a 35-year-old mother via cesarean section due to preterm labor and vaginal bleeding. His birth weight was 2 pounds, 2 ounces (963 g). His mother was given antibiotics and steroids to delay the onset of labor. She was hospitalized and put on bed rest prior to delivery. Complications during her pregnancy included gestational diabetes and twin gestation. Sam's twin sister was discharged at 38 weeks gestation, day of life 72. Sam was discharged at 56 3/7 weeks gestation, day of life 205, with a weight of 12.5 pounds (5690 g).

Medical problems/presenting concerns during Sam's neonatal hospitalization included the following:

- Nutrition: Sam initially required an umbilical artery catheter and umbilical venous catheter, for blood draws and fluid administration. He had a peripherally inserted catheter placed for parenteral nutrition. He received hyperalimentation for 1 month. NG feeds were begun December 7. By mouth (PO) feeds advanced with difficulty and Sam underwent a swallow study on March 27 that showed gastroesophageal reflux and aspiration. A follow-up swallow study on May 29 showed no aspiration. He was discharged on PO/NG feeds and demonstrated oral aversion due to prolonged ventilator support.
- Bronchopulmonary dysplasia: Sam was intubated in the delivery room and given three doses of Curosurf (poractant alfa) for severe respiratory distress syndrome. Antenatal steroids were given. He had a pneumothorax requiring a chest tube. He had pulmonary hypertension requiring therapy with nitric oxide for 5 days. Sam alternated between a high-frequency oscillating ventilator and a conventional ventilator. He was given Decadron (dexamethasone) to facilitate his extubation from the ventilator, which was completed on December 6, and he was put on bubble continuous positive airway pressure (CPAP). Sam was reintubated on December 21 due to a urinary tract infection, which was treated with antibiotics. He self-extubated on December 25 and alternated between bubble CPAP and HFNC for 4 months. At the end of May, he was weaned completely to a HFNC and then weaned to a nasal cannula with 100% oxygen saturation. He was discharged home on a nasal cannula with 2 liters oxygen, an apnea monitor, pulse oximeter, nebulizer equipment, and medications to treat his severe bronchopulmonary dysplasia.
- Sepsis: Sam was initially treated with 7 days of ampicillin and gentamicin.
- Hyperbilirubinemia: Sam was treated with phototherapy for 1 week, with a peak bilirubin of 8.4.
- Hypotension: Sam initially had poor perfusion and was treated with dopamine and a blood transfusion.
- Neurologic: Sam underwent four cranial ultrasounds with asymmetric ventricles noted. He did not have an intraventricular bleed.
- Retinopathy of prematurity: Sam had immature retinas and required repeated eye exams to follow the progression.
- PDA: Sam had a moderate PDA that closed following treatment with two courses of Indocin.
- Anemia of prematurity: Sam required several blood transfusions during his hospitalization due to anemia.
- Apnea: Sam was treated with caffeine for apnea, which resolved in January.
- Infection: Sam had three urinary tract infections, which were treated with antibiotics.
- Hearing screen: Sam's auditory brainstem response was tested on May 31 and he passed for both ears.

Sam's history and medical issues were important to review and be familiar with prior to evaluation because they provided insight regarding therapeutic decision making and impacted Sam's continued intervention plan.

Evaluation Information

Initial Occupational Therapy Evaluation

One of the most important goals of occupational therapy in the NICU is parent education. Initial contact with Sam's parents occurred at an evening NICU parent group on premature infant development presented by the OT, with support provided by the NICU social worker, when Sam was 3 weeks old and critically ill. Although the OT was familiar with Sam's case through attendance at weekly multidisciplinary discharge rounds reviewing all cases in the NICU, Sam did not yet have the medical stability to have an initial OT assessment due to his respiratory compromise. The concepts of developmental differences between healthy and regulated full-term infants and medically fragile and less organized preterm infants were discussed with the parent group. The overall goals of developmentally supportive care and strategies to minimize infant stress including influences of the NICU environment on the infant and his family were presented. The differences between corrected gestational age (GA) and chronological age were discussed. His parents were instructed that developmental milestone expectations would be based on corrected GA rather than chronological age for the first 2 years of age.

Sam's parents were overwhelmed and exhausted with the medical issues their twins were experiencing in the NICU. Their attendance at the parent group allowed them a brief respite from their infant's bedside and provided an opportunity to interact with other NICU parents experiencing the stress and fear of having an infant in the NICU. The NICU was a frightening and unfamiliar environment with unfamiliar procedures, equipment, terminology, and professionals involved in the care of their son. Sam's parents were feeling a loss of control, with uncertainty about the outcome of their son's medical treatment and future development. They were at a loss of knowing how to interact and participate in the care of their son or where to turn for information and advice. The parent group provided an opportunity for them to express their concerns about Sam's development and to begin to understand how they could support his development as his medical status improved.

Another important role of OT in the NICU is consultation. Even during the initial period of recovery, Sam was provided with developmentally supportive positioning within the constraints of his medical care. OT consultation to assist nursing with positioning to promote a balance of flexion and extension, and provide boundaries and containment into flexion, helped minimize the energy expended by Sam as he attempted to seek boundaries in his isolette by extension of his arms and legs. Proper positioning was important in helping Sam to achieve motor stabilization and to prevent musculoskeletal abnormalities, including scapular retraction, neck hyperextension, or wide leg abduction into the supporting surface due to lack of flexor tonus that would have continued to progress in utero.

The NICU staff practiced open communication with the parents, sharing information in a timely and supportive manner, repeating information, and answering questions as often as necessary to achieve an understanding to assist the parents in participating in Sam's care. While Sam's twin sister progressed for her GA and began OT intervention services, Sam's medical stability remained compromised.

Analysis of Occupational Performance

Sam's initial OT evaluation was scheduled around his routine nursing care to avoid interruptions in his schedule and consisted primarily of observations at his bedside. His breathing, overall stability, and spontaneous movement were observed at rest. He was gently unswaddled and the observation continued. Throughout the session, Sam was trying to maintain autonomic stability. However, he demonstrated signs of state disorganization as noted by gaze aversion (looking away and closing his eyes), hyperalertness, and a panicked and worried facial expression. Sam demonstrated abrupt changes between states of alertness (between sleeping and hyperalert states) or remained in a low-level state of alertness with a dull, glassy-eyed look. Initially, he did not have an audible cry. Sam exhibited fluctuations in physiologic function as evidenced by changes in his breathing, with decreases in oxygen saturation and skin color changes. He had frequent tremors and startles.

Sam had difficulty processing tactile, auditory, visual, and kinesthetic stimuli and was easily overloaded. One stimulus at a time was introduced and his tolerance and responses were observed while continually assessing for changes in his baseline color, respiratory rate, heart rate, blood pressure, and oxygen saturation. It was necessary to provide slow and graded handling, with firm support provided to Sam's neck, trunk, and extremities. Sam set the pace for intervention; as he would show signs of disorganization, it was important to assist with reorganization and containment to allow time for recovery before continuing or discontinuing the treatment session. It was also important to remain by the bedside after treatment to evaluate for any delayed response to the treatment and to communicate with the parents and nursing staff regarding what strategies were positive or potentially negative for Sam.

Because of his respiratory status, Sam responded very differently from his twin sister, who achieved medical stability much more quickly. While Sam was still attempting to achieve physiologic stability due to his respiratory compromise, his sister was able to increase interaction with her parents, caregivers, and environment. It was frustrating and confusing to Sam's parents that strategies that worked in calming and interacting with Sam's sister did not work with Sam. Sam's responses were not always predictable and his responses to stimuli sometimes fluctuated each time they were introduced, depending on his recent stressors and the changes apparent in his respiratory/oxygen requirements. Formalized assessment was not appropriate due to Sam's difficulty with state regulation and physiologic stability. Ongoing assessment of his behavioral cues was needed to plan appropriate treatment and caregiving strategies. It was important to help Sam's parents identify Sam's behaviors as indicators of how much stimulation he was able to tolerate and encourage them to provide one mode of input at a time to avoid overstimulation. During treatment, unnecessary stress and fatigue were important to avoid. It was often necessary to conduct or reschedule treatment depending on events that Sam had encountered, such as episodes of bradycardia, frequent oxygen desaturations, lab draws to rule out infection, or testing procedures (e.g., eye exams). These events were stressful to Sam, reduced his energy, and limited his ability to tolerate hands-on intervention. A series of goal areas was selected to support Sam's development in collaboration with his NICU team:

1. Identify the experiences that contribute to Sam's disorganization during caregiving routines.
2. Identify strategies to assist Sam in optimal behavioral regulation and organization.
3. Position Sam in ways that support neuromuscular development.

Sam was followed closely over the following weeks to provide graded, organized sensory input, maintenance of appropriate positioning, continuing evaluation, and continued education to parents. As Sam became more stable and tolerant of input, graded hands-on treatment was initiated. Sam was provided with firm, graded handling and support of his extremities while avoiding sudden changes in his posture. Sam was gradually able to tolerate supported upright positioning with stable oxygen saturation. In coordination with the nursing staff, Sam continued to be positioned in devices to support a more functional flexed posture in supine, prone, and side-lying positions. Parents were encouraged to participate in planning and implementing care strategies for their infants. Sam's parents visited frequently, were eager to participate in his care in any way they could, and were very responsive to any suggestions that were presented by the OT. Sam's parents were encouraged to provide hands-on containment during holding and procedures by bringing Sam's hands to the midline of his body and supporting his head, buttocks, and lower extremities. Sam was swaddled as he became more tolerant of being held with his hands brought to the midline and near his face and mouth, which assisted with regulation and attempts at self-calming.

Reinforcement of Sam's parents' understanding of infant cues, recognizing signs of disorganization, as well as Sam's attempts at self-regulation was provided during each treatment session. Sam's parents were taught signs (behavioral cues) of stress and overstimulation, including limb extension, finger or toe splaying, twitches or startles, arching or limp muscle tone, abrupt color changes, irregular breathing, and gaze aversion. They were also taught signs of relaxation and readiness for engagement. As Sam maintained greater physiological stability, his grasp was facilitated by holding his parents' fingers or a small, lightweight rattle. Sam began to visually fixate briefly with occasional smiles, which were very reinforcing to his parents.

Sam experienced unpleasant and potentially painful stimuli in and around his mouth during his NICU hospitalization. His frequent routine procedures associated with compromised respiratory status included endotracheal and oral suctioning and insertion of oral gastric and NG tubes. These procedures contributed to hypersensitive oral responses, which further contributed to sucking and swallowing difficulties. Sam's parents were encouraged to provide oral care and graded oral input during intubation; as he progressed, graded oral stimulation was provided to promote sucking and non-nutritive sucking in coordination with the speech pathologist.

Following the discharge of Sam's twin sister, the impact of his prolonged hospitalization and chronic condition became more stressful as his parents tried to coordinate their time between their home and the NICU environment. An additional family care conference was scheduled well before Sam's anticipated discharge date to ensure time for training and the opportunity for his parents to ask questions prior to discharge. The interdisciplinary team offered Sam's parents the opportunity to ask questions and voice concerns about Sam's medical and developmental status in an inclusive environment with adequate time provided for updates. Sam's parents were encouraged to verbalize feelings about caring for Sam and his twin sister as well as to discuss challenges they anticipated that could affect healthy bonding and attachment. The role of the NICU follow-up clinic was reviewed. Sam's parents had already attended the NICU follow-up clinic with Sam's twin sister 1 month following her discharge home.

Sam's discharge recommendations were coordinated with the nursing discharge planner. In addition, the social worker facilitated equipment needs for home-based medical support to ensure a smooth transition from the NICU to home for Sam and his family. Sam was discharged with nursing home health visits scheduled 3x per week for 10 visits. He was referred to the home-based state Early Intervention Program for evaluation and initiation of occupational therapy, physical therapy, and speech therapy services due to his delays in development and continued difficulties with feeding. The OT provided written and verbal information about placing Sam on his back to sleep and on his tummy during wakeful periods to continue to promote head control, promote strength of his arms and upper chest, and to optimize the shape of his head and prevent plagiocephaly. The differences between corrected GA and chronological age were reviewed and reminders that developmental milestone expectations are based on corrected GA rather than chronological age were reviewed again with Sam's parents. Written handouts were provided to Sam's parents reinforcing developmental care, including the need for protection from overstimulation, the need for positional support of Sam's decreased muscle tone, and activities to continue to promote his overall endurance for head control, grasp, and reach. Anticipatory guidance of skills that would continue to develop before his first follow-up visit, which would take place in 1 month, were also provided.

Neonatal Intensive Care Unit Follow-Up, First Visit

Sam was seen at clinic at a chronological age of 8 months 2 days and an adjusted age of 5 months 7 days with both parents present 4 weeks after discharge from the NICU. Since his discharge from the NICU, he has had no illness or rehospitalization but remains on 0.5 liters of oxygen continuously. He lives at home with his mother, father, twin sister, and grandparents, who are visiting from India to assist with care of the twins. Sam was evaluated by the state Early Intervention Program and qualified for weekly physical therapy, occupational therapy, and developmental therapy services at home. Weekly therapy services are to be initiated next week.

Sam's physical examination revealed that he weighs 16 pounds (7.25 kg), is 25.75 inches (65.7 cm) in length, and has a head circumference of 36 cm. When plotted on the growth chart for his adjusted age, his weight was at the 25th percentile, his height was at the 25th to 50th percentile, and his head circumference was at the 2nd to 5th percentile.

Sam was assessed with the AIMS. He scored at the 5th percentile, with skills at a 3½ month developmental level for his adjusted age of 5 months 7 days. He has made significant progress since his discharge from the NICU. He is very alert and responsive and less irritable due to the consistency of his parents as his caregivers and the stable environment at home. He has begun to coo and laughs occasionally. He is able to visually track 180 degrees in horizontal and vertical planes. He demonstrates active batting and reach for a toy. He is able to grasp a rattle briefly when it is placed in either hand. Sam is able to bring his hands to midline and to his mouth. Sam demonstrates increased tolerance of prone positioning and is able to lift his head to 45 degrees in prone with forearm support. He exhibits a head lag with pull to sit but is able to demonstrate active neck flexor control when pulled up from supine to sitting with support at his shoulders. Sam is unable to roll from prone to supine or supine to prone. He bears slight weight through both lower extremities with his trunk flexed forward. His parents have been following through with positioning and developmental suggestions that were provided prior to discharge, although it is difficult with the medical care, oxygen requirements, and medical visits Sam requires. Physical and occupational therapy are to be initiated once weekly at home. Sam is primarily fed via an NG tube and is able to take some formula by bottle, but at times he may refuse to take a bottle feeding for 3 to 4 consecutive days. Sam continues to demonstrate significant oral aversion.

Questions to Consider

1. Based on Sam's birthday and his gestational age, determine Sam's due date.
2. Review how to calculate chronological age and gestational age. What are some important tips to remember when completing these calculations?
3. What are some other signs of state disorganization?
4. With a doll, demonstrate ways that you imagine Sam was positioned while he was in the NICU. Consider how he was positioned in supine, as well as in side lying. In addition, demonstrate the containment position for which Sam's parents were provided instruction.
5. What are some signs of a relaxed infant who is ready for engagement and interaction?
6. What are some examples of graded oral stimulation?
7. What is non-nutritive sucking and how could that be facilitated?
8. What is plagiocephaly? How is it treated? How does it influence further development?
9. What are some skills that you anticipate will develop before Sam's first NICU follow-up clinic visit?
10. Write a treatment goal to address Sam's oral aversion. Consider how you could collect data to support the achievement of this goal.
11. Design a home program to address Sam's oral aversion. Consider how the OT would collaborate with the speech and language pathologist to implement this program.
12. Discuss how Sam's feeding difficulties likely impact co-occupations and attachment. Suggest ways to support his participation in age-appropriate co-occupations as well as to support attachment.
13. What is the progression of food textures and how would you begin introducing them to Sam?

Resources

American Occupational Therapy Association. (2007). Specialized knowledge and skills feeding, eating, and swallowing for occupational therapy practice. *American Journal of Occupational Therapy, 61*(6), 686-700.

Hunter, J. (2010). Neonatal intensive care unit. In J. Case-Smith & J. O'Brien (Eds.), *Occupational therapy for children* (6th ed.). (pp. 649-680). St. Louis: Elsevier.

Morris, S., & Dunn Klein, M. (2000). *Pre-feeding skills: A comprehensive resource for mealtime development.* Austin, TX: Pro-ed.

Piper, M., & Darragh, J. (1994). *Alberta Infant Motor Scales.* Alberta: Saunders.

Schuberth, L., Amirault, L., & Case-Smith, J. (2010). Feeding intervention. In J. Case-Smith & J. O'Brien (Eds.). *Occupational therapy for children* (6th ed.). (pp. 446-473). St. Louis: Elsevier.

Marco: Premature Infant/ Neonatal Intensive Care Unit

Mary J. Greer, MOT

History and Background Information

Marco is a small infant boy recently admitted to the NICU. His parents are a young married couple and he is their first child. When Marco's mother went into premature labor, Marco was still 2 months away from his due date. He was born at 32 weeks gestation into a very loud, painful, bright, and stressful environment. The family was unprepared and the few expectations they did have were not fulfilled. Team members, including a neonatologist, nurse practitioners, nurses, respiratory therapist, OT, dietitian, social worker, and case manager, will all be part of Marco's life for a few weeks.

Marco was whisked away from the delivery room quickly and placed on an open warmer bed in the NICU. Very bright lights shone down on him while a team of noisy medical professionals moved quickly within his space. He initially had difficulty breathing on his own and required a ventilator. Another tube, taped to his chin, was inserted through his mouth down into his stomach to vent air. Adhesive pads were placed on his chest to monitor heart and respiratory rates. His foot was wrapped with an oxygen sensor. He was stuck multiple times for routine lab draws and the first newborn vaccinations. IV sites were taped and an arm board was used to maintain elbow extension. As he squirmed, a large hand covered his face while stabilizing the ventilator tubing. When he was medically stable, the activity stopped. Marco was exhausted and fell asleep lying supine with arms and legs spread out flat against the mattress at a time when his body should have been growing larger within a confined space, forcing his trunk and neck to be curled forward, shoulders and hips to be rounded, and extremities to be consistently flexed.

Evaluation Information

Occupational Profile

Sarah and Juan, Marco's parents, live in a rural area about 30 minutes from a hospital. Sarah's primary language is English, but Juan speaks little English. His first language is Spanish; Sarah translates for him when they are at the hospital together. The couple does not visit most days because they share one vehicle. Juan takes the car to work every day, then to night school, where he is earning his welder's certificate. The plan was that he would have finished this educational program by the time Marco was born. Sarah works a few hours per week at a "mother's day out" program through her church. Marco's parents have a strong religious background. Shortly after learning Marco was a boy, they bought a christening gown and invited extended family members to attend the ceremony scheduled for 1 month after the due date. The young couple had been showered with handsome blue clothes and all types of baby toys and gear, from musical rattles to bouncers and swings.

During an obstetrics visit during her 7th month of pregnancy, Sarah was found to be in premature labor and sent straight to the labor and delivery unit. Marco's father was called away from his construction job to be with his wife. Marco's grandparents live out of state. Sarah's mother had a visit scheduled near the expected due date but was unable to come earlier. Many supportive friends and family members are involved in Sarah and Juan's life. However, the NICU visitation policy is that only parents and grandparents are allowed to visit in the unit. In the beginning, when Sarah was still a patient in the hospital, she often sat alone at Marco's bedside. The young couple experienced feelings that Marco belongs more to the hospital because they had no control and were not allowed to touch or comfort their baby during the first 2 days. Despite the strict visitation policy, the unit does encourage parental visits. There is even a fund to help pay for public transportation to and from the unit, but it is not well advertised.

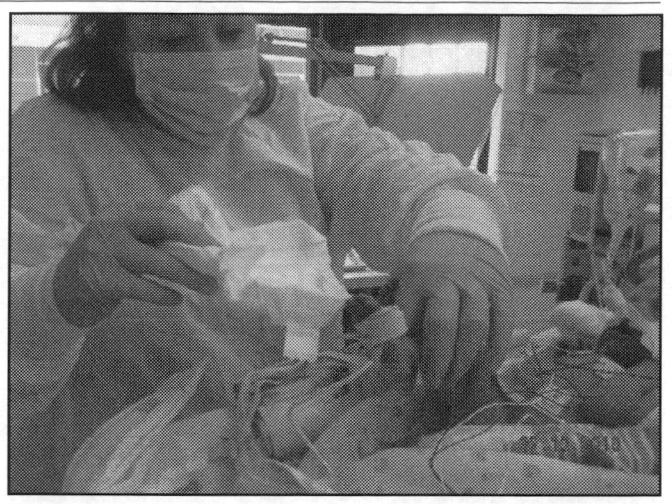

Figure 1-3. Marco's diaper being changed while he is on a ventilator.

Because OT addresses both positioning and feeding, it is the only rehabilitation service provided in the NICU at this hospital. The OT evaluation was not performed during Marco's first week because his medical status was considered highly complex. For the first 2 to 3 days, stimulation of any kind resulted in drops in heart rate and oxygen saturation (Figure 1-3). Once weaned from the ventilator, his respiratory support needs were still significant and he was not tolerating the introduction of breast milk via tube feed. This is not uncommon for premature infants but can become a serious medical issue. By the end of the first week, his respiratory support was weaned and his digestive system began to tolerate tube feedings. Because of staffing issues and needs of the other infants within the unit, Marco's OT evaluation was not performed during the second week in the NICU either. After a long holiday weekend, the OT evaluation was conducted when Marco was 34.5 weeks corrected gestational age (CGA). By this time, he was off the oxygen, had been transferred to an open crib bed, and was being fed with a bottle by the nurses.

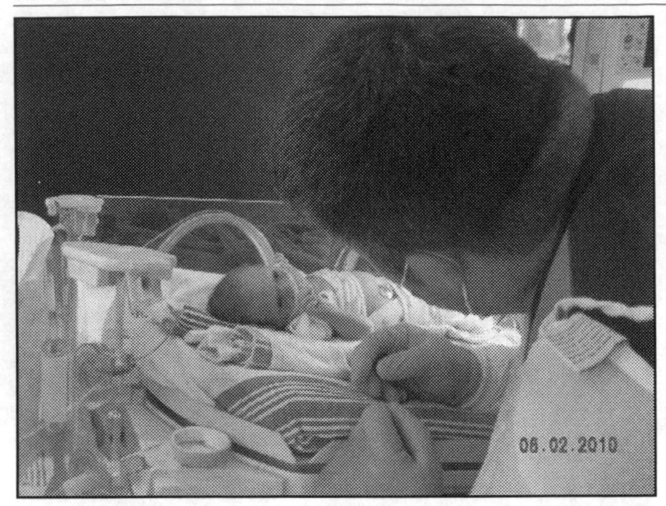

Figure 1-4. Marco in isolette demonstrating eye contact with his dad.

Analysis of Occupational Performance

Client Factors/Body Functions

- Neuromusculoskeletal and movement-related functions: A review of Marco's birth record reveals that his Apgar scores were 7 and 9. His size plotted at the 40th percentile for his stated gestational age of 32 weeks at birth. He initially was noted to have tremors of his arms, legs, and lower jaw whenever he cried. A review of mom's medical history indicated that she smoked almost a pack of cigarettes per day. Mom had an infected tooth but was advised to wait on needed oral surgery until after her baby was born. Mom was given prescriptions for an antibiotic and pain medication to take infrequently until she was able to have dental care. Medically, Marco is doing very well at 34.5 weeks CGA. He has been completely weaned off respiratory support, although nurses document spells of rapid breathing at times, especially during bottle feeds. Marco still has a hep-lock for IV access taped to his ankle for 4 more days of IV antibiotics. He has been out of the warmer bed for 1 week and is able to be dressed and swaddled within the open plastic crib. Marco is fed breast milk when his mom brings pumped milk to the unit, but when it runs out, the nurses feed Marco newborn infant formula. He is tolerating his feeds well now with no digestion concerns.
- As the OT approaches Marco's bed, Marco is lying supine, diapered, and wearing a standard hospital t-shirt. It appears he had been draped with two striped hospital blankets, which he has mostly kicked off. Marco is fussing and wiggling in an asymmetrical tonic neck reflex position, with his head turned to the right, sucking his right hand. When the pacifier is placed in his mouth, he calms down and begins rhythmically sucking the pacifier.
- Upper extremities: The physical evaluation indicates that Marco's muscle tone is low centrally for his age of 34 to 35 weeks CGA. With a slight tug on his upper extremities, he provides almost no resistance and his head lag is completely lax; he does not try to pull his head forward at all when his chest is rising off the mattress. At rest, his lower extremities remain primarily extended and hips in external rotation. When his legs are held in flexion for several seconds, he tries to keep them there momentarily. As the OT brings Marco's hands to midline under his chin, he maintains them in that position for 3 to 4 seconds. In supported sitting, Marco's head control is relatively floppy. With his head supported, he does look around and rotate his neck to the left and right sides. Active movements of extremities are symmetrical, though less than expected. Available range of motion is normal for all joints.
- Vision: Marco's state regulation and endurance for engagement in activity is found to be good for his age. He is able to tolerate brief eye contact (Figure 1-4). Marco is interested in visually exploring the objects and faces that are in his immediate environment. He turns his head in the direction of a voice and tries to physically hold his trunk and head in positions to participate in active observation of his environment. Marco also makes active attempts to calm himself by scooting toward a boundary and mouthing or sucking objects such as his hands, pacifier, or blanket.
- Emotional regulation: He does have difficulty with self-calming and often cries until assistance is provided. Because of Marco's interest in faces and voices and his ability to tolerate social interaction, there is potential for positive bonding experiences with his parents.

Areas of Occupation

Activities of Daily Living

- Bathing: A review of night shift documentation indicates that the nursing staff recently gave Marco a bath with the parents present, but Sarah and Juan only observed. The notes describe Marco flailing about while crying; he was not swaddled for the bath. There are a few videos about swaddling, handling, feeding, and infant care techniques on the unit. One is specifically about developmentally supportive bathing methods to promote state regulation, positioning, and a positive bonding experience. The nursing staff are very busy and do not often use the videos.
- Feeding: Nursing notes that describe feeding quality over the past week indicate Marco is not completing

all of his bottle feeds. Marco is in a very demanding group of infants and the nurse reports that Marco takes too long to eat. In preparation for an occupational therapy feeding assessment, Marco's diaper is changed and he is tightly swaddled into flexion with blankets. Marco's low central tone is noted during handling. Interventions are provided to stimulate jaw and oral tone, promote decreased stimulation, and provide optimal positioning for the feeding. He sucks rhythmically on a pacifier with good tongue protraction and jaw excursion. When the bottle nipple is inserted, Marco initially holds his breath while sucking a long burst. The bottle is withdrawn slightly to force a break in the suck pattern so that Marco will take some breaths. With environmental supports and strategies to facilitate a safe and pleasurable experience, guided by infant demand and comfort, the feed is completed successfully.

- Bowel/bladder management: As part of the evaluation, Sarah is called at home to discuss the OT's findings and impressions. During the conversation, Sarah recalls the first time she was allowed to change Marco's diaper, when he was still on the ventilator, at 2 days old. Since she was discharged from the hospital, she has not been available often. When she is present on the unit, she is passive and waits to be invited to be involved in Marco's care. The nurses believe Sarah is not enthusiastic about meeting her baby's needs and generally disinterested in participating in his care. The OT gathers that Sarah is very concerned about her baby but is unsure of her role and her occupational boundaries within the NICU environment.

Sarah shares that she has been very discouraged about Marco's feedings. Sarah and Juan have not been able to get Marco to take his full bottle and know he cannot come home until he is consistently eating well. Sarah is invited to come to the unit later that day to be instructed on environmental supports, positioning methods, interventions to facilitate flexor tone, feeding strategies, and infant care routines such as bathing and dressing. Sarah explains her lack of transportation. She relies on neighbors to drop her off when they are going to town to run errands. Sarah's weekday visits are usually unscheduled and of inconsistent duration.

As the OT ends the phone call, she overhears the nurse saying that the IV needs to be restarted on Marco. The therapist asks the nurse's permission to support Marco's extremities in flexion and hold the pacifier for Marco during the stressful procedure. These interventions minimize strong extension patterns and facilitate self-calming measures. Starting the IV is difficult, so it is placed in Marco's scalp. This is not uncommon, but it means that a patch of his hair must be shaved off. Knowing this would be important for Sarah and Juan, the OT gathers Marco's cut hair on a long piece of tape and saves it with a "first haircut" note and the date.

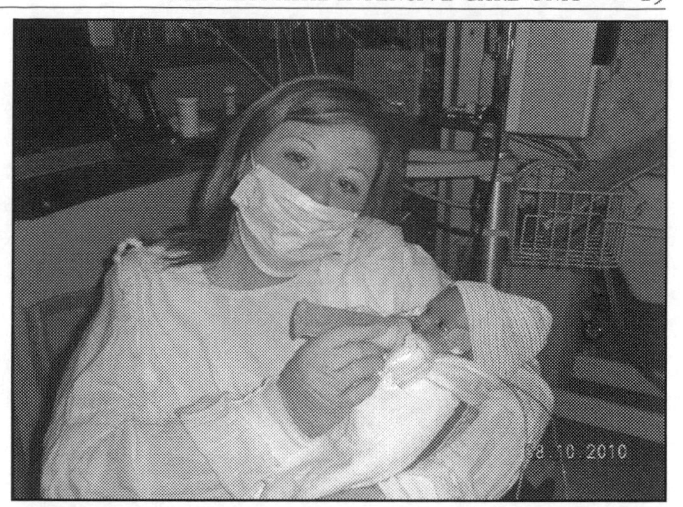

Figure 1-5. Marco's parents are much more involved in his care.

Progress Information

By the end of the third week, Marco's antibiotics are finished. The OT gets to interact with Sarah on three occasions that week. Much discussion, teaching, demonstration, guiding, and supervision take place during those sessions. Marco's parents are more actively involved in his care now (Figure 1-5). As they feel more effective within this environment, their confidence is growing. Juan feels especially proud when he sees Marco wearing the "daddy's boy" outfit he picked out. Sarah and Juan are anxious to take their baby home. They understand that Marco should not be taken out of the home except for doctor's appointments for the first 4 to 6 months due to the risk of respiratory infection. The OT discusses life changes and alterations of roles and expectations for the upcoming months. The cultural expectations for Marco' christening will have to be addressed.

Areas of Occupation

Activities of Daily Living

- Feeding: Because Marco is completing all feeds, half of them very efficiently, the OT is planning to make recommendations today during daily bedside rounds. Marco's weight gain has been borderline and the neonatologist asks the team to consider options of increasing the volume of feeds or sending Marco home to be followed by home health nursing.

Questions to Consider

Goals/Treatment Plan

1. At 34 to 35 weeks CGA, what are Marco's problems that would be addressed by occupational therapy?
2. What are Marco's strengths? What available supports do Marco and his parents have?
3. What are appropriate long-term goals for an infant client in the NICU? How would Marco's parents be involved in the attainment of his long-term goals?
4. What frames of reference will be used to address the problems?
5. Write specific short-term goals for Marco (with his family's involvement) that should be accomplished by 38 to 40 weeks gestational age.
6. Name one or two interventions to address each goal.

Safety Precautions

1. What are the obvious and subtle dangers of ignoring lines and tubing or monitors and alarms in an intensive care setting?
2. What are handling techniques that must be taught to the parents?
3. What are safe feeding techniques that must be taught to the parents?
4. What are the possible dangers to a premature infant in an environment filled with excessive stimulation?
5. What are specific ways infants communicate their needs?
6. How would the team address education needs in light of the father's limited English?

Self-Care/Work/Leisure

1. What are basic infant care skills about which a first-time parent may need to be educated?
2. What are items that may be needed for a minimal-stimulation infant bath?
3. What are infant cues showing that Marco is ready to interact socially with his parents?
4. What are appropriate responses by Marco's parents when Marco becomes tired and fussy?
5. What are work tasks of a very young infant?
6. How can Marco's parents use routine to provide temporal structure for Marco? What environmental objects and cues would be used?

Equipment/Adaptations

1. What specialized equipment or adaptations to current equipment would you recommend the parents use for the first few weeks they are home?

Neuro/Musculoskeletal

1. How does tone develop as a premature infant grows and matures to term age?
2. What are aspects of typical NICU environments and care that present hindrances to normal biomechanical development that ultimately affect muscle tone?
3. Regarding tonal concerns, how would you describe future implications of the lack of development of normal muscle tone?
4. What interventions are appropriate for a small infant who exhibits lower central tone than expected? How would these be incorporated into routine activities in which the child is involved and is learning to participate?
5. How would meaningful parent-infant interactions be affected or changed by incorporation of these interventions?

Cognition/Perception

1. Generally, what are a premature infant's cognitive and perceptual capacities?
2. What behaviors are exhibited by a preterm infant who is ready for and able to accept meaningful social interaction with parents?
3. What behaviors are exhibited by a preterm infant who is overwhelmed or overstimulated by the environment?
4. What type of stimulation is appropriate to provide during activity or interaction with a 34- to 36-week CGA infant?

Psychosocial

1. How would the OT incorporate meaningful activities and interactions between parent and infant into a treatment plan?
2. What are some objects from home that can be used within Marco's space to personalize it for the family?
3. What family supports can the OT provide or obtain to promote the mother's involvement in Marco's care?
4. When are occasions when the OT would call the parents at home to discuss Marco's performance and progress?
5. What are "firsts" that the OT would or would not want to tell the mother over the phone?

6. What parent instruction is appropriate about allowing friends and family members to interact with Marco after he gets home?

Situations

1. When you arrive in the unit early on Monday morning during shift change, you notice Marco is crying. He has scooted himself up so that his head is pressed against the plastic side of the open crib and his electrodes are pulling. Do you speak to the nurse, and what interventions do you provide?
2. During feeding, Marco no longer has a fast respiratory rate and seems organized and alert for the duration of the feed. You change him from a slow-flow nipple to a standard nipple and advise the nurse of the change. The next day, you notice the nurses are not being consistent with the nipples used during feeds. How do you address this issue?
3. As Marco gets older, he can tolerate a bath and dressing. You know Marco's mother is not planning to visit until the night shift. As the OT, you need to teach the parents how to bathe Marco safely with regard to minimizing stimulation and monitoring his behaviors. How do you arrange to meet with the mother? What is your plan for the session?
4. Because the NICU is part of an acute care hospital, the care is usually reimbursed in the same manner as a diagnosis-related group. Because services are not individually billed, how would you document a 45-minute session that involved support and reassurance to the mother as you addressed concerns she had about home routines with Marco?

Discharge Planning

1. In light of Marco's tonal issues, are there particular baby toys or equipment at home that Sarah and Juan should be discouraged from using? How would you suggest supporting Marco differently with typical baby equipment or devices?
2. Because Marco was born at 32 weeks gestation, he qualifies to have a developmental clinic appointment at 6 weeks after discharge. What activities and play experiences could be suggested to keep Marco on target with developmental milestones until his next checkup?

Resources

American Occupational Therapy Association. (2006). Specialized knowledge and skills for practice in the neonatal intensive care unit. *American Journal of Occupational Therapy, 60*(6), 659-668.

Hunter, J. (2010). Neonatal intensive care unit. In J. Case-Smith & J. O'Brien (Eds.), *Occupational therapy for children* (pp. 649-677). Maryland Heights, MI: Mosby.

Pablo: Premature Infant/ Neonatal Intensive Care Unit

Sonia F. Kay, PhD, OTR/L and Marvieann Garcia-Rodriguez, MHS, BHS, OTR

History and Background

Pablo is a premature baby boy born at 25 weeks gestation via emergency cesarean section due to placental abruption and nonreassuring heart rate. Apgar scores at birth were 3 at 1 minute, 5 at 5 minutes, and 10 at 10 minutes. At delivery, the baby required stimulation, oral suctioning, supplemental oxygen via facemask, chest compressions (brief), and endotracheal tube ventilation on a conventional ventilator. Pablo's heart rate came up quickly to > 100 beats per minute. Birth weight was 2.01 pounds (0.913 kg). Neurological testing at 7 days of age via head ultrasound was negative for an intraventricular hemorrhage. The baby was started on prophylactic antibiotics and IV fluids for hydration and nutrition. The NICU team for Pablo included nurses, care assistants, a neonatologist, nurse practitioner, OT, physical therapist, audiologist, social worker respiratory therapist, and lactation specialist.

Pablo is the first child of a 20-year-old woman who lives approximately 2 hours from the hospital. The parents are of Latino descent and live together but are not married. Both parents are high school graduates and are employed. In fact, the mother continued to work after the delivery to save maternity leave time for when the baby is discharged home. Pablo's mother would like to stay home with the baby and eventually breastfeed. She has started to pump and save her milk in the freezer at home. When the parents visit the hospital, mom leaves expressed breast milk for the baby in the unit freezer for the nurses to use for gavage feedings. There is extended family on both sides in their hometown that are supportive and will be involved with Pablo's care after discharge. The parents maintain daily contact by telephone and try to come to visit once a week on the weekend. On the last visit, they placed a small cross at the bottom of the isolette.

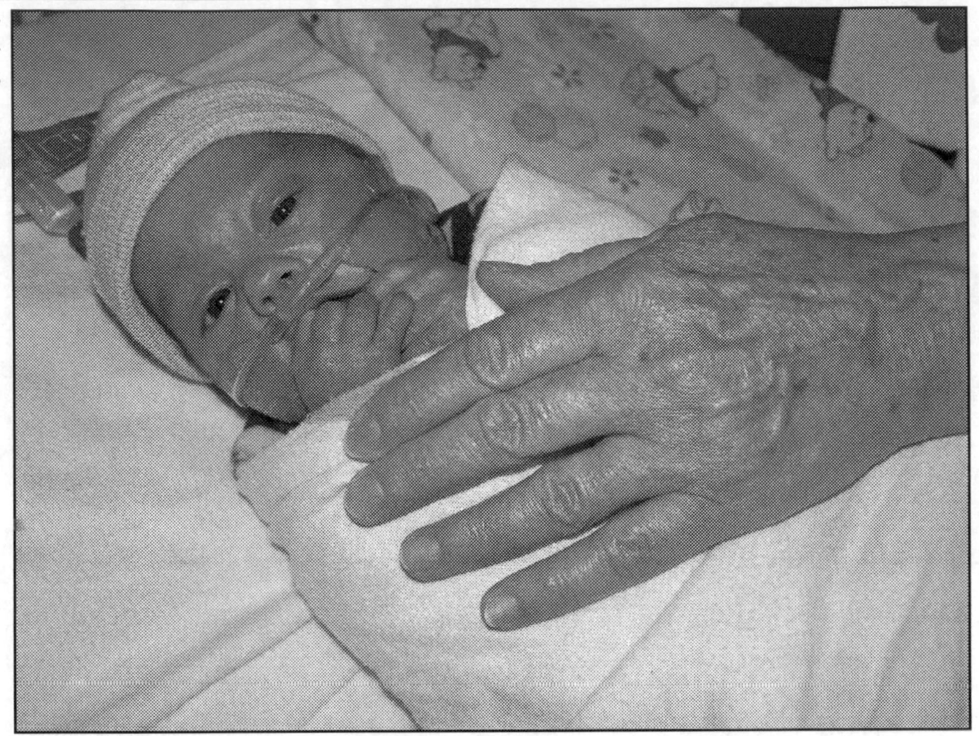

Figure 1-6. Pablo being swaddled so that he has an opportunity to experience boundaries and suck.

Evaluation Information

Neonatal Intensive Care Unit Evaluation

Occupational Profile

After receiving the referral for an OT evaluation of Pablo (25 weeks corrected age), the OT checked with the nurse to determine the best time to see him during regular nursing care. This initial OT assessment was observational and was conducted during the nurse's daily assessment. This included temperature, vitals, abdominal girth, and diaper change. The OT observed how many times the nurse touched the child during care to determine how this impacted the infant's ability to manage the stress of care. After observing, the therapist suggested that additional tactile and positional input be given to the child to decrease the stress of the procedures.

The OT based the evaluation on the five subsystems described by Als in the Synactive Theory of Behavioral Development (1982). This assessment examined Pablo's functioning in the areas of physiological status, state behaviors, self-regulation, movement, method of feeding, any attempts at visual interaction, and response to movement and touch during nursing care and/or by the therapist. For the evaluation, Pablo was positioned supine. He could not be positioned prone because of contraindications related to the umbilical line. He had an oxygen saturation monitor on his foot, was on a conventional ventilator, an IV for fluids, and an NG tube for gavage feedings. No bilirubin lights were required. The primary IV was an umbilical line that was placed at the delivery. His color was pink and he progressed from a sleep state to a drowsy state. Pablo opened his eyes momentarily but did not orient or focus on faces. Hearing appeared intact because the baby quieted when the therapist spoke softly, but this will be confirmed with a hearing test by the audiologist at a later date. The baby was briefly interested in the pacifier. The baby was extubated at 28 weeks to nasal CPAP. The therapist made recommendations to the nurse to create an environment with close boundaries and to provide the baby with opportunities to suck (non-nutritive suck; Figure 1-6). When the IV umbilical line is removed, prone positioning can be implemented.

Analysis of Occupational Performance

At 32 weeks corrected age, the Neonatal Neurobehavioral Examination (Morgan, Koch, Lee, & Aldag, 1988) was used with the following results. Overall tone was slightly low with extension noted more in the upper extremities than the lower extremities. Some jitteriness was noted in the arms. Arm recoil was noted but sluggish. There was little resistance to the scarf sign and popliteal angle was near zero. The baby rooted to the pacifier, Moro reflex was positive, weak grasp reflex was present bilaterally, and plantar grasp was present bilaterally. The baby was noted to have indwelling thumbs toward the palm of the hand. Pablo was NPO due to feeding intolerance, but he did suck on the pacifier intermittently when awake and encouraged. Fifteen minutes into the evaluation, he started crying and displayed finger splaying, tongue thrusting, and some arching. In addition, heart and respiratory rates increased. Pablo required swaddling and deep pressure by the therapist's hands to calm down. He was positioned on the tummy (prone) with boundaries to encourage a tucked, flexed posture. The therapist suspected that there was a medical reason for the baby's arching. She shared this thought with the nurse. The evaluation was ended at that point.

Progress Information

At the next session a few days later, the OT discovered that the nurse practitioner had placed Pablo on an anti-reflux medication, which did decrease his tendency to arch and cry. The OT had fabricated splints for Pablo's indwelling thumbs (Figure 1-7) and provided the nurse with a wearing schedule. A repeat ultrasound was negative for an intraventricular hemorrhage. He resumed gavage feedings through an NG tube without abdominal distention. When Pablo was offered the pacifier, he actively sucked with traction on the nipple. The therapist noted that he was corrected to 35 weeks 3 days and spoke to the neonatologist about starting oral feedings. The nurse agreed. The OT and the nurse discussed a plan for advancing bottle feeding and will share this with the parents when they come in on the weekend.

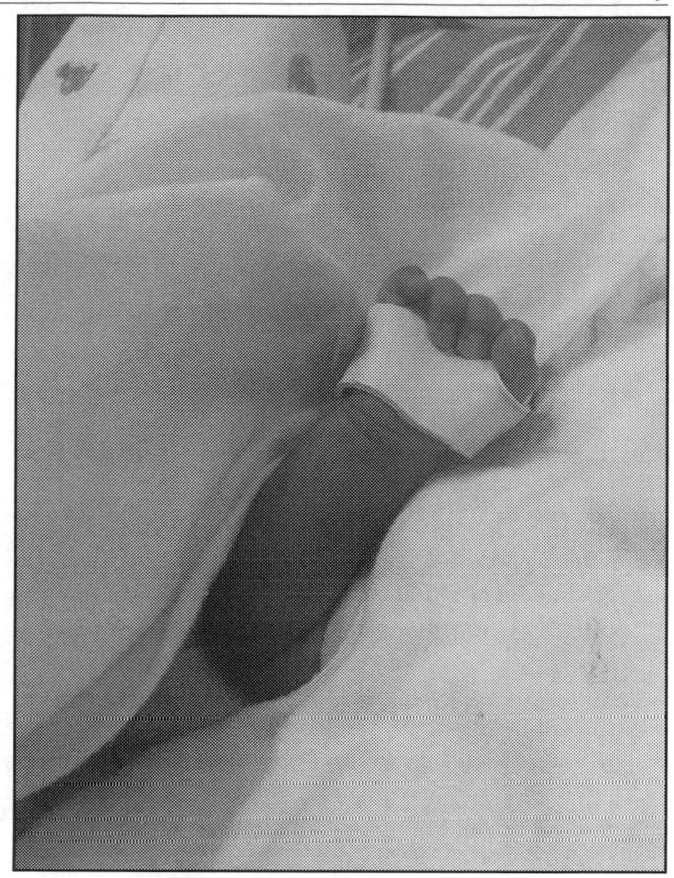

Figure 1-7. Splint for indwelling thumb.

Planning for Discharge

Pablo was progressing nicely and it was time for discharge planning. The OT called on the social worker to arrange a time during the week to discuss Pablo's care with his professional team. During this meeting, the mother expressed the desire to breastfeed. The lactation specialist was brought in to meet with her and discuss the process of getting the baby to the breast. The mom noted that Pablo appeared to want to move his head to the right more than the left. The OT and the nurse validated this observation. He appeared to be using his hands more with the thumbs out of the palms, which pleased everyone. The nurse made the final arrangements for the parents to learn CPR and to use a car seat that would help them to safely transfer Pablo home.

Questions to Consider

Goal Areas and Treatment

1. Go to the AOTA website. Describe the requirements for an OT working in the NICU in terms of knowledge, skills, and experience. http://www.aota.org/practitioners-section/children-and-youth/highlights/39462.aspx?ft=.pdf (In order to access this document, the student will have to be a member of AOTA.)
2. Using the principles of family-centered care, what further information does the OT need to find out from the family and other staff members? What are some ways that the OT might be able to do this? What other team members will the OT need to collaborate with to maximize the effectiveness of therapeutic interactions?
3. The NICU environment includes many pieces of equipment that are necessary for the well-being of the child. Describe the purpose of the following pieces of equipment found in the NICU: isolette, CPAP, oxygen saturation monitor, NG tube, bilirubin lights, and radiant warmer.

Safety Precautions

1. Preterm infants are very fragile. What would be the primary safety concerns of the therapist when working with Pablo? How will the team work together to address these concerns?
2. Premature infants are at risk for many medical conditions, including retinopathy of prematurity, respiratory distress syndrome, necrotizing enterocolitis, and intraventricular hemorrhage, among others. What are these conditions and how would they impact the infant's development?

Intervention Plan

1. From the evaluation information, what would you deem as Pablo's and his family's strengths and needs for participation in occupation?
2. Premature infants in the NICU will receive an individualized developmental care plan. What are the elements of this plan and how can they be implemented in the NICU for Pablo?
3. The NICU unit is a very busy place. One of the OT's roles is to provide input for positioning and environmental adaptations. Discuss the goal of positioning for premature infants and give three examples of adaptations to the environmental context that will maximize Pablo's sensory regulation.
4. How could Pablo's prematurity impact his social emotional development? What suggestions would be helpful to Pablo and to his family to decrease stress and foster infant mental health?
5. Write three long-term goals for Pablo and your first set of short-term objectives. Describe how you will involve the family in establishing and meeting these goals.
6. Discuss the frames of reference that would be applicable to this case. Give two examples of an intervention that would be tied to the frames of reference you have chosen. Provide one source of evidence for these interventions.
7. Pablo required some time to develop before he could tolerate oral feedings. What would be the progression of intervention to facilitate oral feedings and what are physiological signs the therapist will need to monitor?

Planning for Discharge

1. From the vantage point of supporting occupation, what functional abilities does Pablo need to achieve and what skills does Pablo's family need to have learned before discharge? What topics should the OT include in the parent education and home program?
2. After Pablo is discharged, the OT might need to facilitate services that support Pablo and his family. What federal laws will assist in providing these services? What are the criteria for eligibility and service provision?
3. What impact could the premature delivery have on Pablo's development in the future? What areas of function would need to be monitored?

References

Als, H. (1982). Toward a synactive theory of development: Promise for the assessment of infant individuality. *Infant Mental Health Journal*, 3, 229-243.

Morgan, A., Koch, V., Lee, V., & Aldag, J. (1988). Neonatal neurobehavioral examination: A new instrument for quantitative analysis of neonatal neurological status. *Physical Therapy, 68*(9), 1352-1358.

Resources

American Occupational Therapy Association. (2006). Specialized knowledge and skills for practice in the neonatal intensive care unit. *American Journal of Occupational Therapy, 60*(6), 659-668.

Garcia-Rodriguez, M. (2013). Lecture on Occupational Therapy in the NICU. Personal Collection of M. Garcia-Rodriguez, Nova Southeastern University, Ft. Lauderdale, FL. Presented at Nova Southeastern University.

Hunter, J. (2010). Neonatal intensive care unit. In J. Case-Smith & J. O'Brien (Eds.). *Occupational therapy for children.* (pp. 649-677). Maryland Heights, MI: Mosby.

Chapter 2

Introduction to Early Intervention

Early intervention (EI) describes services for children from birth to 3 years of age who have a developmental delay, have a diagnosed disability that has a high likelihood of causing a developmental delay, or, at a state's discretion, are at risk of developmental delay. The purpose of EI services is to meet the *developmental* needs of an infant or toddler in one or more of the following areas: physical development (movement), cognitive development (learning), communication development (interaction), social or emotional development (behavior), or adaptive development (use of existing skills).

Legislation

The Individuals with Disabilities Education Act (IDEA) Part C provides the policies and regulations for EI programming. IDEA Part C supports participating states with federal grants in order to operate a comprehensive statewide program of EI services for infants and toddlers with disabilities and their families. Refer to the U.S. Department of Education website (http://idea.ed.gov) for further information about IDEA Part C.

Natural Environments

Part C of IDEA states that "to the maximum extent appropriate to the needs of the child, EI services must be provided in natural environments, including home and community settings in which children without disabilities participate." (34 CFR §303.12[b])

Natural environments include the home and community settings and programs that are available to all young children. The use of natural environments helps family members and caregivers to enhance a child's learning opportunities through everyday activities and routines in typical settings.

Goals of Early Intervention

One of the primary goals of EI is to support families in promoting their children's optimal development in family and community activities. This includes the active participation of family members and caregivers throughout the EI process. The success of EI depends on building partnerships, which includes equal participation of all collaborators, including the family and service providers. Intervention is linked to specific, family-centered goals and is built into family routines and everyday activities.

For example, EI focuses on the following:

- Supporting the relationship between the child and parent/caregiver
- Empowering parent/caregiver understanding and confidence
- Building child-adaptive capacities
- Enhancing family functioning within the natural environment

Early Intervention Services

EI services are based on the needs and priorities of the child and family. The Individualized Family Service Plan (IFSP) is a family's written plan of EI services. The IFSP is developed by family members and service providers and identifies functional outcomes and the services needed to address those functional outcomes.

EI services may include one or more of the following areas:

Cahill SM, Bowyer P, eds. *Cases in Pediatric Occupational Therapy: Assessment and Intervention (pp 25-45).*

- Assistive technology/aural rehabilitation
- Audiology
- Developmental therapy/special instruction
- Family training and support
- Health consultation
- Medical services (only for diagnostic or evaluation purposes)
- Nursing
- Nutrition
- Occupational therapy (OT)
- Physical therapy (PT)
- Psychological/counseling services
- Service coordination
- Social work
- Speech language
- Transportation
- Vision

Role of Occupational Therapy in Early Intervention

IDEA Part C identifies OT as a primary service in EI. This means that OT can be provided as the only service a child and family receive or in addition to other services. OT practitioners work with the team to support and build the family's capacity to care for their child and be successful in everyday routines. OT practitioners may also adapt the environment or modify activities to promote participation. This could include selecting or making assistive devices to facilitate development. OT practitioners use a family-centered model in EI practice, which places importance on family strengths. Respecting differences in beliefs, values, culture, and priorities is key to providing successful EI services.

Occupational Therapy Process in Early Intervention

The OT process can be used to guide EI practice. Throughout the process, collaboration with the family and team is highlighted to promote successful outcomes. Evaluation in EI includes screenings, formal and informal assessments, parent/family interviews, and observations in natural environments. Intervention includes developing and implementing the IFSP and incorporating evidence-based practice. Outcomes are used to promote parent/caregiver empowerment and to meet the family and child's identified goals, needs, and priorities.

Questions to Consider

1. Who is the "client" in EI?
2. Where is the EI "setting"?
3. How can OT practitioners address the needs of the entire family rather than focusing only on the child's delays or deficits?
4. How does the OT process in EI differ from other pediatric settings?
5. What are some challenges to implementing the OT process in EI?

Reference

Individuals with Disabilities Education Improvement Act of 2004, 20 U.S.C. §1400 et seq. (2004). http://idea.ed.gov

Royce: Developmental Delay/Early Intervention

Ashley Stoffel, OTD, OTR/L and
M. Veronica Llerena, MS, OTR/L

History and Background Information

Royce is 18 months old and is currently receiving OT services through EI. She is the only daughter of two working professionals. Her mother works as an engineer and her father as a pediatric OT. They both have extended family members who live nearby and provide support. Royce's maternal grandmother cares for her on weekdays while both parents work. The family lives in a first-floor condominium in a residential neighborhood in a large city. The family is Filipino. Royce's parents speak English, and Royce's grandmother speaks both English and Tagalog.

Brief Medical History and Developmental Considerations

Royce experienced some complications at birth. Her umbilical cord was wrapped around her neck, causing her distress. She was delivered full-term via cesarean section. She was diagnosed with bilateral hip dysplasia, more pronounced in the left hip. She wore a pelvic harness for 1 month, then a hip abduction brace for the following 5 months. The braces restricted movement. At 2 months, Royce was diagnosed with strabismus and had bilateral eye surgery, followed by eye patching for a couple of months.

Royce began receiving clinic-based PT when she was 8 months old due to her physical and visual concerns.

Royce also had a history of slow weight gain, and the family tried to feed her higher calorie foods. Because of her slow progress with gross motor skills and increasing concerns in other areas of development, the family sought out EI services when Royce was close to 18 months old. Royce's first OT transferred her case to a new therapist when she went on maternity leave.

Occupational Profile

Royce's parents describe her as a happy, easygoing child. They also report that she smiles often, gives hugs, and loves to snuggle and read books. The OT notes that Royce shows interest in others and her surroundings. Royce is easily distracted, and she does not appear to visually examine objects. She often looks at people rather than at objects. Royce also has low muscle tone and lacks stability in her joints, which impacts her motor skills. Royce just started crawling and demonstrates low endurance in supported standing. She is able to use a fisted grasp to secure objects in her palm but cannot manipulate objects much beyond that. Based on standardized assessment results, Royce's developmental age is between 8 and 10 months.

Royce has many toys and books. She shows a preference for books and soft dolls. She has a favorite doll named Bibsy. Royce participates in toddler classes at the public library and the park district. Her grandmother takes her for walks daily. There are a couple of playgrounds near the family's home.

Royce wears an eye patch over her right eye periodically throughout the day. Royce's PT has provided some equipment for Royce. She wears Hip Helpers (snug lycra shorts; Enabling Development, Inc) to provide hip stability. She also uses bilateral ankle-foot orthoses and a stabilizing pressure input orthosis to further enhance gross motor stability. Because her father has experience with Kinesio Taping, Kinesio Tex Tape is used on her shoulders, back, and abdomen to promote postural control.

Royce's parents are concerned that she is not yet standing independently. One of their main goals is for Royce to walk. They also want Royce to be able to play with toys in a variety of ways and use words or gestures to communicate. Royce's dad especially wants to focus on increasing her strength and postural stability as primary strategies toward the family's goals. He hopes that by increasing her strength and endurance, Royce will have a better foundation to build cognitive, fine motor, and communication skills.

A Typical Session With the New Occupational Therapist

The OT arrives at Royce's home and is greeted by Royce and her grandmother. The OT reads the note left in the communication notebook by Royce's father, detailing progress during the week and any new concerns or insights. Royce's father notes that Royce tried to stack her snack cups this week. He also notes that the family is encouraging Royce to use more supported sitting positions such as sitting on a low bench versus the floor.

Typical activities during the initial sessions included the following:

- Pulling her favorite doll, Bibsy, from the couch or up from the ground while prone over her therapy ball
- Pushing the ball, bouncing on the ball, and maintaining sitting balance on the ball while the ball is moved
- Reaching overhead for favorite objects like beads, stuffed toys, or gel clings stuck on a glass door
- Removing objects from plastic containers, toy purses, cardboard boxes, large empty juice containers, or peanut butter jars

After 3 months, Royce maintains supported standing for longer, pulls to stand on her own, and is visually exploring objects more consistently. She is self-directed in play and has limited persistence with overly challenging tasks. The OT and Royce's grandmother work together to identify a variety of strategies to maximize Royce's attention and participation. For example, her grandmother will bounce her on the ball prior to a seated task.

Progress Information

Summary of Royce's 6-Month Individualized Family Service Plan Meeting

During EI, the IFSP is reviewed at least every 6 months. A meeting is generally set up with the family and service providers to discuss progress and any changes needed to the IFSP.

The team and family discuss Royce's goals and progress. After 6 months of therapy, Royce is beginning to walk, though unsteadily. She pulls out the contents of the kitchen cabinets and her toys off of her toy shelves. She shows more intentionality in her play and sometimes imitates the actions of others.

The meeting begins with the family describing their perspectives, which gives the parents a chance to relay how they feel about Royce's progress. Both parents are pleased that Royce is walking and, in general, seems more purposefully engaged in her environment. Royce's father recognizes many incremental gains made by his daughter, including more attempts to communicate and more purpose in her play. He, perhaps more than anyone, recognizes how hard Royce works. Despite these gains, he acknowledges that progress is slow. Royce's mother expresses her interest in making sure that, to the extent possible, Royce will be able to participate in the typical activities of children her age. She relates that it is not always easy to find community toddler classes that are a good match for Royce. Despite this, the family continues to seek opportunities for Royce to be engaged in activities outside the home where she can be around peers.

One of the outcomes of the 6-month IFSP meeting is an idea to start play dates with Royce and a pair of twins who live a block away. The twins are just a few months younger than Royce and also receive EI services. The OT works with both families. Both families are experiencing challenges accessing "typical" environments and settings used by their children's peers. Therapeutic play groups were a possibility, but space was often limited because few of these groups were offered.

Without disclosing information about the twins, the OT asks Royce's parents if they are interested in play dates with a pair of neighborhood children also receiving EI services. The family is interested in this idea, and they give the OT permission to speak with the twins' parents about Royce. The twins' parents are delighted by the idea of having play dates with a neighborhood child and likewise give the OT permission to move forward in organizing a time for the children to play.

The twins' parents are Mexican immigrants who met working in a factory. After the twins were born, their mother left her job to care for them. The twins' father continued working and also attends school in the evenings. The twins' maternal grandmother helps with their care. The family primarily speaks Spanish. The twins have a diagnosis of CHARGE syndrome. They have mild to moderate hearing loss and each has functional vision in one eye, but not the other. They are very active toddlers who, like Royce, have just started walking. They have strong fine motor skills and, unlike Royce, often choose to engage in play with puzzles, blocks, and other manipulatives. Unlike Royce, they shy away from children at the park, often clinging to their mother with fear. The twins have not had much exposure to structured play opportunities with peers. The twins' parents are also looking ahead to when their children will enter school, and they are seeking ways to increase successful interactions with peers.

Royce's family agrees to the play dates knowing that their daughter is social and will genuinely enjoy the company of peers. They also welcome the idea of using the home environments for these social opportunities. Unlike the park district playgroups or neighborhood parks, the home environment provides more focused opportunities for interaction, the support of an OT and parents, and familiar resources. The twins' family is also interested in the idea of a controlled environment to help the twins be more open to interacting with peers. For these two families, the home environment is also free of the judgments and unpredictability that could go along with other settings.

The First Play Date

Because of the twins' social anxiety, the first play date takes place at the twins' home. They live in a first-floor apartment in a six-flat building. The living space is not large but ample enough for the three children to play on the wooden floor. Both mothers and maternal grandmothers accompany the children on this first play date. The OT is also present. This meeting is loosely structured to allow the children to explore being together and the space. While shy and watchful at first, the twins quickly warm up to Royce and follow her as she explores many new objects. She gives the twins hugs and explores the shelves and drawers of toys around the room, rarely pausing for any length of time with one single toy. The children engage mostly in parallel play (Figure 2-1). The families deem the play date successful and worth another try. A schedule is established with play dates occurring twice a month at alternating houses. Royce will host the next one.

After 3 months, session routines are established at each of the family's homes.

The following is a list of typical activities that the children do together when they play at Royce's condo:

- Taking turns pushing and pulling one another in the diaper box "train" that Royce's father fashioned by attaching a long strap to one of the box handles and fastening a towel to the bottom so it could easily glide across the floor
- Playing social games such as ring-around-the-rosie (Figure 2-2)
- Playing basketball with Royce's hoop and balls
- Taking turns going down her slide
- Looking at books
- Engaging in visual motor tasks like puzzles side by side or cooperatively (e.g., taking turns stacking nesting blocks to build a tower; Figure 2-3)

At the twins' home, the following are typical activities:

- Taking turns jumping on a mini trampoline
- Taking turns riding and pushing one another on a ride-on toy
- Singing songs with finger plays
- Pretending to have "picnics" with stuffed animals
- Playing with messy textures such as play dough, fingerpaint, and pudding

Questions to Consider

1. What are some strengths of Royce and her family?
2. Based on the information given so far, what might you anticipate to be the family's main concerns?
3. What are the priorities and concerns that Royce's family has identified?

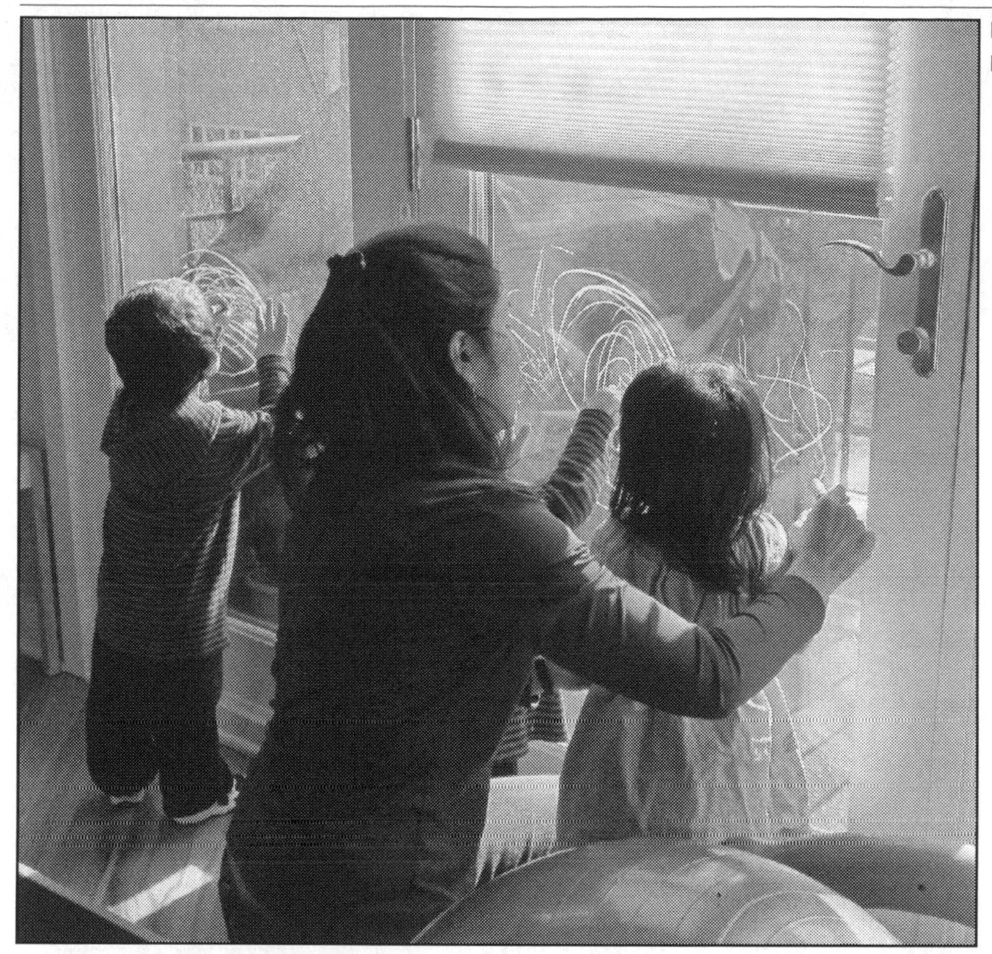

Figure 2-1. Children engaged in parallel play.

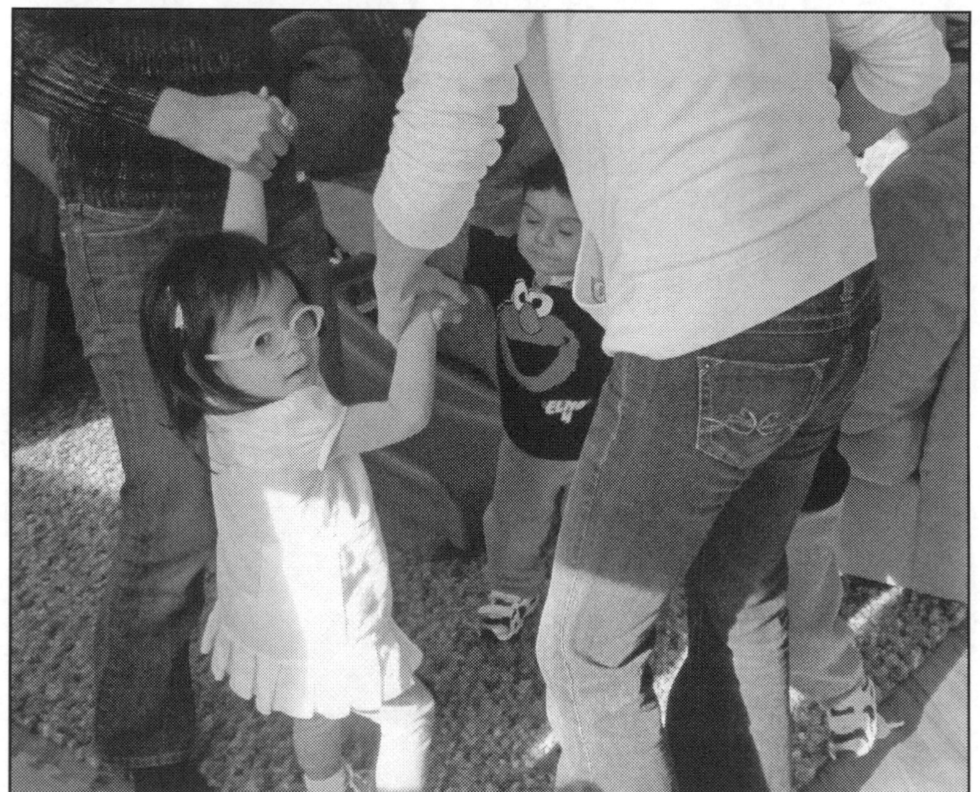

Figure 2-2. Play date where children are playing ring-around-the-rosie.

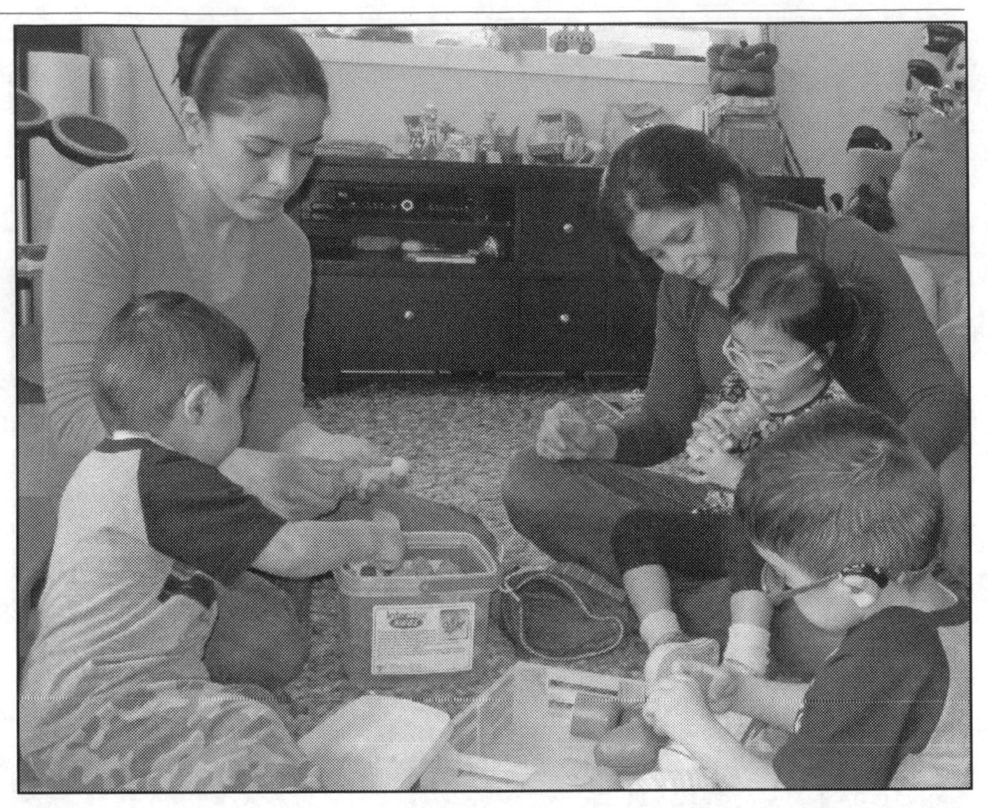

Figure 2-3. Children engaged in visual motor activities and cooperative play.

4. What remaining questions do you have that you would hope to address during the initial sessions?
5. After the initial sessions with the new OT, what strengths do you identify?
6. What are the priorities and concerns that Royce's family has identified after a few months of services?
7. Based on information from the 6-month IFSP meeting and using EI principles, what changes would you make to the intervention, if any?
8. A natural environment is not a particular place. Providing EI services in a natural environment does not mean providing services only in the child's home. Natural environments include home *and* community settings in which children without disabilities participate. Could natural environments be used to address the concerns and priorities identified during Royce's 6-month IFSP review?
9. What are some examples of natural environments that might be applicable to this case? What are some of Royce's natural environments?
10. What are some challenges to using natural environments in EI?
11. How did the intervention with Royce's neighbors look different from the initial sessions?
12. What were the benefits of including Royce's neighbors in the intervention?
13. Can you identify any potential concerns regarding including Royce's neighbors in the intervention from the OT's perspective? Can you identify any concerns regarding this type of intervention from the family's perspective?
14. How was the concept of natural environments utilized in this case?
15. What were the benefits of using everyday activities during the play dates?

Resources

Goode, S., Diefendorf, M., & Colgan, S. (July, 2011). The importance of early intervention for infants and toddlers with disabilities and their families fact sheet. The National Early Childhood Technical Assistance Center (NECTAC). Available at: http://www.nectac.org/pubs/pubs.asp

Individuals with Disabilities Education Improvement Act of 2004, 20 U.S.C. §1400 et seq. (2004). Available at: http://idea.ed.gov

Myers, C. T., Stephens, L., & Tauber, S. (2010). Early intervention. In J. Case-Smith & J. O'Brien (Eds.). *Occupational therapy in children* (6th ed.). (pp. 681-712). St. Louis: Elsevier.

Workgroup on Principles and Practices in Natural Environments. (November, 2007). *Agreed upon mission and key principles for providing early intervention services in natural environments.* OSEP TA Community of Practice-Part C Settings. Available at: http://www.nectac.org/topics/natenv/natenv.asp

Catherine: Agenesis of the Corpus Callosum/Early Intervention Transition

Deborah K. Anderson, PT, MS, PCS

History and Background Information

Catherine, age 2.5 years, has a diagnosis of agenesis of the corpus callosum (AgCC). She was born full-term via cesarean section weighing 9 pounds, 8 ounces. Catherine was diagnosed with AgCC at birth and underwent a series of tests that also identified a small hole in Catherine's heart. AgCC is a rare congenital brain abnormality that occurs when the corpus callosum fails to develop as it should early in the prenatal period. AgCC refers to either complete or partial development of the corpus callosum, which is an important midline structure of the brain. Catherine, through magnetic resonance imaging, was found to have partial development of the AgCC. This diagnosis may result in multiple developmental disabilities. At 2.5 years old, Catherine presents with significant delays in gross motor, fine motor, and speech development. Catherine also exhibits delays in cognition and social/emotional behavior but has shown tremendous growth in these areas and has almost achieved age-appropriate skills. Catherine receives weekly OT, PT, and speech and language therapy.

Occupational Profile

Catherine lives with her parents and younger sister in the heart of a Midwestern suburban community. Catherine's parents are both professionals who work outside of the home. Catherine's dad is an engineer who works for a local technology company with mostly traditional daytime work hours and the need to attend a few evening events. Her mom is a nurse who drives approximately 45 minutes to a hospital in one of the surrounding communities. Catherine's mom has worked at this hospital since before Catherine and her sister were born and has been able to negotiate flexible work hours to manage work and daycare arrangements around both her and her husband's schedule. Because of Catherine's parents' work schedules, therapists provide EI services at either Catherine's home or the home of her daycare provider. Catherine's sister, Mae, is 6 months old and has no known birth or developmental problems.

Catherine and her family live in a two-story Victorian house. The family bedrooms are all on the second floor, with the kitchen, living room, dining room, bathroom, and play room occupying space on the first floor. Catherine's therapies take place mostly on the first floor of the family home, which provides open floor space, changing floor surfaces, and access to toys. Catherine and Mae have a variety of toys serving large and small motor play as well as coloring utensils, paper, and books for more sedentary play. A screened-in porch off of the living room houses a small play set that can be used in all but the coldest weather. A large collie named Lucy is the only family pet. Lucy is typically in the basement during therapy sessions.

In contrast to Catherine's home environment, the daycare environment has limited floor space for movement. The daycare provider, a 60-year-old woman, provides daycare for up to six children in her home. Catherine and Mae are the youngest children, with the others spending most of their day at the local grade school. Daycare is provided in a small 900-square-foot ranch-style house. Bins of toys are accessible to both children and therapists in the front room of the home.

Catherine enjoys looking through books, coloring, and engaging in imaginative play with a small kitchen set. Motivation for motor play has frequently included "shopping" for plastic food items placed around the living room. Rocking with a favorite doll in a small child's rocking chair has become a favorite activity for Catherine, especially when she is tired.

Current Individualized Family Service Plan Goals

- Parents want Catherine to be independently mobile in all environments.
- Parents want Catherine to be able to communicate her wants and needs with less frustration.
- Parents want Catherine to be able to safely eat a variety of foods.
- Parents want Catherine to assist with self-care needs.

Progress Information

At this time, Catherine walks independently on level surfaces and is still somewhat unsteady on outdoor surfaces. Catherine negotiates stairs by crawling up them on her hands and knees. Catherine is able to climb onto her couch at home and safely turns herself around to lower feet first from the couch back to the floor. Catherine has fallen off the couch and chairs in the home environment because she frequently sits on the very edge of the furniture. Catherine enjoys playing at the local playground. She crawls through tunnels and maintains sitting when moving down the slide. Despite multiple attempts by parents, daycare worker, and therapists, Catherine does not enjoy swinging.

Catherine speaks in short, two- to three-word sentences and communicates her wants and needs using words.

Catherine turns pages of books, assembles six-piece puzzles, and scribbles on paper using large crayons. Catherine starts most coloring tasks with her right hand; however, she often switches hands rather than cross her midline. Catherine has not yet been exposed to scissors. Catherine sits at the table with her parents and infant sister for mealtime in a wooden Tripp Trapp chair (Stokke AS), which provides support for her feet and a seat belt for safety. She is able to finger feed and uses a spoon to bring food to her mouth. Catherine is beginning to be able to spear food with a fork. She requires cues to wipe her mouth with a napkin and often needs assistance to thoroughly clean her face. Catherine is able to eat a general diet; however, she has self-limited her food choices, as she does not like certain textures and flavors. Catherine prefers to eat white bread, bagels, chicken nuggets, and plain pasta. She will also eat bananas and other pieces of ripe fruit. Catherine does not like vegetables, other types of meat, casseroles, or crunchy snacks (e.g., cereal or crackers). Catherine is able to take off her socks but not her shoes. She assists with dressing by placing her head, arms, and legs in the holes of the garment when they are presented to her. Catherine continues to wear diapers and has little awareness of when she is wet. She does communicate discomfort when she has had a bowel movement. Catherine does not enjoy bath time because she is fearful of getting her hair rinsed. Despite Catherine's easygoing demeanor, when frustrated, she will scream, cry, or lie on the floor. When Catherine is upset, she requires an adult's assistance to calm down. Strategies that work to help Catherine calm down include bear hugs, slow rhythmic rocking, and looking at picture books.

Preparing for Transition to School

When Catherine turns 3 years old, she will no longer qualify for Part C services of IDEA (Myers, Stephens, & Tauber, 2010). Part C services are those that have been provided through the state's EI program since Catherine was 3 months old. At 3 years of age, Catherine's educational and therapeutic needs will be regulated by Part B of IDEA if she is found eligible to receive these services. In order to determine eligibility for Part B services, the following needs to happen between today, when Catherine is 2.5 years old, and her third birthday:

- Parents make contact with the special education coordinator in their local school district.
- Catherine's service coordinator through the EI program requests updated progress reports from the EI therapists to send to the school system.
- Catherine is evaluated by the school psychologist and the school therapists through her school district.
- Parents visit local school.
- The IFSP team develops a transition plan.
- The IFSP team holds a transition meeting with Catherine's family and school personnel.

Questions to Consider

1. What is the function of the corpus callosum and how might AgCC impact Catherine's development?
2. What strategies might be necessary for the therapists to maintain communication about Catherine's therapeutic needs?
3. What challenges might the home or daycare environment present for the therapists? What are the benefits of providing services in these environments? Based on what is known about Catherine and her IFSP goals, develop a 60-minute OT session for Catherine that takes place in her home. Develop another session that would take place at the daycare center. How are these sessions the same? How are they different?
4. Develop a co-treatment session with either the PT or the speech therapist. Describe how the role of each professional is unique as well as times when a transdisciplinary approach may be used.
5. Give examples of strategies or techniques that the OT could use to support Catherine's parents and her daycare teacher in working with Catherine to make progress toward her goals. Describe how these strategies or techniques would be incorporated into one of the treatment sessions that you developed above.
6. What examination tools would help the OT evaluate Catherine's development and provide the school system with important information about her educational needs?
7. What types of accommodations and modifications would the OT recommend for Catherine at school? Consider transitioning into the classroom from the bus, snack time, art, music, and field trips into the community.
8. What information might the school OT contribute to the transition meeting?
9. How will Catherine's OT services in school be different from those that she received in EI? How will her services be the same?
10. What concerns might Catherine's family have about transitioning to the school system?
11. What are some ways in which the school therapists could ease Catherine's transition into the school system?

Reference

Myers, C. T., Stephens, L., & Tauber, S. (2010). Early intervention. In J. Case-Smith & J. O'Brien (Eds.). *Occupational therapy in children* (6th ed.) (pp. 681-712). St. Louis: Elsevier.

Resource

Paul, L. K., Brown, W. S., Adolphs, R., Tyszka, J. M., Richards, L. J., Mukherjee, P., & Sherr, E. H. (2007). Agenesis of the corpus callosum: Genetic, developmental and functional aspects of connectivity. *Nature Reviews Neuroscience, 8*(4), 287-299.

Tommy: Sensory Dysmodulation and Dyspraxia/Early Intervention

Kimberly Bryze, PhD, OTR/L and Roberta K. O'Shea, PT, DPT, PhD

History and Background Information

Tommy, age 2 years, was referred to OT and PT through the state EI (Part C) system. Tommy lives with his parents in a small townhouse in Chicago that is conveniently located two doors away from his paternal grandmother, who serves as his babysitter during the week.

Tommy was born full-term without complications. He learned to roll from his stomach to his back by 4 months of age and reportedly "hated tummy-time," preferring to sit in his bouncer or infant seat and "watch the world around him." He sat independently at 8 months, crept for a very short period of time, and pulled to stand using furniture by 9 months of age. Once in a standing position, Tommy would stand for long periods of time and not transition back to sitting, seemingly "getting stuck" and unable to return to a sitting position on the floor. Tommy did not walk without handheld guidance or the support of furniture until he was 15 months of age.

Tommy did not babble or speak any words until 18 months of age. His parents and grandmother were not worried about his speech-language development because "other children always speak for him" and "he didn't have much to say." His parents reported that Tommy was always a quiet child, never causing "any trouble," and that he had been a "very good baby." However, when he was approximately 18 months old, he began to express his dislike of self-care tasks such as bathing, having his hair washed or cut, nails cut, and teeth brushed. Tommy's parents chose to keep his hair close-cropped to eliminate the need to brush his hair more than once a day. Although dressing and undressing were unpleasant, his parents chose several outfits that were less problematic in which to dress Tommy, such as soft jersey knits and pullover cotton shirts rather than blue jeans and buttoned shirts.

Tommy's parents were concerned about his picky eating and general avoidance of foods. He had difficulties transitioning from breast to bottle, to pureed foods, to thicker textures, and then to finger foods without gagging, choking, and avoidance of eating by pursing his lips. Tommy's mother expressed her concern that Tommy never seemed to be hungry, reportedly never fussing, gesturing, or indicating his need for food and reluctantly eating only when food was presented to him. He preferred foods that were bite-sized, dry and crunchy, or salty and was averse to foods that were sticky, lumpy or of mixed texture, or pudding-like. His diet revolved around French fries, crackers, cubes of cheese, corn puffs, bites of hot dog or lunch meats, and chips. He refused all fruits, yogurt, cereals (both dry with milk and hot cereals), and most green vegetables; the vegetables he would eat included some green beans and cooked carrot sticks that he would pick up with his hands. At 2 years of age, Tommy did not use any utensils for eating, preferring to pick up food with his fingers. If the pieces of food were too small to grasp easily, he would not feed himself but would receive the food if someone fed him.

The referral to EI was initiated by Tommy's parents after prompting by Tommy's pediatrician, who expressed concern with his delays in speech and language, slow weight gain, and general passivity to movement. The EI team determined that Tommy would benefit from weekly developmental therapy, OT, PT, and speech therapy services through his transition to school-based services when he turned 3 years of age.

Evaluation Information

Initial Occupational Therapy Evaluation

Tommy was evaluated using a team-based, transdisciplinary approach in which the PT took the lead to administer the gross- and fine-motor sections of the *Peabody Developmental Motor Scales*, and the OT took the lead to interview his parents and administer the *Infant-Toddler Sensory Profile* (Dunn, 2002). Tommy's parents were present throughout the evaluation session and were the primary reporters from whom the team gathered much of the previously reported developmental history and insight into the family's daily life. The developmental therapist facilitated various play interactions with Tommy using the *Transdisciplinary Play-Based Assessment* (Linder, 2008).

Table 2-1

Infant/Toddler Sensory Profile

	LESS THAN OTHERS			MORE THAN OTHERS		
Sections	**Section Raw Score Total**	**Definite Difference**	**Probable Difference**	**Typical Performance**	**Probable Difference**	**Definite Difference**
General Processing	No section raw score total is calculated for the General Processing Section					
Auditory Processing	47/50	50---x-------48	47-----------44	43-----------35	34-----------31	30-----------10
Visual Processing	23/35	35-----------32	31-----------28	27------x----20	19-----------16	15-----------7
Tactile Processing	22/75	75-----------68	67-----------62	61-----------48	47-----------42	41-------x---15
Vestibular Processing	12/30	25-----------30	26-----------24	23-----------18	17-----------15	14---x-------6
Oral Sensory Processing	15/35	35-----------33	32-----------30	29-----------21	20-----------17	16-x---------7

Peabody Developmental Motor Scales- 2

Domain	**Raw Score**	**Age Equivalent**	**Percent Delay**	**Standardized Score**
Stationary	38	18 months	25%	8
Locomotion	81	16 months	33%	3
Object Manip	9	15 months	37%	5
Grasping	38	12 months	50%	5
Visual Motor Integration	40	14 months	42%	7

Tommy's Gross Motor quotient: 53 (average is 85 to 115)
Tommy's Fine Motor quotient: 76
Tommy's Motor quotient: 70

Assessment Results

Infant-Toddler Sensory Profile

Results of the Infant-Toddler Sensory Profile were obtained through observation, interview, and discussion with Tommy's parents. Each item was rated according to the standardized scale in the manual and data on the following categories of sensory processing functions were obtained: auditory processing, visual processing, tactile processing, vestibular processing and oral sensory processing. As noted in Table 2-1, all but one category, visual processing, indicate that Tommy has difficulty processing sensory inputs in his daily life. His visual processing appears to be a relative strength, and some concerns are noted with his ability to process auditory information. However, he demonstrates significant difficulty processing tactile, vestibular, and oral-sensory inputs, which impact the ease and efficiency by which he is able to play, perform self-care tasks, and interact with others in his daily life.

Administering the Infant-Toddler Sensory Profile as part of an interview format proved to be helpful for Tommy's parents because they were able to discuss Tommy's relative strengths and challenges and provide examples of ways in which his apparent sensitivities impact the quality of his daily life. They were able to make connections and discuss the ways in which some sensory challenges affected other sensory situations (e.g., when Tommy was in a noisy and busy environment he was unable to eat without increased tendency toward gagging or aversion; in environments that were visually stimulating or with many people, such as a mall or the food store, Tommy was less willing to walk independently and would prefer/need to be carried). Moreover, in the course of discussion, his parents became increasingly aware of the ways in which they had adapted their routines to avoid the sensory challenges Tommy faces on a daily basis. Specifically, his parents identified sensory-driven choices they had made, such as their choice of certain clothing textures that Tommy tolerates, the provision of certain foods that they know he would eat (although admittedly not as nutritionally balanced as they would like), and declining social opportunities to join other young parents at the zoo for the day.

Tommy's scores on the Infant-Toddler Sensory Profile are shown in Table 2-1.

Observations of Play

Tommy was offered several developmentally appropriate gross- and fine-motor toys with which to play, including puzzles, balls of various sizes, a riding toy propelled by pushing with both feet, an indoor climbing and slide structure, and a water table that was filled with uncooked navy beans and various toys through which to pour the beans as well as scoops and containers. Tommy's approach to this sensory- and movement-rich environment was one of caution and occasional confusion. He stood in the center of the large room for several minutes taking in all the possibilities with his eyes but not initiating interaction with any objects until the developmental therapist brought him to the bean table. She demonstrated how to use a cup to scoop and pour the beans into a second cup and into the "waterwheel," allowing the beans to flow through an opening to a wheel where they turned and dropped back into the pool of beans. The examiner gave Tommy the cup and when he did not make any movement except to look at her, she used hand-over-hand guidance to help him scoop up beans and pour them into the wheel. After at least five attempts, Tommy began to initiate the scooping but maintained his forearm in supination while reaching for the wheel toy; the examiner had to help him pronate and pour the beans into the wheel.

Tommy was led to the large wooden ramp in the room and shown how the ball could be rolled down the ramp. He smiled and appeared to understand the game, but when encouraged to position himself at the top of the ramp on the large platform to roll the ball down, Tommy was unable to creep or walk up the ramp without support from the examiner. He was unable to shift his weight forward to balance as the surface angled upward. After several unsuccessful attempts, the examiner held him by the arm and walked with him up the ramp. Tommy was then able to sit at the top of the ramp and roll the ball down to the examiner at the bottom of the ramp. The OT sat behind Tommy on the ramp to help him "catch" the ball as it was rolled up to him. Tommy's anticipation of the ball's trajectory never improved and consistent assistance was offered to him to catch and then roll the ball.

When presented with one-piece and three-piece puzzles, Tommy was able to successfully insert the one-piece, circular form into the form board with a little difficulty. He was able to position each of the three-piece forms near the appropriate spaces in the form board, indicating his visual perception of their shapes and placement, but could not rotate or manipulate the forms to insert them successfully into their spaces. When presented with crayons and paper, Tommy was able to scribble a few circular patterns while holding the crayon in a palmar grasp. He was unable to imitate a vertical or horizontal line, reverting to scribbles.

Analysis of Occupational and Physical Therapy Assessment Results

Results of the evaluation indicate that Tommy experiences delays of greater than 30% in both gross- and fine-motor skill development, which is the cutoff for eligibility for EI services in the state. His gross-motor difficulties impact his ability to navigate within his physical environment for play, mobility, and general exploration. Further, he is unable to grasp and manipulate tools and materials that he needs in everyday task performances, such as using utensils during mealtime, playing with a wide variety of toys and puzzles, and helping with performing self-care tasks as would be expected of a 2-year-old child (e.g., pulling off socks, helping with donning his pullover shirts, assisting with managing the toothbrush during toothbrushing). Moreover, Tommy experiences significant challenges in his ability to effectively process sensory information from his body and the environments in which he lives and plays. His sensory processing difficulties appear to impact his ability to use sensory information in adaptive and appropriate ways for social play with other children, tolerance and performance of tactile-rich self-care tasks, and exploration of new toys and environments offered to him (Bundy, Shia, Qi, & Miller, 2007; Parham & Mailloux, 2010).

Further, based on observations of play during the evaluation session, Tommy demonstrates significant difficulty with the planning and sequencing of motoric actions needed to interact with objects in play and exploration. Although he was obviously interested in managing the large ramp in the room, he was not able to figure out how to position and move his body in order to scale the ramp while creeping or walking without considerable assistance from an adult. He was unable to anticipate the movement of the ball toward him to capture the ball in his hands and roll it back to the examiner. Not until he was seated on the floor and the ball was rolled directly to him was he able to play "catch" with the examiner. He likewise had difficulty with fine-motor manipulation and rotation of objects in space to manage the puzzles, beans, and drawing tasks.

Parent Goals

Given the results of the assessments and the evaluation session, Tommy's parents expressed interest in several areas in which they identified their greatest need and hopes for Tommy. The goals for the EI team were shared by all team members, as is consistent with EI practice. Tommy's goals for EI were as follows:

- Tommy will use a spoon to feed himself soft foods during mealtimes.
- Tommy will actively participate in daily self-care task performances without distress or aversive responses, specifically bathing, toothbrushing, and dressing.
- Tommy will play with developmentally appropriate toys such as stacking large blocks, propelling ride-on toys, turning pages of board books one by one, and rolling and kicking a ball.

- Tommy will independently and safely climb and play on toddler playground equipment such as the steps, tunnels, moving bridge, and short slide.

Focus of Intervention

Occupational and physical therapy services were provided twice per week. One session consisted of a 2-hour, transdisciplinary, center-based, multi-child session, and one additional session was provided as a home-based, cotreatment session. This center-based session included a time each week for free play, music and circle time, gross-motor exploration, fine-motor, sensory and craft work, and snack time before dismissal. The parent(s) were included in the session with up to 10 children, ages 18 to 36 months. During these sessions, occupational, physical, speech, and developmental therapies were provided in a playful, child-centered setting.

Tommy received a second weekly 90-minute in-home session with both OT and PT. This session was held in the late afternoon/early evening after his parents returned home from work and retrieved Tommy from his grandmother's home. The focus of this session included gross-motor play designed to improve motor skill development and provide sensory-motor opportunities through which he could learn new ways of moving his body in play to facilitate the development of praxis and motor learning. On warm summer evenings, therapy sessions included movement opportunities at the local park rather than in the rowdy home environment. Tommy became highly motivated to play and engage in gross-motor activity, and therapy built in repetition of skills with enough variation to keep the challenge level just enough while maintaining the fun factor. Initially, the gross-motor time also included games that included blowing horns and playing kazoos; this served to desensitize his mouth in readiness for meal times.

Included in each session was a mealtime in which specific attention was directed to Tommy improving his ability to use a spoon to feed himself. The OT began using a short-handled toddler spoon and within a few months, Tommy was able to use a "grown-up teaspoon," although he held the handle close to the bowl of the spoon for additional control. By the time he turned 3 years of age, he was able to use a small fork safely and independently to spear soft solid foods such as waffles, green beans, and small bites of softer meats consistent with early 3-year-old skill development.

Over time, the textures of foods he readily ate were graded slowly to include softer foods (e.g., mashed potatoes rather than french fries) and expand his tolerance for foods with varying textures (e.g., simple casserole of cheesy potatoes with peas or macaroni and cheese). The inclusion of yogurt for expanded opportunities for his lunches, and his previous choice of crunchy foods gradually gave way to rice crackers with peanut butter and eventually sandwiches. As Tommy developed increasing skill with holding and manipulating the spoon, his willingness to try new foods and textures also increased. Improved skill development, mastery, and confidence in one area facilitated skill development in another area (Schuberth, Amirault, & Case-Smith, 2010).

With the rough-and-tumble, rowdy gross-motor play offered twice per week, Tommy's ability to tolerate touch input to his body seemed to improve (Anzalone & Lane, 2012; Bundy et al., 2007). He also began to develop the initial "me do" attitude consistent with most 2 year olds, which furthered his sense of control over self-care tasks involving considerable tactile inputs (e.g., brushing his hair, washing his hands, attempting to brush his own teeth while watching his actions in a mirror at his face-level). Several sessions also included an after-meal bath time and playing with the OT, who brought new boats to float and colored soap crayons for the sides of the tub and his arms and legs.

Recommendations for regular follow-through of sensory-friendly strategies for integration into his daily life at home and at grandma's house were offered at each session. Upon reevaluation of the Infant-Toddler Sensory Profile and Peabody Developmental Motor Scales just before he turned 3 years of age (Table 2-2), improvements in several areas of development were noted.

Tommy improved in all areas of the Peabody. As he learned to tolerate and modulate sensory input, he was able to learn basic and advanced play skills and developmentally important motor skills. He also learned coping strategies and problem-solving strategies that were age appropriate and successful. As he gained confidence and control, the adverse and ineffective behavioral strategies he initially used were extinguished.

Questions to Consider

1. In what ways does the Transdisciplinary Play-Based Assessment approach complement the sensory-based approach to assessment?
2. In what ways did physical gross-motor play contribute to improvements in Tommy's eating skills, both oral motor and fine motor?
3. Using principles from sensory integration theory, describe how rough-and-tumble play improved Tommy's tactile hypersensitivity.
4. Identify several authentic, natural ways in which the OT's methods could be carried over by Tommy's parents throughout the week (without developing and prescribing a "home program").
5. What is the relationship between play/playfulness and sensory integration?

TABLE 2-2

INFANT/TODDLER SENSORY PROFILE

		LESS THAN OTHERS			MORE THAN OTHERS	
Sections	**Section Raw Score Total**	**Definite Difference**	**Probable Difference**	**Typical Performance**	**Probable Difference**	**Definite Difference**
General Processing	No section raw score total is calculated for the General Processing Section					
Auditory Processing	44/50	50-----------48	47---------x-44	43-----------35	34-----------31	30-----------10
Visual Processing	24/35	35-----------32	31-----------28	27-----x-----20	19-----------16	15-----------7
Tactile Processing	46/75	75-----------68	67-----------62	61-----------48	47--x---------42	41-----------15
Vestibular Processing	17/30	25-----------30	26-----------24	23-----------18	17-x---------15	14-----------6
Oral Sensory Processing	28/35	35-----------33	32-----------30	29-x---------21	20-----------17	16-----------7

PEABODY DEVELOPMENTAL MOTOR SCALES 2

Domain	**Raw Score**	**Age Equivalent**	**Percent Delay**	**Standardized Score**
Stationary	42	35 months	3%	9
Locomotion	137	33 months	8%	10
Object Manip	29	34 months	5%	9
Grasping	44	34 months	5%	9
Visual Motor Integration	111	34 months	5%	9

Tommy's Gross Motor quotient: 96 (average is 85 to 115)
Tommy's Fine Motor quotient: 74
Tommy's Motor quotient: 94

6. What is praxis? How were Tommy's difficulties with praxis identified?
7. What is the relationship to tactile, proprioceptive, and vestibular sensory processing to praxis dysfunction?
8. Describe ways in which the Transdisciplinary Play-Based Assessment, the Infant-Toddler Sensory Profile, and the Peabody Developmental Motor Scales complemented each other to provide an understanding of Tommy's strengths and needs.
9. Tommy's initial food choices are somewhat common for children with oral-motor sensitivity. Describe why they commonly might be seen in children with oral sensory difficulties.
10. What might you consider to be the benefits of both group/center-based EI services and individualized, home-based EI services for Tommy?

References

Anzalone, M. E., & Lane, S. J. (2012). Sensory processing disorders: Feels awful and doesn't sound very good, either! In S. J. Lane & A. C. Bundy, Eds. *Kids can be kids: A childhood occupations approach* (pp. 437-459). Philadelphia: F. A. Davis Co.

Bundy, A. C., Shia, S., Qi, L., & Miller, L. J. (2007). How does sensory processing dysfunction affect play? *American Journal of Occupational Therapy, 61(2),* 201-208.

Dunn, W. (2002). *Infant-Toddler Sensory Profile.* San Antonio, TX: Pearson Publishing.

Linder, T. (2008). *Transdisciplinary Play Based Assessment.* Baltimore, MD: Paul H. Brookes Publishing.

Parham, L. D., & Mailloux, Z. (2010). Sensory integration. In J. Case-Smith & J. Clifford O'Brien, *Occupational therapy for children* (pp. 325-372). Maryland Heights, MO: Mosby Elsevier.

Schuberth, L. M., Amirault, L. M., & Case-Smith, J. (2010). Feeding intervention. In J. Case-Smith & J. Clifford O'Brien, *Occupational therapy for children* (pp. 446-476). Maryland Heights, MO: Mosby Elsevier.

Resources

American Occupational Therapy Association. (2007). Specialized knowledge and skills in feeding, eating, and swallowing for occupational therapy practice. *American Journal of Occupational Therapy, 61*(6), 686-700.

Bundy, A. C., Lane, S. J., & Murray, E. A. (2002). *Sensory integration: Theory and practice* (2nd ed.). Philadelphia: F. A. Davis Co.

Folio, M., & Fewell, R. (2000). *Peabody Developmental Motor Scales* (2nd ed.). Austin, TX: ProEd.

TABLE 2-3

SCORES FROM COOPER'S EARLY INTERVENTION EVALUATION

HAWAII EARLY LEARNING PROFILE SCORES		
Subtest	**Age Range**	**Percent Delay**
Cognitive	1-2 months	50-75% delay
Gross Motor	1 month	75% delay
Fine Motor	1 month	75% delay
Expressive Language	1-2 months	50-75% delay
Receptive Language	1-2 months	50-75% delay
Social-Emotional	1-2 months	50-75% delay
Regulatory/Sensory Organization	2 months	50% delay
PEABODY DEVELOPMENTAL MOTOR SCALES		
Subtest	**Age Equivalency**	**Percent Delay**
Grasping	1 month	75% delay
Visual-Motor	1 month	75% delay
Reflexes	4 months	No delay
Stationary	2 months	50% delay
Locomotion	2 months	50% delay
Object Manipulation	—	Not tested

Cooper: Developmental Delay/Early Intervention

Susan M. Cahill, PhD, OTR/L

History and Background Information

Cooper was born full-term via cesarean section due to breech presentation and weighed 7 pounds, 10 ounces at birth. Cooper's mom's pregnancy was largely unremarkable. However, his mom was hospitalized around 22 weeks gestation because of a virus and low blood pressure. Before leaving the hospital, after his pediatrician noticed a hip click, Cooper was diagnosed with bilateral hip dysplasia. The pediatrician recommended double diapering to keep his hips in proper alignment until he could be seen by an orthopedic specialist. Cooper was discharged home from the hospital 4 days after birth.

Cooper lives with his mom, who is a special education early childhood teacher, and his dad, who is a computer programmer. Cooper also has a sister, who is 2 years old and attends daycare. Cooper was born in the early spring and his mom was planning to stay home with him for 5 months. However, now that Cooper is 4 months old, his mom is worried that he isn't developing in the same way that his sister did. Cooper's family lives in a three-bedroom ranch-style home in a suburb of a major metropolitan area. Cooper has a large extended family with many cousins ranging in age from 2 months to 17 years. Two of Cooper's older cousins sometimes babysit him and his sister. Cooper and his sister have many toys. Since he has been home, Cooper has spent time in a baby swing and a bouncy seat. Cooper also has a Bumbo seat (Bumbo International) and an Exersaucer (Evenflo), although his parents do not think that he is ready for them yet. The family has two large dogs and Cooper often cries when they bark. Cooper's family has begun to try to keep Cooper separated from the dogs and will often place Cooper supine in a foldable play yard when the dogs are in the same room with him.

Cooper's mom contacted the local EI agency to schedule an evaluation because of her concerns with his overall development.

Evaluation Information

Initial Multidisciplinary Evaluation

The EI team came to evaluate Cooper when he was 4 months and 10 days old. The team was composed of the OT, the PT, and the developmental therapist. In addition, an EI case worker was present at the end of the evaluation and to conduct an initial IFSP meeting.

Cooper was evaluated using the Hawaii Early Learning Profile and the Peabody Developmental Motor Scales (Table 2-3).

Observations and Information From Interview

Cooper appeared to be a happy boy, although his mom reported that he might be getting hungry. Cooper was able to tolerate touching different textured objects and temporarily grasped most toys that were placed in his hand. Cooper was not yet able to reach for toys that were presented to him, although he did look at them. Cooper seemed particularly interested in toys that made music and less so in toys with flashing lights. Cooper was able to track an object in all planes; however, he did not look when his name was called. Cooper tolerates tummy time for 15 minutes or longer and is able to turn his head from side to side when on his belly. However, Cooper does not maintain neck extension and will generally place his head down on the floor while on his tummy (Figure 2-4). Cooper is not yet able to roll over. Cooper sometimes gets frustrated and cries when he wants to roll over. Cooper quickly calms down when comforted by his mom or dad. He sometimes quiets down when being distracted by his older sister. Cooper is able to mouth his hands and has an easier time doing this when his head is turned to the side. Cooper fatigues easily and appears to present with decreased strength. He is able to, yet seems to struggle, to bring his hands and his head to midline. In addition, he is not able to maintain a midline position with hands or head for more than 30 seconds. During the observation, reciprocal kicking and arm movements were not observed. When Cooper was pulled to sit, he demonstrated a full head lag. When positioned in a highchair or stroller, Cooper cannot maintain an upright position unless the device is tilted. Even when the device is tilted, he needs repositioning frequently.

Cooper's mom reports that Cooper is breastfed and that he is able to eat well. She has noticed that much of the milk dribbles out of Cooper's mouth and wonders if he is making a tight enough seal with his lips when he is eating. However, she is not concerned at this time as Cooper is growing adequately and gaining weight. Cooper has not yet been exposed to finger foods, rice cereal, or other baby food. Cooper does have a highchair and his mom has tried to position him in it when the family eats dinner. However, Cooper is not able to sit in the highchair for very long, even when it is tilted. Cooper's mom reports that she will usually bring the foldable play yard into the kitchen during dinner so Cooper can lie in it and be close to his family.

Cooper's mom indicated that Cooper's hip dysplasia has resolved. The family last followed up with the orthopedic specialist approximately 2 weeks ago. This physician remarked that Cooper no longer has bilateral hip clicking and x-rays suggest that his hips are in proper alignment. The family should no longer double diaper Cooper, and the physician suggests that his mild hip dysplasia should not have interfered with his development in any way.

Eligibility Determination

Cooper was found to be eligible for EI services because of delays of more than 30% in several areas of development. The multidisciplinary team recommended that he receive weekly OT and developmental therapy sessions and that he be reevaluated for PT services after 6 months.

Team Goals

Cooper's parents discussed the evaluation results with the team and determined the following priority areas for treatment:

- To improve mobility so that Cooper can roll over independently
- To improve grasping so that Cooper can hold toys and begin to self-feed

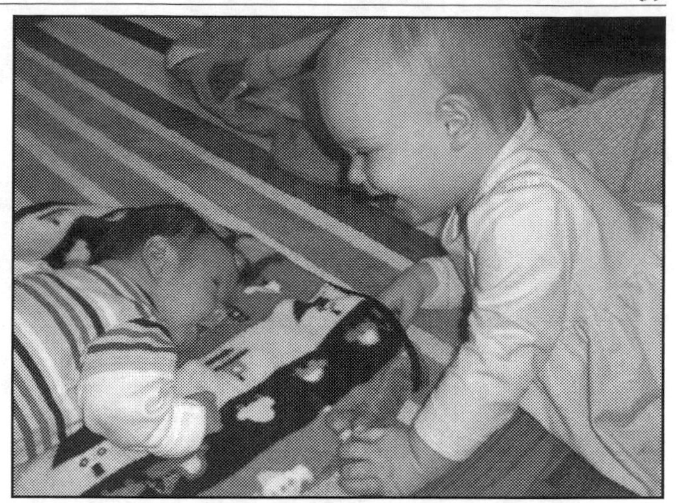

Figure 2-4. Cooper during tummy time with his sister.

- To improve sitting so that Cooper can ride in the stroller or sit in a highchair for 10 minutes

Questions to Consider

1. What other information would you like to know from Cooper's parents?
2. What other assessment tools would provide Cooper's EI team with information about his development? Why might an OT choose one assessment tool over another?'
3. Cooper had a multidisciplinary evaluation. Describe how you think the different clinicians negotiated their roles for assessment administration.
4. What are the pros and cons of having a multidisciplinary evaluation?
5. Are Cooper's parents' goals and expectations developmentally appropriate? Explain your answer.
6. What are Cooper's strengths?
7. Develop three measurable goals that are aligned with Cooper's team goals.
8. Develop a 60-minute home-based intervention plan for Cooper that targets one or more of his team goals. Be specific about how you would arrange the space, as well as what materials you would need.
9. Describe three to four recommendations that you have for Cooper's parents. Explain how these recommendations could be incorporated into the family's typical routines.
10. What are the developmental milestones that children Cooper's age should have already mastered?
11. What are the developmental milestones that children Cooper's age will typically master within the next 6 months?

12. Cooper is to be reevaluated for physical therapy in 6 months. Assuming that he gets OT services, what are some indicators that the OT might observe that would indicate that Cooper might need a reevaluation sooner? What are some indicators that the OT might observe that would suggest that Cooper might need a speech and language evaluation?

Resources

Danto, A., & Pruzansky, M. (2011). *1001 pediatric treatment activities: Creative ideas for therapy sessions.* Thorofare, NJ: SLACK Incorporated.

Myers, C. T., Stephens, L., & Tauber, S. (2010). Early intervention. In J. Case-Smith & J. O'Brien (Eds.). *Occupational therapy in children* (6th ed.) (pp. 681-712). St. Louis: Elsevier.

Ricky: Developmental Delay and Sensory Processing Disorder/ Early Intervention

Robin Elaine Fogerty, OTD, OTR/L; Thelma Haydee Montemayor, MOTS; and Patricia Bowyer, EdD, MS, OTR, FAOTA

History and Background Information

Ricky is a 20-month-old Hispanic boy with a history of developmental delays. Ricky's parents report that he began missing developmental milestones at 2 months of age. They recently visited their pediatrician and shared concerns about Ricky's overall development. Specifically, Ricky has a history of failure to thrive due to his refusal to eat. He is just starting to walk and shows little interest in social interactions and play. Ricky also becomes fearful when exposed to loud sounds and unfamiliar environments/activities. The pediatrician has referred Ricky to an EI agency due to atypical development and sensory processing disorder.

Ricky lives at home with his mother, father, and two sisters (ages 6 and 8 years). Spanish is the only language spoken at home. Ricky stays at home during the day with his mother. His father works long hours on a commercial farm. His sisters attend school during the day. Ricky's mom reports that they spend most of their time inside their home. Ricky spends most of his time in his pack and play, where he is most comfortable. His mom takes care of a few animals outside when Ricky is napping. They go to the store weekly and to the occasional doctor appointments. Friends and family visit Ricky's home each day. However, because of Ricky's adverse reactions to new environments, the family rarely visit other people's homes.

The goal priorities expressed by Ricky's parents include the following:

1. Ricky will eat more foods and successfully join the family at mealtimes.
2. Ricky will tolerate everyday sounds.
3. Ricky will be able to play on his own.
4. Ricky will play with his sisters and other children.
5. Ricky will enjoy participating in family activities, and stop crying/screaming all the time.
6. Ricky will be able to talk.
7. Ricky will be able to walk around by himself.

Early Intervention

Upon admission to Easter Seals EI, Ricky received a comprehensive evaluation that included the following: OT, PT, speech therapy, and case management. EI therapy services will be primarily provided at the family's home. Ricky will receive OT twice per week for 60-minute sessions.

Occupational Therapy Evaluation

The OT selected the Short Child Occupational Profile (SCOPE) to guide the overall assessment and intervention planning process. The SCOPE (Bowyer et al., 2008) is a theory-based assessment tool that provides information about a child's occupational participation based on the major concepts of the *Model of Human Occupation* (Kielhofner, 2008). The goal of the SCOPE is to provide a strengths-based assessment to guide interventions that support a child's participation in valued roles, and the occupations associated with them (Bowyer et al., 2008). The SCOPE allows for varied data collection methods (observation, interview, records review, and other assessment tools) to determine item ratings. Ricky's SCOPE ratings are based on following data sources: parent interviews (SCOPE and sensory history), Infant/Toddler Sensory Profile (Dunn, 2002), and the Pediatric Volitional Questionnaire (Semonti, Kafkes, Schatz, Kiraly, & Kielhofner, 2008). Ricky's SCOPE ratings appear in Figure 2-5.

Volition

Ricky's mom reports that he prefers to sit and watch others rather than actively explore the environment through touch or movement. He is interested in watching others from a distance. Ricky spends most of his day in his pack and play; this is where he is most content. He does not initiate solitary or joint exploration of objects or environments

Ricky's SCOPE Ratings Summary

SCOPE Rating Key

F	Facilitates	Facilitates participation in occupation
A	Allows	Allows participation in occupation
I	Inhibits	Inhibits participation in occupation
R	Restricts	Restricts participation in occupation

Domain	Item	Rating
Volition	Exploration	F A (I) R
	Expression of Enjoyment	F A I (R)
	Preferences & Choices	F A (I) R
	Response to Challenge	F A I (R)
Habituation	Daily Activities	F A I (R)
	Response to Transitions	F A (I) R
	Routine	F A (I) R
	Roles	F A (I) R
Communication & Interaction Skills	Non-Verbal Communication	F (A) I R
	Verbal/Vocal Expressions	F A (I) R
	Conversation	F A (I) R
	Relationships	F A (I) R
Process Skills	Understands & Uses Objects	F (A) I R
	Orientation of Environment	F A (I) R
	Plan & Make Decisions	F A I (R)
	Problem Solving	F A (I) R
Motor Skills	Posture & Mobility	F A (I) R
	Coordination	F A (I) R
	Strength	F (A) I R
	Energy/Endurance	F A (I) R
Environment: Home	Physical Space	F A (I) R
	Physical Resources	F (A) I R
	Social Groups	F (A) I R
	Occupational Demands	F A (I) R
	Family Routine	F A (I) R

Figure 2-5. Ricky's SCOPE ratings. (Adapted from *A User's Manual for The Short Child Occupational Profile (SCOPE)*, by P. L. Bowyer et al., 2008, Chicago: University of Illinois at Chicago, Department of Occupational Therapy, School of Applied Health Sciences. Copyright 2005 by Model of Human Occupation Clearinghouse, University of Illinois at Chicago, Department of Occupational Therapy, School of Applied Health Sciences. Adapted with permission.)

on his own. Ricky's mom shared that if she gets on the floor with him and initiates play, Ricky will imitate her actions with some toys. However, he does not really seem interested and does not persist. He used to like a stuffed toy; however, he has lost interest over the last few months. Similarly, he used to express excitement and joy when a cartoon was played. However, he seems ambivalent about this activity today. During observations, he clung to mother and did not leave her lap. He sustained visual attention with watching others manipulate materials; however, he did not reach toward or manipulate materials with his own body. Ricky is reported as being fussy and appears fearful during most interactions with people/objects/environments. He is happiest when he is riding in the car or riding in a stroller during neighborhood walks. Although he does not express enjoyment during these activities, he is calm and happy in his demeanor. Ricky's volition is negatively impacted by self-regulation and sensory processing differences. According to the ITSP information, Ricky is easily overstimulated by sensations. Ricky has difficulty processing touch, vestibular, auditory, and oral sensations (Table 2-4). As a result, he tends to avoid sensory exploration, and demonstrates an overall fearful disposition. Ricky expresses fearfulness and discomfort when exposed to busy environments, when placed on the floor around other children, when others move quickly around him, when he attempts to move through the environment, when exposed to loud

TABLE 2-4

RICKY'S INFANT/TODDLER SENSORY PROFILE SUMMARY

QUADRANT SCORES	
Low registration	Typical performance
Sensation seeking	Probable difference (less than others)
Sensory sensitivity	Probable difference (more than others)
Sensation avoiding	Definite difference (more than others)
SENSORY PROCESSING SECTION SCORES	
Visual processing	Typical Performance
Auditory processing	Probable difference (less than others)
Vestibular processing	Probable difference (less than others)
Tactile processing	Definite difference (more than others)
Oral processing	Definite difference (more than others)

Table 2-5

Ricky's Pediatric Volitional Questionnaire Results

	SPONTANEOUS	*INVOLVED*	*HESITANT*	*PASSIVE*
Shows curiosity	x			
Stays engaged	x			
Shows preferences			x	
Tries new things			x	
Tries to produce effects			x	
Task-directed				x
Initiates actions				x
Expresses mastery pleasure				x
Tries to solve problems				x
Practices skill				x
Seeks challenges				x
Organizes/modifies environment				x
Pursues activity to completion				x
Uses imagination/symbolism				x

sounds, and when exposed to foods. The PVQ was also administered to help inform SCOPE ratings in the area of volition. The PVQ scores are summarized in Table 2-5.

Habituation

Ricky demonstrates strength in understanding and anticipating routines. However, he has marked difficulty with participating and cooperating in many daily routines. For example, in the morning he wakes up and sits by the pack and play waiting to be placed inside. He prefers to sit inside the pack and play and have his bottle while his family gets ready for school and work. They have breakfast at the table in the morning; however, Ricky becomes extremely distressed at mealtimes and this is too disruptive when there is limited time to get ready for the day. During other mealtimes, Ricky is fed by his mother while in his high-chair. He will cry and refuse to eat; she persists because he needs to gain weight. Meal times are described as stressful for both Ricky and his family. Ricky also has difficulty with the family bedtime routine. After about 1 hour of trying to lay Ricky down, he is finally loaded into the car and driven around until he falls asleep. Ricky also has tantrums during diaper changes. He does anticipate and cooperate with the routine of getting into a stroller and going for a walk and getting into the car seat when going for a car ride. Ricky has difficulty with transitions because he seems to anticipate any change with fear. He does not persist in tasks so he does not participate in termination of tasks. In addition, he cannot regulate arousal effectively to handle the transition to something new.

In the area of role participation, Ricky is most successful in his role as a child/son with his mother. He meets some expectations in his role as child/son; he looks to his mother for reassurance that situations are safe and follows his mother's lead and instructions when he is able to achieve self-regulation that allows task tolerance. At this time, Ricky does not demonstrate actions associated with being a sibling or a friend, which limits his ability to develop social interaction skills and develop relationships. He primarily displays fear and withdrawal behaviors with other children because of his sensory processing difficulties. He is fearful of others when they are moving quickly in his proximity and cannot tolerate the typical noise level of other children.

Communication and Interaction Skills

Ricky demonstrates relative strengths in his nonverbal communication skills. He points to items he wants, pushes away unwanted items, reaches toward his mom when he wants to be picked up, and waves goodbye to express that he either wants to leave or wants others to leave him alone. He also communicates physically by pulling his mother toward or away from things. He shakes his head "no" in response to anything he does not like. Ricky can verbalize three words: "mama," "no," and "ju" for juice. He asks for juice only when juice is visually present. He verbalizes "mama" and "no" across many situations; some are appropriate and some are not. Many of Ricky's vocal sounds are made when he's upset; he makes sounds to demonstrate protest and discomfort. When Ricky is calm and content, he tends to be very quiet and relies more on physical communication. It is likely that Ricky is frustrated by his limited communication skills, contributing to his frequent meltdowns. Ricky's ability to build relationships with other children is limited. He is frightened by other children and becomes increasingly upset as other children try to interact with him. However, he does show social interest when children are at a safe distance; he watches them with curiosity. He clearly distinguishes between different people. He responds well with physical touch or handling by his parents only. He demonstrates strength in responding reciprocally with his mother when they are alone at home. He will watch his mother's face and imitate her expressions, imitate her actions, and look back at his mother to see her reactions to his actions.

Process Skills

Ricky demonstrates the ability to appropriately select and try to use objects. During observations, he imitated his mother by attempting to place a shape in a shape sorter. He correctly chose the shape from other nonrelated objects and knew this object was supposed to go into the hole. When given a marker, he held the tool in an expected manner and tried to imitate scribbling by tapping the marker on paper. However, Ricky does not initiate selection or object use until after he is prompted by his mother's actions. Ricky demonstrates an awareness of the people, objects, and activities occurring in his environment. Due to his sensory hyper-sensitivities, he appears to be hyper-aware and fearful as people move and interact around him. His reactions to changes in the environment can be extreme. For example, he quickly notices the vacuum and will cover his ears and begin crying upon its appearance in the room. When he is playing with mom, he becomes distressed when his siblings praise and clap as a result of his accomplishments. At this time, he does not demonstrate the ability to initiate and carry out a plan of action to completion. He relies on his mother to select activities and initiate manipulation. Even with support and encouragement, his interaction with objects is fleeting. Ricky tends to look at objects placed in his proximity. If objects are simply placed in his hand, he will quickly discard them. Owing to his decreased volition in the areas of showing interest, exploration, and persistence, he does not attempt problem solving at this time. He primarily imitates actions that are prompted by adults; attempts are momentary. He does show attempts to ask for assistance. For example, after trying to place a shape into a shape sorter, he either disengaged from the task or handed the object to his mother.

Motor Skills

Ricky demonstrates adequate trunk stability when seated; he is able to freely use hands and arms in any seated position. He has recently started walking and is able to walk across flat surfaces without assistance; however, he keeps arms positioned in high guard and appears fearful of falling. He will not attempt to walk or stand when other children are present. Rather, he clings to his mother or sits down and begins crying. Ricky's development of fine-motor coordination is likely impacted by his lack of experience with interacting with the objects in his environment and limited play exploration/participation. Overall, Ricky's motor movements are slow and hesitant. He is able to grasp medium-sized objects with a tripod or pincer grasp. He can coordinate bilateral actions such as tapping objects together or holding a cup with one hand while removing objects with the other. Ricky appears to have adequate strength to hold body positions, grasp, and move against objects with resistance. He is still developing lower-body strength and coordination needed for stable walking. Ricky displays a very uneven energy pattern throughout the day, swinging from agitated states, to more passive lethargic states. He takes two naps during the day; one nap is over 2 hours in length. If left to his preference, Ricky will sit and watch his environment, rather than engage in movement.

Environment

At home, Ricky is provided with a safe environment. The use of the pack and play provides boundaries that help Ricky with self-regulation when the environment becomes overwhelming to him. However, the pack and play does not provide solutions for when the environment becomes too noisy. Additionally, the use of the pack and play for extended periods of time does not afford Ricky the opportunity to learn to walk, explore his environment, or begin to socially interact with other children. Ricky does have access to safe and appropriate toys when in and out of his pack and play. However, he does not have access to alternative forms of communication. He also lacks any type of support to practice walking around his environment without fear of falling (for example, a push toy.) Ricky's social environment is supportive. Although his responses to sensations limit the family's activities outside of the home, Ricky has access to family and peer interactions daily while at home. However, the demands of these interactions currently exceed his ability level and result in meltdowns/withdrawal/avoidance. Some elements of both occupational demands and the family routine may also be limiting Ricky's participation. For example, quieter periods of family interaction may not occur, which would support Ricky's ability to get out of the pack and play and interact with siblings. Noisy, busy, and rushed mealtimes may also contribute to Ricky's distress during mealtimes.

Questions to Consider

Goal Areas and Treatment Focus

1. Using the OT evaluation data, develop a list of strengths and challenges for Ricky.
2. Review the SCOPE, ITSP, and PVQ score summary tables and determine which SCOPE and/or sensory factors need to be addressed during intervention.
3. Develop intervention goals and intervention strategies for each item listed in #2. Refer to the SCOPE Goal and Intervention Planning Chart (Table 2-6) for guidance and examples.
4. How can you establish trust and rapport with Ricky and his family?

Intervention Plan

1. Describe the following types of interventions you could use with Ricky:
   a. Occupation-based
   b. Sensory-based
2. Describe the role of OT in a group for sensory processing. Would a mom and child group facilitate development and education? How?
3. In what other environments can therapy take place?
4. How does culture play a role in intervention planning?
5. How can you incorporate the family into treatment?
6. How can you answer the following parental concerns?
   a. "What does sensory processing mean?"
   b. "Will it affect him later in life?"
   c. "Will he always have this?"
   d. "How does (intervention strategy) help him?"
   e. "How is OT different than other therapies in helping my child?"
   f. "When is it okay to stop?'

Safety Precautions

1. What safety issues might you discuss with Ricky's family?

Planning for Discharge

1. What do you need to consider for transition to school-based services?
2. Describe what home modifications you can suggest.
3. What are inexpensive strategies parents can utilize for continued development?

References

Bowyer, P., Kramer, J., Ploszaj, A., Ross, M., Schwartz, O., Kielhofner, G., & Kramer, J. (2008). *A user's manual for The Short Child Occupational Profile (SCOPE; version 2.2)*. Chicago: University of Illinois at Chicago, Model of Human Occupation Clearinghouse, Department of Occupational Therapy, College of Applied Health Sciences.

Dunn, W. (2002). *The Infant Toddler Sensory Profile*. San Antonio, TX: Psychological Corporation.

Kielhofner, G. (2008). *Model of Human Occupation: Theory and application*. (4th ed.). Philadelphia: Lippincott, Williams, and Wilkins.

Semonti, B., Kafkes, A., Schatz, R., Kiraly, A., & Kielhofner, G. (2008). *The Pediatric Volitional Questionnaire (PVQ; Version 2.1)*. Chicago: University of Illinois at Chicago, Model of Human Occupation Clearinghouse, Department of Occupational Therapy, College of Applied Health Sciences.

Table 2-6

SCOPE Goal and Intervention Planning Chart

SCOPE ITEM	KEY WORDS FOR GOAL WRITING	EXAMPLE GOAL	STRATEGIES FOR INTERVENTION	THEORETICAL REASONING	FAMILY INVOLVEMENT
VOLITION: Exploration	• Investigates • Attempts • Explores • Tries new things • Examines • Shows curiosity • Seeks • Shows interest • Responds Touches • Engages	• Child will investigate 2 new objects when they are placed within reach with verbal cues. • Child will show interest in an object by visually attending to that object when placed in front of him/her.	• Provide child with opportunities to explore new objects and encourage free play in a safe, appropriate environment. • Provide physical support when needed to enable the child to demonstrate exploration of new activities. • Provide the child with various types of toys (musical, interactive/cause and effect, texture, sports/games) to encourage identification of interests.	When a child explores he/she: • develops interests • learns about the environment • learns about his/her abilities.	• Provide the child with new play options and settings (toys, playgrounds, objects, groups, or programs). • Support the child to try a range of home chores and self-care tasks. • Learn physical positioning/support techniques to facilitate the child's optimal engagement with objects.
HABITUATION: Routine	• Coordinates • Structures • Sequences • Anticipates • Initiates • Follows • Completes	• Child will follow all steps of a 4 step routine when using a picture schedule 90% of the time. • Child will demonstrate awareness of the beginning of lunch time by sitting in his seat when the food cart is brought to the room.	• Help family identify activities/times at home in which a routine could be integrated. • Have a routine/sequence for therapy sessions. • When there is a change in a daily routine, be sure to let the child know the changes and what is expected of him/her. • Help the child to practice engagement in a school/home routine by working on those tasks in therapy.	Routines: • help a child to understand what is expected of him/her • provide structure and predictability • facilitate participation through more efficient and effective use of time and skills.	• Have the child work on homework every day for 30 minutes immediately after supper. • Have the child initiate the bedtime routine at the same time every school night • Have the child prepare his/her backpack for school each night before bed.

Adapted from *SCOPE Goal and Intervention Planning Chart* by P.L. Bowyer et al., 2008, Chicago: University of Illinois at Chicago, Model of Human Occupation Clearinghouse, Department of Occupational Therapy, College of Applied Health Sciences. Adapted with permission.

Chapter 3

Introduction to School Systems

School systems practice includes services for children between 3 to 22 years of age. Historically, school-based occupational therapy (OT) services were provided only to children who were found eligible for special education and/or related services or those who needed special supports to gain physical access to the school building or the educational curriculum. More recently, school systems practice has grown to include children in general education as well as opportunities for occupational therapists (OTs) to participate in program development.

Special Education and Related Services

OT is recognized as a related service. Special education and related services are designed to enable students with disabilities to obtain functional, developmental, and academic gains within school curricula. Special education services are typically provided as part as an Individualized Education Program (IEP). The IEP is a legal document that provides detailed information on the child's specific needs and outlines the goals, services, and accommodations and modifications that the child will receive. The IEP is reviewed annually, and children must be reevaluated for special education and related services at least every 3 years.

Legislation

The Individuals with Disabilities Education Act (IDEA) is the federal law that ensures specialized educational services to children with disabilities. Part B of IDEA governs the provision of services to children ages 3 to 21. IDEA began as the Education for All Handicapped Children Act in 1975 and was most recently amended by Congress in 2004. This important legislation guarantees access to a free, appropriate, public education for children with disabilities. According to this law, educational services must be provided in the least restrictive environment (LRE).

Least Restrictive Environment

IDEA requires that children with disabilities participate in their educational program in the LRE:

To the maximum extent appropriate, children with disabilities, including children in public or private institutions or other care facilities, are educated with children who are not disabled, and special classes, separate schooling, or other removal of children with disabilities from the regular educational environment occurs only when the nature or severity of the disability of a child is such that education in regular classes with the use of supplementary aids and services cannot be achieved satisfactorily (IDEA, 2004).

The special education team works together to determine the LRE based on individual student needs. The educational placement is an important component of the IEP and is reviewed annually and may be changed if warranted.

The Individualized Education Program Team

The IEP team always includes the child's parents, a regular education teacher, a special education teacher, and a representative of the local educational agency. Based on the child's needs, the IEP team may also include related service professionals such as the following:

Cahill SM, Bowyer P, eds. *Cases in Pediatric Occupational Therapy: Assessment and Intervention (pp 47-88).*

- OT
- Physical therapist (PT)
- Speech-language pathologist/audiologist
- Psychologist
- Adaptive physical education teacher
- Counselor
- Orientation and mobility specialist
- Nursing or medical specialist
- Social worker

The Role of School-Based Occupational Therapy

Like OTs in other areas, OTs in the school setting focus on functional participation in work, self-help, and leisure activities. The work of students is learning, which is a complex process that includes many factors, including attending to instruction, accessing the learning environment, working collaboratively with peers, accessing educational materials, and demonstrating knowledge. The OT provides services that enable the student to more fully participate in his or her role as a learner, classmate, and friend. Common self-help skills the OT may address in school include eating/feeding, dressing, or toileting. Leisure skills in an educational environment may include accessing the playground, engaging in social and cooperative play, and participating in sports.

School-based OT services must be functionally, developmentally, and/or educationally relevant. It is important that the OT work closely with the special education teacher and other team members to determine the child's needs and provide OT services that are related to the student's educational programming.

School-Based Occupational Therapy in Response to Intervention

OT practitioners are increasingly providing services to students in general education under Response to Intervention (RtI). RtI is a multi-tiered problem-solving model designed to support students in general education who struggle with learning or behavior. Schools that have adopted RtI provide an evidence-based curriculum and use sound instructional methods. They also regularly and systematically collect data related to student outcomes. These data are used to determine if students require more intensive support to achieve grade-level academic expectations.

Questions to Consider

1. What are some key factors associated with school-based practice?
2. How can OTs collaborate with the rest of the IEP to provide quality services to students with special needs?
3. How is the OT process different in school systems practice from other pediatric settings?
4. What are some challenges and opportunities to implementing the OT process in school-based settings?
5. Read the *AOTA Practice Advisory on Occupational Therapy in Response to Intervention*. What is the difference between traditional school-based OT services and RtI services?

References

American Occupational Therapy Association. (2012). AOTA Practice Advisory on Occupational Therapy in Response to Intervention. Retrieved from: http://www.aota.org/Practice/Children-Youth/School-based/RTI.aspx

Individuals with Disabilities Education Improvement Act of 2004, 20 U.S.C. §1400 et seq. (2004). Available at: http://idea.ed.gov

Denny: Autism and Attention Deficit Hyperactivity Disorder/School Systems

Meghan Suman, MS, OTR/L, BCP

History and Background Information

Denny, a 6-year-old first-grade student, lives in a suburban area with his father, mother, and 11-year-old sister. Denny's extended family resides in Poland. Denny's mother and father completed college in Poland. His father works in technology and his mother stays at home. Denny's older sister, Marta, was diagnosed with autism at age 2 and attention deficit hyperactivity disorder (ADHD) at age 8. Denny's father reports that the family enjoys hiking, watching television, and attending community events. The parents report that they primarily speak Polish in the home but are trying to speak English to Denny and Marta as much as possible.

Denny was born at 7 pounds, 8 ounces via elective cesarean section following a full-term, healthy pregnancy. At birth, he was diagnosed with an incomplete cleft of the soft palate, clubfoot on the right side, and borderline microcephaly. Feeding was initially difficult, but Denny was eventually able to feed successfully with a Haberman nipple.

Denny's club foot was in a cast continuously for his first 6 months of life. Surgical correction was completed around his first birthday and he continued to wear an ankle-foot orthosis (AFO) at night until age 3. Reconstructive surgery to correct Denny's cleft palate was completed at age 15 months. Denny experienced recurrent ear infections throughout his first 2 years and had bilateral tubes placed at age 20 months. Ear infections were not eliminated but decreased in frequency to one to two infections each year. Denny had four teeth removed at age 3 years due to dental decay caused by sleeping with a bottle in his mouth.

Denny's parents report that his motor milestones were delayed because of the cast on his right leg and subsequent corrective surgery. They report that the surgeon recommended PT following the surgery, but Denny did not receive therapy due to insurance issues. Denny achieved his developmental milestones as follows:

- Sits up: 9 months
- Crawls: 15 months
- Walks: 20 months
- Feeds self: 15 months (finger foods)
- Toilet trained: 6 years
- Imitates sounds: 14 months (inconsistently)
- First word: 6 years ("bubbles")

Denny began receiving in-home early intervention (EI) services at age 30 months. Denny was referred for EI services by his pediatrician. In the EI program, Denny received speech-language therapy twice a week and developmental therapy twice a week. He was evaluated by an OT at age 33 months but did not start services before transitioning to the school district. The Early Intervention Individual Family Service Plan (IFSP) identified differences or delays in the areas of sensory processing, fine-motor skills, self-help, communication, and behavior. The OT who evaluated Denny through EI recommended that his parents pursue a medical diagnostic assessment from a developmental pediatrician or pediatric neurologist to rule out autism, but Denny's parents did not pursue this option.

When Denny turned 3, he transitioned from EI to the public preschool system. The evaluation team at the preschool included a psychologist, special education teacher, speech-language pathologist, PT, and OT. Denny separated from his parents without difficulty and entered the testing area with the team. He darted around the room and explored several objects before choosing a glittery baton and standing on his toes near the window. Denny waved the baton back and forth and vocalized, although the team was unable to discern any words. The team attempted to complete the Peabody Developmental Motor Scales, but Denny did not engage in adult-directed activities and was unable to complete this standardized assessment. The speech-language pathologist engaged directly with Denny and offered him a variety of play options, but he struggled to transition away from the baton. When the therapist blew bubbles, Denny vocalized loudly, laughed, and jumped. The team used play-based observations, parent interview, and the Hawaii Early Learning Profile (HELP; Parks, 1992) to complete their evaluation. In the parent interview, Denny's father expressed concern that Denny was continuing to demonstrate delays resulting from his early medical history, especially the cleft palate and ear infections. He reported that Denny and Marta were very different children in personality and development.

The school-based team met with Denny's parents and his EI providers to review the evaluation results and develop an IEP for Denny. The team determined that Denny was a child with an educational disability and was eligible for an IEP. The team found that "developmental delay" was the category that best described Denny's disability. The team considered and discussed two educational placement options for Denny, including a self-contained special education classroom and a general education preschool classroom with additional supports from a special education teacher and related services. Denny's EI providers and parents expressed concern that Denny had little exposure to typically developing children, as he had spent most of his time at home with Marta. The IEP team chose a general-education setting for Denny, where he would attend preschool in a classroom with peers from the community and have the support of a special education teacher, OT, and speech-language pathologist. The team hypothesized that daily exposure to highly verbal peers and typical classroom routines would assist Denny in meeting his goals and achieving developmental milestones. Denny's IEP goals addressed fine-motor and prewriting skills, toileting, communication, play, early literacy, and early numeracy skills.

In the general education preschool classroom, Denny rarely remained in his workspace and required hand-over-hand assistance to follow basic classroom routines such as hanging up his jacket. He did not eat during snack time. He demonstrated negative behaviors, including pulling peers' hair and clothes, spitting, and throwing. The team paired Denny with positive peer models and provided visuals and social stories for a variety of school behaviors. The OT and classroom teacher created a sensory "cool down" space within the classroom and color coded his materials and workspace to provide boundaries. The team developed a behavior reward system in which a staff member would blow bubbles when Denny earned five tokens. Even with these supports, Denny's classroom performance remained problematic and he was unable to participate in the curriculum in the general education classroom.

After 10 weeks, the school team met with Denny's parents to discuss a change in placement. The IEP team discussed the available options for Denny and decided that the LRE that would meet Denny's needs would be a self-contained special education classroom within the same school building. This would allow Denny to spend most of his day in a smaller classroom with five other students with similar needs. He would participate in an individualized curriculum with direct instruction on language and functional independence. Denny continued to join his general education class on the playground with assistance and supervision from a teacher's aide. He was more successful accessing the curriculum in the self-contained classroom. Although his behavior remained significantly discrepant from that of his typical peers, he began to make slow progress toward his IEP goals.

Denny continued to receive his educational programming and related services in a self-contained special education classroom within a regular elementary school throughout kindergarten and first grade. The OT developed a fine-motor and prewriting program that Denny completed daily with his teacher or teacher's aide. She set up an individualized sensory program for him in the school's sensory room and provided sensory supports within the classroom. She collaborated with the speech-language pathologist to set up a system for Denny to identify and communicate his toileting needs, and collaborated with the team to develop a formal behavior support plan.

Evaluation Information

In first grade, Denny's team held a meeting to plan his reevaluation. Denny's parents attended the meeting and shared their concerns. They reported feeling confused about the cause of Denny's developmental delays. They asked how long speech development typically takes after cleft palate surgery, because Denny repeats only one or two words. The speech-language pathologist explained that global communication delays such as Denny's do not typically result from cleft palate and that the team may want to look more closely at the nature of Denny's disability beyond his early medical history. The psychologist suggested that parents and teacher complete the Gilliam Autism Rating Scale (Gilliam, 1995) to determine if Denny meets the educational criteria for autism. The parents expressed that Denny is very different from his sister, who has autism. They also asked why Denny would have such difficulty learning while Marta demonstrates high-level skills in math and reading. The team explained that the skills and abilities of children on the autism spectrum vary greatly. The psychologist also suggested completing IQ testing to determine if Denny has a cognitive disability that may be impacting his rate of learning. The team determined that the speech-language pathologist would complete informal observations to evaluate Denny's language skills and would also work with the special education teacher and OT to complete the Verbal Behavior Milestones Assessment and Placement Program (VB-MAPP; Sundberg, 2008). The VB-MAPP is an assessment tool that focuses on early language milestones and barriers to language development. In order to consider the educational disability categories of autism and cognitive disability, the team needed information on sensory processing and adaptive behavior. The team determined that the OT would complete classroom observations and administer the Sensory Profile-School Companion (Dunn, 1999) to assess sensory processing. The team considered both the Vineland Adaptive Behavior Scales (Sparrow et al., 2005) and the School Function Assessment (SFA; Coster, 1998) to assess adaptive behavior, and chose the SFA based on its relevance to goal setting in the school environment. The team agreed that the OT and social worker would work together to administer the SFA.

The OT began the evaluation process by conducting a short parent interview. The concerns Denny's parents shared at the reevaluation planning meeting were primarily related to Denny's diagnosis. Because the OT evaluation would assess Denny's performance in a wide array of tasks in school, the therapist wanted to be sure to gather information from the parents to ensure that she addressed areas that were of concern to Denny's family. The following are some of the questions the OT asked and a summary of the responses from Denny's father:

OT: *When he is at home, what is Denny best at doing?*

Denny's father: *Playing by himself. Choosing toys he likes.*

OT: *What is the most difficult part of the day for you taking care of Denny?*

Denny's father: *Mealtime. Denny is very picky. He likes yogurt and pudding, but only if we feed it to him. This takes a lot of time. The only things he feeds himself are crackers, cookies, and chips. He is very messy when he eats these things.*

OT: *What chores does Denny help with at home?*

Denny's father: *My wife and I take care of the house. We don't need help. We always keep our house very clean.*

OT: *Does Denny ever put his own dishes in the sink or put his clothes in the laundry basket?*

Denny's father: *No. My wife and I do those things. Denny and Marta don't need to do that.*

OT: *What places do you like to go as a family?*

Denny's father: *We go hiking. We go to the store as a family.*

OT: *What are some difficulties you face taking Denny and Marta to events in the community?*

Denny's father: *Denny doesn't like to close the bathroom door. That's probably our fault because we don't make him do it at home. That makes it hard to stay anywhere very long because he will need a bathroom break and then we have to go home. Also, mealtime is a problem. It's hard to eat in a restaurant. Denny only likes certain things, he is so messy, and he always wants us to scoop the food into his mouth. Marta gets very loud. People don't like us in restaurants. We always eat at home now. If we are too far from home, we eat in the car.*

TABLE 3-1

DENNY'S SP SCHOOL COMPANION SCORES

	MUCH LESS THAN OTHERS	LESS THAN OTHERS	SIMILAR TO OTHERS	MORE THAN OTHERS	MUCH MORE THAN OTHERS
Quadrants	***Definite Difference***	***Probable Difference***	***Typical performance***	***Probable Difference***	***Definite Difference***
Registration	*				X
Seeking	*	*			X
Sensitivity				X	
Avoiding	*	*		X	
Factors					
School Factor 1	*	*			X
School Factor 2	*			X	
School Factor 3	*	*		X	
School Factor 4	*	*		X	
Sections					
Auditory	*			X	
Visual	*				X
Movement	*	*		X	
Touch	*	*			X
Behavior	*			X	

*No Probable or Definite "Less than others" score is ever given for this category

Explanation of Terminology on Sensory Profile- School Companion

-Quadrant Summary-
Registration—measures the student's awareness of all types of sensation available.
Seeking—measures the student's interest in and pleasure with all types of sensation.
Sensitivity—measures the student's ability to notice all types of sensation.
Avoiding—measures the student's need for controlling the amount and types of sensations available at any time.
-School Factor Summary-
School Factor 1—measures the student's need for external supports to participate in learning.
School Factor 2—measures the student's awareness and attention in the learning environment.
School Factor 3—measures the student's range of tolerance for sensory input within the learning environment.
School Factor 4—measures the student's availability for learning in the learning environment.

OT: *Have you ever tried getting Denny to feed himself with a spoon?*

Denny's father: *Not really. After the cleft palate surgery, we were very happy to have him eat anything. Now he just insists on eating this way.*

After the parent interview, the OT administered the Sensory Profile-School Companion to the special education teacher and completed classroom observations of sensory processing. Results of the Sensory Profile-School Companion indicated that Denny was demonstrating atypical responses to visual and touch sensations and that he demonstrated low registration and sensory seeking behavior patterns. In the area of vision, the teacher indicated that Denny has difficulty staying organized, avoids eye contact, watches others as they move around the room, and looks away from tasks to notice all other activity in the room. In the area of touch, she noted that Denny doesn't notice when his face and hands are soiled, plays or "fiddles" with objects and school materials, and is fidgety or disruptive when standing in line or close to other people. The items on the Sensory Profile-School Companion related to "low registration," included missing oral and demonstrated directions, appearing not to hear the teacher, seeming oblivious within an active environment, and showing little emotion regardless of the situation. Denny's full scores on the Sensory Profile-School Companion are documented in Table 3-1.

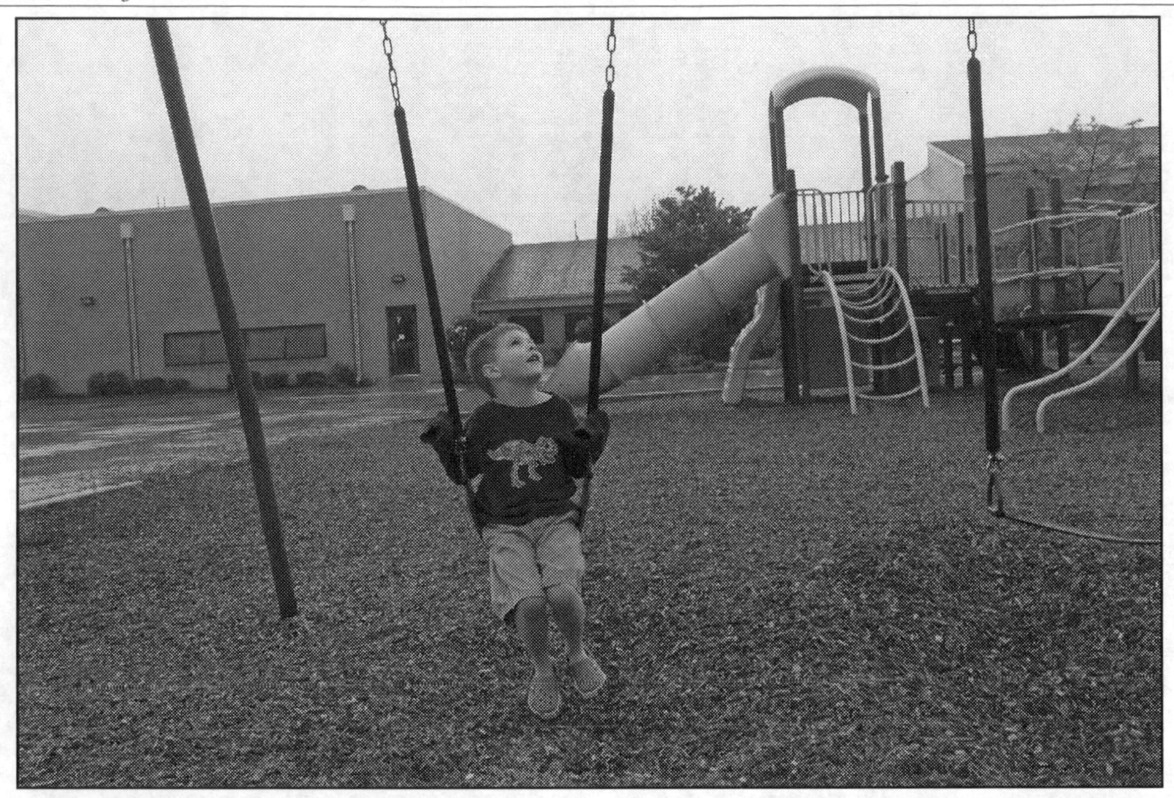

Figure 3-1. Denny on the swing at recess.

The OT observed Denny in several settings and noted the following:

- Morning calendar group: Denny is seated at a table with his teacher and four peers. He has his Picture Exchange Communication System (PECS) book with him. He is shaking his head back and forth and blowing upward, moving his hair with each blow. The teacher places two PECS cards on his strip, sunny and rainy. She tells the group that the weather today is sunny. She says, "Give me sunny" and holds out her hand. Denny continues to blow on his hair. The teacher's aide gives Denny hand-over-hand assistance to take the correct picture. He begins to wave the picture in his peripheral vision. The aide physically prompts him to hand the card to the teacher. The teacher opens the window blinds as she talks about the weather. Denny begins to spit on the table. The teacher's aide moves his chair back so he is further from the table. Denny begins to shake and blow on his hair again. The teacher prompts another student to answer a question. Denny reaches out and pulls the hair of the student next to him. Denny is removed from the group. He sits in the "cool down" area as the group finishes, alternately blowing on his hair and spitting toward the window.
- Lunch: Denny is seated in a relatively quiet classroom with four peers. The lights are dimmed. He opens his lunch bag, screams, closes his lunch bag, and pushes it off his desk. The teacher prompts him to pick up his bag. He does but refuses to unpack his lunch, so his teacher helps him. She takes out his yogurt container and sets it on his desk. Denny knocks it to the floor. He screams whenever it is placed on his desk. Eventually, his teacher puts it back in his backpack. Denny sits quietly at his desk eating crackers. After each bite, he crumbles a bit of cracker, holds it above eye level, and sprinkles it to the floor.
- Recess: Denny goes to recess with his special education class. His teacher's aide reports that he uses only the swings at recess (Figure 3-1). On this day, Denny swings and occasionally spits into the air while swinging. He pulls his sleeves over his hands while holding onto the swing chains.
- Restroom: Denny waits outside the restroom while the teacher's aide makes sure it is empty. He uses the restroom without closing the door. The OT prompts Denny to close the door, but he does not respond. The OT closes the stall door. Denny screams and pulls the door open again. He remains in the stall for more than 5 minutes kicking his feet and watching his shoes light up. The teacher's aide prompts him verbally several times to "finish up" and then steps inside the stall to assist him. Once she enters the stall, Denny stands up independently and quickly dresses. He moves to the sink. He runs the water but does not wet his hands. He obtains some foam soap from the dispenser and begins to flick it onto the mirror. The teacher's aide

prompts him to finish washing his hands. He turns off the water and wipes the soap from his hands on a paper towel. Denny and the aide exit the restroom.

- Fine-motor centers: Denny rotates through a variety of "centers" within the special education classroom designed to provide opportunities for fine- and visual-motor development. Denny has practiced printing his name 3x each day since beginning kindergarten. In the observation, he receives hand-over-hand assistance to print his name. When the teacher removes this assistance, Denny draws a series of counterclockwise loops across the paper. Denny grasps his pencil using a static four-finger grasp. During cutting tasks, he does not attend to shapes or lines but rather cuts straight across the paper. He continues to pick up pieces of paper, cutting each in half across the middle, until the teacher assists him to move to the next station. He strings beads without difficulty, pausing frequently to swing the string of beads in his peripheral vision.

Based on clinical observations, the OT concluded that Denny is seeking visual sensory stimulation by spitting into the sunlight, flicking soap onto the mirror, and waving objects in his peripheral vision. He is demonstrating tactile avoiding behaviors by avoiding contact with the chains on the swing and avoiding getting his hands wet when washing. His "low registration" behaviors, however, were not consistent with clinical observations. Children with low registration typically have a high threshold for sensation, resulting in stimuli going unnoticed. Denny does notice and respond to the sensory stimuli in his environment, but his very low language skills and atypical social interactions caused his scores on the Sensory Profile-School Companion to fall in the low registration range. Based on both the results of the Sensory Profile-School Companion and clinical observations, the OT was able to conclude that Denny demonstrates both visual sensory seeking and tactile sensory avoiding behaviors, but he does not truly present as a child with low registration.

The OT and social worker met to create a plan for completing the School Function Assessment (SFA). The SFA is a criterion-reference rating scale for children in kindergarten through sixth grade. The scale has three parts: participation, task supports, and activity performance. Subsections are further broken down into physical and cognitive/behavioral elements. In Denny's case, the OT completed the physical elements as well as items within the "personal care awareness" and "safety" sections. The results of the SFA indicated that Denny was demonstrating delays in all areas. His areas of relative strength were travel, maintaining and changing positions, and recreational movement. The areas where he demonstrated the greatest discrepancy were written work, functional communication, and behavior regulation.

Reevaluation Meeting

The team met with Denny's parents to review the results of the reevaluation. The psychologist found a nonverbal IQ of 54 and skills falling primarily in the 12- to 20-month range on the HELP. The speech-language pathologist and the special education teacher found that most skills on the VB-MAPP fell in the 0- to 18-month range. Based on the assessment results outlined above, the OT was able to document differences in sensory processing and significant delays in adaptive behavior. The team discussed these results with the parents at the meeting. They found that Denny continued to be eligible for special education as a child with both autism and a cognitive disability. Denny's parents indicated that this helped them understand why Denny's learning style and academic progress was so different from Marta's. His parents also expressed sadness that his disability was more significant than they had originally thought. Denny's mother described feeling worried about planning for the future for two children with special needs, especially in a country where they have no family. The OT shared resources with the family regarding a local support group for parents of special-needs children.

Individualized Education Program Meeting

Upon completing the reevaluation meeting, the team began working with Denny's parents to build an IEP for Denny. The special education teacher proposed goals related to early literacy and numeracy skills. The speech-language pathologist proposed a goal for imitating verbal sounds and a goal for the use of an augmentative communication device for requesting preferred items. The social worker proposed a goal for reducing the number of aggressive behaviors (e.g., hair pulling) through the use of an individualized behavior support plan.

The OT took into account Denny's educational history, information from the reevaluation, and parent concerns when designing the OT goals. She explained to Denny's parents that these were beginning steps toward greater independence for Denny at school. She encouraged Denny's parents to take small steps toward increasing his independence at home as well by allowing him to take a greater role in household management and self-care activities. The IEP goals proposed by the OT are listed below:

- Given visuals and incentives as needed, Denny will independently close the stall door when using the restroom on 5 out of 5 opportunities.
- Given visuals, incentives, and verbal prompts as needed, Denny will use a spoon to independently feed himself at least five bites of a preferred food within a 20-minute lunch period on 3 out of 5 school days.

- Given visuals as needed, Denny will mark his name on a variety of projects and worksheets using a self-inking name stamp.
- Given an individualized sensory program and environmental sensory supports in the classroom, Denny will engage in more than 2 minutes of functional play with three different classroom toys without demonstrating repetitive behaviors in one 30-minute play period.

The OT worked with the team to determine what types of supports and accommodations should be listed in the IEP. The final list included an individualized sensory program, environmental modifications to limit visual distractions during instruction, increased physical space during instruction and transitions, visual supports in the restroom to encourage privacy, daily practice with self-inking name stamp for classroom work, and fading assistance with feeding. The OT proposed modifying the classroom environment to introducing a study carrel rather than working at an open table. She created visual supports related to feeding and restroom use using the computer program Boardmaker (Mayer-Jonson). She also created a series of worksheets Denny could use to practice using his name stamp. Denny's parents were very pleased with the goals and programming proposed by the OT and the team.

Questions to Consider

1. Locate resources that could have been provided to Denny's parents by the EI therapists to help them better understand typical development.
2. What additional questions might the OT ask Denny's father during the interview? How would information gained from these questions be used?
3. What other assessment tools might be appropriate to administer to Denny? Describe your rationale for selecting different tools.
4. Polish is Denny's parents' first language. What steps should be taken at the IEP meeting to ensure that they are fully able to participate and to understand what is being shared about their son?
5. What are some of Denny's strengths?
6. Review the accommodations recommended by the OT. Describe in detail how these accommodations would be implemented.
7. Describe the type of coordination and collaboration that would be needed between the teacher and the OT to maximize Denny's progress towards goals.
8. Develop a data collection sheet for one of Denny's goals. Be specific as to who would collect the data, how often it would be collected, and how it would be shared with the IEP team.
9. Develop or locate a visual support to help Denny during feeding or going to the bathroom.
10. Assume that Denny receives 45 minutes per week of OT services at school. Describe in detail how the OT could spend this time in Denny's classroom to support him in meeting his goals. Consider treatment activities, as well as ways that the OT could be integrated into the general classroom routine.
11. Besides a name stamp, what are some other examples of personal supports, tools, or equipment that might benefit Denny?
12. Describe in detail how the OT could communicate Denny's progress to his parents in both formal and informal ways.

References

Coster, W. (1998). *The school function assessment manual.* San Antonio, TX: The Psychological Corporation.

Dunn, W. (1999). *Sensory profile school companion manual.* San Antonio, TX: The Psychological Corporation.

Gilliam, J. (1995). *The Gilliam autism rating scale: Examiner's manual.* Austin, TX: Pro-Ed.

Parks S. (1992). *Inside HELP – Administration and Reference Manual for the Hawaii Early Learning Profile (HELP).* Palo Alto, CA: VORT Corporation.

Sparrow, S., Cicchetti, D., & Balla, D. (2005). *Vineland-II: Vineland adaptive behavior scales* (2nd ed.). San Antonio, TX: Pearson.

Sundberg, M. L. (2008). *VB-MAPP verbal behavior milestones assessment and placement program: A language and social skills assessment program for children with autism or other developmental disabilities.* Concord, CA: AVB Press.

Resources

Miller Kuhaneck, H., & Watling, R. (2010). *Autism: A comprehensive occupational therapy approach* (3rd ed.). Bethesda, MD: AOTA Press.

National Dissemination Center for Children with Disabilities. (2010). Building the legacy: A training curriculum on IDEA 2004. Available at: http://nichcy.org/laws/idea/legacy

Donovan: Emotional Disturbance/Middle School

Heather Roberts, MHA, OTR/L

History and Background Information

Donovan, age 12 years, was first diagnosed with an emotional disturbance due to bipolar disorder, ADHD, and oppositional defiant disorder 4 years earlier in elementary school. He has a history of multiple inpatient hospitalizations due to his out-of-control and aggressive behavior. He lives with his mother, who adopted him at birth. At school, he has a history of being off task, verbally threatening to peers, demonstrating poor social skills, and becoming overly upset about things. He has difficulty with anger control and impulsivity. Donovan's general intellectual ability was determined to be average, with a score of 97. Donovan attends middle school in a social adjustment classroom on a reduced day and receives psychological and counseling services.

Donovan was referred to OT by his middle school teacher. The teacher's concerns included poor pencil grasp, difficulties with handwriting, and difficulties with clothing fasteners.

Evaluation Information

Occupational Profile

Donovan has an emotional disturbance. This is his second year in middle school. He has worked up to attending school on a half day schedule. He was very cooperative with the OT during evaluation; however, it is reported that he has difficulty following directions and listening to his teachers and has frequent outbursts resulting in visits to the principal's office. Donovan participates in adaptive physical education. This is the only class Donovan attends that is not in the social adjustment classroom. Donovan reports that he enjoys drawing and creating video games on the computer. He currently lives with his mother and has two small dogs.

Analysis of Occupational Performance

The Beery VMI is a developmental sequence of geometric forms to be copied with paper and pencil. It is designed to assess the extent to which individuals can integrate their visual and motor abilities. Standard scores are interpreted as 85 to 115 being average. There are three parts to the VMI:

1. The visual motor integration piece required Donovan to copy different shapes. Donovan received a standard score of 69, which is below average.
2. On the visual perception piece, Donovan pointed to shapes that were the same. He received a standard score of 94, which is in the average range.
3. On the motor coordination part, Donovan was asked to copy shapes and stay within the lines. He received a standard score of 78, which is below average.

Areas of Occupation

Instrumental Activities of Daily Living

- Classroom activities: Donovan ambulates around the school, including outside, the cafeteria, and the gymnasium independently. He changes positions; gets on/off chair, toilet, and floor. He picks up items off of the floor and carries items while walking. His gait is slower than that of his peers and appears to be an odd shuffling gait. Donovan uses his right hand and expressed a keen interest in art and drawing. He demonstrates a tripod grasp on a pencil.

Performance Skills

- Use of materials: Donovan opens/closes books, turns pages in a book, and uses writing utensils to draw/write on paper.
- Setup and cleanup: Donovan disposes of his trash in a trash receptacle, removes materials from large containers, puts objects in small containers (jar), uses a sponge to wipe up a spill, takes out materials to work on, obtains objects out of his backpack, and passes out materials. He opens sealed bags and sandwich bags.

Activities of Daily Living

- Eating and drinking: Donovan eats regular food without choking, gagging, or spillage. He drinks from a cup and straw, uses forks and spoons, and accesses the water fountain. In addition, he wipes his hands and face with a napkin.
- Hygiene: Donovan washes his hands and toilets independently. This includes clothing management and all activities in the bathroom.
- Clothing management: Donovan removes and puts on his jacket and raises/lowers his pants for toileting; he is independent with buttons/snaps on a dressing vest. He zips/unzips but is unable to thread the zipper. He dons/doffs his shoes and hangs up his jacket and backpack on a hook. He wears sweatpants or elastic shorts, pullover sweatshirts, and only shoes with Velcro (Velcro USA) daily to school.

Activity Demands

- Computer use: Donovan operates the computer and uses the keyboard and mouse to carry out functions. He inserts discs into the computer and navigates various school-approved websites. He reports that he loves being on the computer and hopes to work in the video gaming industry when he is older. He is not currently using the keyboard for his written output.

Donovan shows great interest in the activities the OT presented to him during the evaluation. He asks intuitive questions and expresses a strong desire and enjoyment in drawing and photography. He reports that he gets to go home from school at noon and will play video games until dinner. He reports that he never has homework and does not perform any chores at home. Donovan demonstrates delays in regard to his emotional state; his inability to control his emotions leads to poor and aggressive behavior.

Questions to Consider

Goals/Treatment Plan

1. Write out a problem list for Donovan.
2. What are Donovan's strengths and how can they be used to help him achieve his goals?
3. What are your goals for Donovan?
4. What recommendations to the teacher and staff would you make?
5. If you think the teacher has unrealistic expectations for Donovan producing written output, how would you handle this?
6. What frames of reference will you use? What would a typical treatment session entail?

Safety Precautions

1. What are the primary safety concerns that should be addressed with Donovan?

Self-Care/Leisure/Work

1. What would you identify as Donovan's self-care deficits?
2. What are some suggestions you have for Donovan's teachers in regard to his written output?
3. How can you use Donovan's interests to improve his behavior in the classroom?
4. What are some ideas you have that Donovan can do when he is at home?
5. What might you work with mom on at home?

Equipment/Adaptations

1. What type of environmental adaptations might need to be made in the classroom for Donovan to be more successful?
2. If Donovan were to begin taking a class with the general education students, what modifications might he need to ensure he was successful?

Neuromusculoskeletal

1. What can be done to improve Donovan's visual-motor and motor coordination deficits? What compensatory strategies or modifications could you use if there is no improvement?

Psychosocial

1. What are some activities you could work on with Donovan to improve his ability to control his emotions?

Teacher/Staff Education

1. How will you work with Donovan's teacher and psychologist on his behaviors?
2. What would you include in your conversation with Donovan's teacher about his need to interact more with peers?

Dismissal

1. How long would you plan to work with Donovan and his teacher?
2. What would your dismissal criteria be for Donovan?
3. If you recommend continued services into high school, what future goals might you have for him?

Resources

Bazyk, S., & Case-Smith, J. (2010). School-based occupational therapy services. In J. Case-Smith & J. O'Brien (Eds.). *Occupational therapy for children* (6th ed.) (pp. 7173-743). St. Louis: Mosby/Elsevier.

Beery, K., Buktenica, N., & Beery, N. (2010). *Beery-Buktenica developmental test of visual-motor integration* (6th ed.). San Antonio, TX: Pearson.

Serena: At Risk for Learning and Social Emotional Disabilities/School Systems

Susan M. Cahill, PhD, OTR/L

History and Background Information

Serena, a fourth-grade student, moved into this school district 2 weeks after the start of the second quarter. Serena was referred to the school's RtI problem-solving team (PST) by her teacher, Ms. K, after she had been in her class for 3 weeks.

Prior to attending the PST meeting, Ms. K completed the PST Referral Form (Table 3-2) and routed it to the school social worker, who coordinated the problem-solving team. The referral form provided basic demographic information, the reason for the referral, and a list of professionals who could be invited by the teacher to attend the meeting.

After the social worker received the referral, she invited the OT to come to Serena's PST meeting. The social worker felt that the OT might have something to contribute to the case because she and the OT had collaborated before to support other students who struggled with making friends and turning in assignments on time.

Table 3-2

PST Referral Form

Student Name: Serena W	**Grade:** 4	**Date of Referral:** December 2
Referring Teacher: Ms. K		
Reason for referral: Serena recently moved into our district. I have been unable to get past records from her mother and Serena has reported that this is the third school that she has gone to this year so far. She seems totally lost in my class. She can't keep up, she has turned in only about half of her assignments, and she doesn't seem to be making friends.		
Team members requested at meeting: X Assistant Principal X Social Worker____Nurse____Speech & Language Pathologist ____Occupational Therapist____Special Area Teacher:____________		

First Problem-Solving Team Meeting

During the first meeting, Ms. K, the assistant principal, the social worker, the OT, and two other grade-level teachers were present. The PST members asked Ms. K probing questions in an effort to identify patterns in Serena's behavior, as well as performance discrepancies between Serena and her classmates. In addition, they asked about Serena's strengths and needs.

Ms. K identified that Serena had strong oral reading skills compared to her peers and that when she was paying attention, she could orally answer comprehension questions. Serena was also able to do basic math computation in her head and was often the last student out in the math flash card game that they played every Friday. Ms. K told the PST team that Serena had the most difficulty completing independent assignments in class and turning in her homework. The assignments that she did turn in were of poor quality (e.g., items missing, copying errors). Most often, however, Serena failed to turn in assignments at all; this included assignments that Ms. K had witnessed her working on and completing in class. Serena did not perform well on tests and had stated several times that she didn't study because she was out late at her aunt's house. Ms. K described Serena as a sweet, well-behaved, kind young lady who seemed to want to do well and was very willing to stay in during lunch recess to make up assignments that she had lost. When asked about Serena's difficulty making friends, Ms. K indicated that she thought that there weren't many opportunities for her to interact with other students. Serena often arrived a few minutes late to school, which meant that she missed out on playing with and talking to peers on the playground before the morning bell. She also was often picked up by her mother a few minutes before the dismissal bell.

The PST discussed Ms. K's concerns and determined that Serena's difficulties did not appear to be related to academic difficulty but rather organization. For this reason, they decided not to include her in a Tier 2 reading or math group. The PST suspected that Serena's difficulties turning in homework assignments were a result of poor organizational skills and that her difficulties with making friends had to do with a limited ability to socialize with them in informal situations.

The OT asked about previous interventions that had been tried to help Serena. Ms. K shared how she had repeatedly provided Serena with extra copies of worksheets and the number to the school's homework hotline. She also allowed Serena to stay in during lunch recess to complete missing assignments. Ms. K also moved Serena's desk twice so that she would be able to sit with different groups of students in the effort to help her get to know her classmates better.

The PST determined that they needed more information before they could make recommendations to support Serena. The team developed an action plan that included the following steps:

1. The social worker will follow up with Serena's mom regarding late dropoffs and early pickups.
2. The OT will observe Serena during class to gain insights into the habits and routines that she uses related to organization.
3. The social worker will collaborate with the teacher to identify two to three peers that Serena could eat lunch with in the social worker's office at least once a week.

The team agreed to implement the action plan and to meet to discuss Serena's needs in 4 weeks.

Following the First Problem-Solving Team Meeting

The social worker had difficulty setting up a time to meet with Serena's mom due to her work schedule. When the social worker did get a chance to speak with Serena's mom over the phone, she learned that Serena's mom worked two jobs and that Serena spent many afternoons and evenings at her aunt's house. While she was at her aunt's house, Serena was expected to complete her homework, help with cooking dinner, and clear the dinner dishes. Serena also had the opportunity to play with her 2-year-old twin cousins, whom she adored. Serena's mom was apologetic about the late dropoffs and early pickups. She reported that she often had to pick Serena up early so that she could make the evening shift at the retail store where she worked. Serena's mom also shared that both she and Serena often had a difficult time waking up in the morning. Serena's mom's evening shift at the retail store ended at 10:30 PM, at which time she would leave to pick Serena up from her aunt's house. Serena was often asleep on the sofa and had to be roused in order to collect her belongings and get in the car for the 20-minute drive home. Once Serena and her mom were back home, Serena was expected to wash up, brush her teeth, put on her pajamas, and get her clothes ready for the next day. Serena sometimes had difficulty getting back to sleep and awoke sleepy most mornings. Serena's mom described their morning routine as "a quick dash out the door" in an effort to get to school on time.

The OT observed Serena in Ms. K's class for approximately 15 minutes on two separate occasions. During the first observation, the OT observed Serena completing a math assignment in which Serena had to copy even-numbered problems from her textbook onto notebook paper. She also had to complete the problems by showing how she arrived at her answers. The OT noted that Serena completed the assignment at a very fast pace, which impacted the quality of her performance because she ended up skipping problems and forgetting to show her work several times. The OT did note, however, that Serena's answers to the problems were correct. During the math assignment, Serena readily and consistently maintained task focus and she used goal-directed task actions that were focused on completing the math assignment. Serena was not distracted by the chatter produced by other students and reluctantly answered one of her peer's questions after the peer interrupted her two times. Serena continued working on the math assignment, even after Ms. K had instructed the class to put it away and to take out their math homework from last night to turn it in. Serena did not attend to Ms. K's instructions and continued working on her math assignment while the rest of the class turned in their homework assignments. Serena continued to work on her math assignment until Ms. K said that it was time for the students to gather their lunch tickets from their desks and head to lunch. At this time, Serena quickly put her notebook paper and her math book in her desk and began searching for her lunch ticket. Serena used a random pattern to search her desk. She started searching in the right upper quadrant, then moved to lower left quadrant, then to the upper right quadrant, and then to right lower quadrant. While she was searching, the other students began getting in line. Serena raised her hand and Ms. K came over to assist her. Ms. K located Serena's lunch ticket under the math book in the upper left quadrant of her desk. Serena lined up for lunch and the observation ended.

During the second observation, the OT observed Serena on the playground during lunch recess. Serena was observed to ask a group of students in the third grade if she could join into their game of jump rope. The students said yes. Serena waited in line behind four other girls for her turn to jump. During that time, the other students were singing a rhyme as one of the girls jumped. Serena appeared to not know the rhyme, but she clapped and cheered for the girl who was jumping as the tempo of the song went faster. By the time it was her turn, Serena was singing the rhyme as she jumped. The other girls playing jump rope cheered her on. While Serena was playing jump rope with the third graders, most of the girls in her class were playing four square. When the recess monitor called the different classes to line up, Serena approached the school building with the third graders and then stood near the door waiting for her grade to be called. The observation ended as Serena was lining up with her class to go into the school building.

The social worker collaborated with Ms. K to find two girls and one boy in Serena's class to have lunch with Serena in the social worker's office. During lunch, the two girls, the boy, and Serena got along well. However, all of the children were anxious to finish eating so that they could go to the playground for lunch recess. The social worker did not want to force the children to stay in her office, so she dismissed them.

Second Problem-Solving Team Meeting

During the second PST meeting, the social worker and the OT shared the data that they had collected over the past 4 weeks. The PST discussed this data in light of the information that they already knew about Serena. The rest of the meeting focused on developing a new working hypothesis to explain the reasons behind Serena's concerns and evidence-based recommendations to support her at school. The team also had to develop goal statements so that they could collect data to determine if Serena was making progress with the recommendations they were suggesting. Finally, the PST made a plan to meet again in 6 weeks to discuss Serena's progress.

Questions to Consider

1. The social worker attributed Serena's difficulty with turning in assignments to be related to poor organizational skills. What other "red flags" might a PST identify as OT concerns?
2. What are the different RtI tiers? What are some examples of ways that OTs could support students at each tier?
3. What do you see as the pros and cons of the interventions that Ms. K initially tried with Serena?
4. If you had the opportunity to speak with Serena's mom over the phone, what additional questions would you ask?
5. If you had the opportunity to speak with Serena, what questions would you ask?
6. Imagine that you are part of the PST. What are some new working hypotheses that could explain why Serena is experiencing challenges? Use evidence from the case to support your answers.
7. Do you believe that Serena needs short-term direct OT intervention? Why or why not? If so, what would be the focus of this intervention?
8. What are some recommendations that you have for Serena's teacher?
9. What are some recommendations that you have for Serena's mother?
10. What are some recommendations that you have for Serena?
11. Write two measurable goals related to Serena's challenges.
12. Describe in detail how data would be collected for these goals. Consider what the data collection form would look like, who would collect the data, and how you anticipate Serena's progress to change over time.
13. Search the evidence to find support for two of the recommendations that you made and summarize it.
14. Describe why you selected two of the recommendations that you did based on principles from theories or OT frames of reference.
15. Discuss how the PST might respond if Serena did not make progress after 6 weeks of the recommendations being implemented.

Resources

Bazyk, S. (2007). Addressing the mental health needs of children in schools. In L. Jackson (Ed.), *Occupational therapy services for children and youth under IDEA* (3rd ed.). (pp. 145-166). Bethesda, MD: AOTA Press.

Bazyk, S., & Case-Smith, J. (2010). School-based occupational therapy services. In J. Case-Smith & J. O'Brien (Eds.). *Occupational therapy for children* (6th ed.) (pp. 7173-743). St. Louis: Mosby/Elsevier.

Cahill, S. M. (2007, September). A perspective on response to intervention. *School System Special Interest Section Quarterly, 14*(3), 1-4.

Cahill, S., Clark, G., Csani, C., Ivey, C., Jackson, L., McClosky, S., ... Ray, S. (2012). Response to intervention: Your questions answered. *OT Practice, 17*(3), 18-20.

Kendra: Cerebral Palsy

Robin Elaine Fogerty, OTD, OTR/L; Meagan E. Wisniewski, BS; and Patricia Bowyer, EdD, MS, OTR, FAOTA

History and Background Information

Kendra, age 8 years, was diagnosed with cerebral palsy. She has moderate spastic hemiparesis that affects the left side of her body. She is able to walk independently, with the aid of a left AFO. Her left upper extremity is more severely affected than her lower extremity. She has had many surgeries on her left hand to help with the spasticity. Her hand has limited functional movement.

Kendra is an only child. She lives with her mother, who works as hairdresser to support their single-income family. Kendra enjoys swimming and playing the Nintendo Wii with her friends. She is very competitive and does not like to lose. Kendra's main responsibilities at home are to clean her room and pick up her toys. She occasionally helps her mom prepare dinner.

Kendra's typical school-day routine involves taking the bus to and from school, attending class, homework, playing video games for 1 hour, and reading with her mom before bed. On the weekends, Kendra usually spends time with her extended family. Weekend activities involve going to church, having picnics, or playing with her grandparents' dog.

Kendra is in the third grade at a public elementary school near her home. Previous educational testing reveals that Kendra has typical cognitive and academic achievement abilities. She is in mainstream classes with typical peers. However, she experiences difficulties with school tasks, especially those that involve the use of two hands. Kendra was referred for an OT evaluation.

Evaluation Information

Occupational Profile

Short Child Occupational Profile (SCOPE)

The OT selected the SCOPE to guide the overall assessment and intervention planning process. The SCOPE (Bowyer et al., 2008) is a theory-based assessment

Kendra's SCOPE Ratings Summary

SCOPE Rating Key

F	Facilitates	Facilitates participation in occupation
A	Allows	Allows participation in occupation
I	Inhibits	Inhibits participation in occupation
R	Restricts	Restricts participation in occupation

Domain	Item				
Volition	Exploration	(F)	A	I	R
	Expression of Enjoyment	(F)	A	I	R
	Preferences & Choices	(F)	A	I	R
	Response to Challenge	F	A	(I)	R
Habituation	Daily Activities	(F)	A	I	R
	Response to Transitions	F	(A)	I	R
	Routine	(F)	A	I	R
	Roles	(F)	A	I	R
Communication & Interaction Skills	Non-Verbal Communication	(F)	A	I	R
	Verbal/Vocal Expressions	(F)	A	I	R
	Conversation	(F)	A	I	R
	Relationships	(F)	A	I	R
Process Skills	Understands & Uses Objects	(F)	A	I	R
	Orientation of Environment	(F)	A	I	R
	Plan & Make Decisions	(F)	A	I	R
	Problem Solving	F	A	(I)	R
Motor Skills	Posture & Mobility	F	(A)	I	R
	Coordination	F	A	I	(R)
	Strength	F	A	(I)	R
	Energy/Endurance	F	A	(I)	R
Environment: School	Physical Space	F	(A)	I	R
	Physical Resources	F	A	(I)	R
	Social Groups	F	(A)	I	R
	Occupational Demands	F	A	(I)	R
	Family Routine	(F)	A	I	R

Figure 3-2. Kendra's SCOPE Rating Form. (Adapted from *A User's Manual for the Short Child Occupational Profile (SCOPE)* by P. L. Bowyer et al., 2008, Chicago: University of Illinois at Chicago, Department of Occupational Therapy, School of Applied Health Sciences. Copyright 2005 by Model of Human Occupation Clearinghouse, University of Illinois at Chicago, Department of Occupational Therapy, School of Applied Health Sciences. Adapted with permission.)

tool that provides information about a child's occupational participation based on the major concepts of the Model of Human Occupation (MOHO; Kielhofner, 2008). The goal of the SCOPE is to provide a strengths-based assessment to guide interventions that support a child's participation in valued roles, and the occupations associated with them (Bowyer et al., 2008). The SCOPE allows for varied data collection methods (observation, interview, records review, and other assessment tools) to determine item ratings. Kendra's SCOPE ratings are based on classroom observations, teacher interviews, and student interview. Kendra's SCOPE ratings appear in Figure 3-2.

Child Occupational Self-Assessment

The Child Occupational Self-Assessment (COSA) is a MOHO-based self-assessment tool (Keller, Kafkes, Basu, Federico, & Kielhofner, 2005). The COSA was administered to better understand Kendra's perspective of occupational competence. The COSA data are included below in the SCOPE ratings and narrative.

Volition

Kendra actively explores familiar and unfamiliar environments, tasks, and objects. She regularly attempts new activities and is motivated to participate in the same activities as her peers. She also wants to complete activities in same manner as her peers and easily gets frustrated when she cannot. Once frustrated, Kendra frequently turns down offers for help from her teacher and classmates. Occasionally, she completely shuts down and refuses to participate in the activity any further. She values the praise of others for her accomplishments and expresses enjoyment by smiling, verbalizing, and showing others her accomplishments. Kendra expresses her preferences clearly. During her interview, Kendra listed many activities that she prefers and stated that she "hates going to art class." She added that art is "stupid" and a "waste of time." After further investigation, it was discovered that Kendra is very frustrated during art because she is unable to successfully meet the motor demands. Figure 3-3 gives an example of the scoring on the Response to Challenge item. Underlining is used to capture items considered in the rating for the item.

Additional information about Kendra's perspectives of self-efficacy and competence were obtained during her COSA assessment. Kendra noted that she was really good at *dress myself, do things with my friends,* and *follow classroom rules.* Kendra noted her biggest problems were in *use my hands to work with things, make my body do what I want it to do, think of ways to do things when I have a problem,* and *keep working on something when it gets hard.* All of these problems were marked as being really important, with *make my body do what I want it to do* as most important.

Volition

Response to Challenge

The child engages in new activities and/or accepts the opportunity to achieve more, or perform under condition of greater demand.

F	The child spontaneously seeks and persists in new or more challenging activities.	***Comments:*** *Spontaneously engages in new tasks. Easily frustrated. Quickly gives up. When encouraged or offered an alternative, she states "I can't do it." Refuses to attempt once her initial attempts are unsuccessful. Initiates but difficulty with persistence.*
A	The child spontaneously attempts new or more challenging activities, but is easily frustrated and/or needs some support in order to persist.	
(I)	The child usually requires significant support to engage in new and more demanding activities and to overcome frustration and persist during such activities	
R	The child avoids new or more challenging activities because they elicit a high level of frustration.	

Figure 3-3. An example of the scoring on the SCOPE *Response to Challenge* item. (Adapted from *A User's Manual for the Short Child Occupational Profile (SCOPE)* by P. L. Bowyer et al., 2008, Chicago: University of Illinois at Chicago, Department of Occupational Therapy, School of Applied Health Sciences. Copyright 2005 by Model of Human Occupation Clearinghouse, University of Illinois at Chicago, Department of Occupational Therapy, School of Applied Health Sciences. Adapted with permission.)

Habituation

Kendra knows the steps and sequences involved in everyday self-care, school, and leisure activities. She easily anticipates and cooperates with daily routines. For example, she independently enters the classroom, gets out homework folder, puts away backpack, turns in folder, goes to desk, and begins her bell work. Kendra's mother has purchased pull-on clothing, which allows Kendra to dress independently. Kendra independently recognizes cues in the environment at times of transition. For example, when the teacher retrieved the lunch cards from the classroom entrance, she smiled and said "time for lunch!" to a peer. She does well with the majority of transitions during the school day. However, she needs cues at times to stop a current task when it is time to move onto a different activity. She will continue to try and quickly finish and will say "wait" and "I am not finished." Kendra will respond to cues but appears frustrated because it takes her longer to complete motor tasks (e.g., writing). Kendra easily demonstrates and verbalizes what it means to be a friend and a student. She understands activities that are safe for children her age as well. She is known to quickly point out role-related rules. For example, after another student acted out in class, Kendra looked to her nearby peer and said "not supposed to talk back to the teacher!" Figure 3-4 gives an example of the scoring on the *Routines* item.

Communication and Interaction Skills

Kendra's teacher and mother report that she excels in peer and adult interactions. Kendra also self-reports this as an area of strength. She demonstrates appropriate verbal and nonverbal skill abilities. She is able to join in, follow, and participate in conversations. Kendra enjoys joining peers in a variety of activities and is very competitive. However, she will become upset when she loses or is on the losing team. Kendra does encounter difficulties with joining in due to motor differences. Sometimes, Kendra feels embarrassed by this. At other times, she will attempt to hide her disability and participate in activities despite potential safety concerns. Kendra really enjoys interacting with friends and joining them in physically active games. She would like to fully participate in all of these activities.

Process Skills

Kendra's teacher and mother report that Kendra excels in cognitive tasks. She easily selects the appropriate materials for tasks, and uses them appropriately (within her motor abilities). She recognizes and appropriately adapts to environmental cues. Kendra also demonstrates strength in her ability to plan and make decisions. For example, Kendra enjoys planning elaborate play schemes with her friends, such as pretending a secret operation on the playground that ends in chasing down and capturing a suspect.

Kendra is able to problem solve tasks that are not motor related. For example, she can generate alternative ideas

Habituation

Routine

The child has an awareness of routines and is able to participate effectively in structured daily routines.

Rating	Description	Comments
(F)	The child demonstrates an awareness of the sequence and structure of a regular routine, and can anticipate, initiate, and/or cooperate with activities related to these routines.	**Comments:** *Initiates and carries out classroom routines as expected. Observed multi-step morning routine, put away back pack, put away home work, went to desk, started working. Anticipated lunch routine when she saw teacher retrieve lunch cards.*
A	The child requires occasional cueing and redirection in order to cooperate with the regular sequence and structure of routines in his/her life.	
I	The child is often unable to participate in the sequence and structure of regular routines.	
R	The child does not demonstrate an awareness of the sequence and structure of regular routines; does not anticipate, cooperate, and/or initiate routine activities.	

Figure 3-4. An example of the scoring on the SCOPE *Routines* item. (Adapted from *A User's Manual for the Short Child Occupational Profile (SCOPE)* by P. L. Bowyer et al., 2008, Chicago: University of Illinois at Chicago, Department of Occupational Therapy, School of Applied Health Sciences. Copyright 2005 by Model of Human Occupation Clearinghouse, University of Illinois at Chicago, Department of Occupational Therapy, School of Applied Health Sciences. Adapted with permission.)

when peers do not agree on game selection. However, her ability to generate alternatives to motor challenges inhibits her ability to either participate in tasks, or participate efficiently, effectively, or safely. She wants do things the same way as her peers. When she is limited by her physical differences, she tends to repeatedly try the same strategy until she either accomplishes her goal, or gives up completely. She does not ask for help, generate alternative approaches, or select a different role within the tasks that better match her abilities. For example, when playing catch on the playground, Kendra has experienced facial abrasions when trying to catch a basketball (which she cannot do). Softer types of balls are available, and she is much better at kicking and chasing. She has repeatedly been hurt on the playground from such tasks. Kendra also attempts to climb monkey bars at recess and needs an adult to prompt her about safety. During art class, Kendra does not generate alternative approaches to tasks and requires an adult to intervene with alternatives well before she becomes frustrated. During the COSA assessment, Kendra self-reported the "*think of ways to do things when I have a problem*" item as one of her biggest problems.

Motor Skills

Kendra's motor skills are her area of greatest challenge; her motor skills do not support her participation in many activities that occur across the school day, including writing, art class activities, physical education, and recess/playground tasks. Her greatest area of strength in motor skills is in her postural and mobility skills. She is able to sit unassisted in regular classroom chairs, sit on the floor with good sitting balance, get up and down off of the floor using right hand to assist, and she is able to access all areas in her classroom/school building. She is also able to run and walk on flat and uneven playground surfaces. She tends to run well behind peers and falls with minor scrapes when outside. She has learned to carry her own tray at lunch by using her left forearm under the tray. Although she is able to sit at a desk unsupported, decreased postural control does result in a propped, forward flexion position on the desk top, and this likely contributes to her handwriting difficulties.

Motor coordination is her area of greatest difficulty. She is unable to complete many two-handed tasks due to spasticity and weakness in her left hand. At rest, her muscle tone does relax. However, upon exertion her hand takes on a fisted position, her elbow flexes, and her forearm is held in a pronated position. This position does allow Kendra to use her left hand as a functional helper to hold and stabilize items; however, she needs to be cued to do this. For example, her paper slides under her right hand as she writes. With a cue, she stabilizes the paper with her left hand. After a period of time, her left arm was removed and she did not replace it when she began writing again. Motor coordination difficulties were also noted in her right (unaffected) limb. Kendra demonstrated difficulty with calibrating graded movements (force and speed). This greatly impacted her ability to form smooth lines and to start/stop lines effectively. During a writing observation, it was clear that Kendra understands how to form letters, but her poor motor control makes execution difficult. Her writing legibility was 50% in print and less than 10% in cursive.

Decreased strength is also noted during grasping tasks. Items such as markers and glue sticks slipped from Kendra's right and left hands as she attempted to open them. At times, she used her teeth in place of her left hand, and her right hand continued to slip. Kendra is able to grossly grasp and hold light items with her left hand. However, she

Motor Skills

Coordination

The child exhibits effective gross and fine motor movements during activities.

F	The child effectively coordinates body parts to achieve fine and gross motor movements.	***Comments**: Can grossly grasp with LUE; Delays/fails to use LUE to stabilize task items; Diff. grading movements (speed & force) during writing tasks (RUE).*
A	The child exhibits uncoordinated movement during some fine and/or gross motor activities.	
I	The child has difficulty coordinating fine and/or gross motor movements during most activities.	
(R)	The child is unable to coordinate, manipulate, and use fluid movements.	

Figure 3-5. An example of the scoring on the SCOPE *Coordination* item. (Adapted from *A User's Manual for the Short Child Occupational Profile (SCOPE)* by P. L. Bowyer et al., 2008, Chicago: University of Illinois at Chicago, Department of Occupational Therapy, School of Applied Health Sciences. Copyright 2005 by Model of Human Occupation Clearinghouse, University of Illinois at Chicago, Department of Occupational Therapy, School of Applied Health Sciences. Adapted with permission.)

does not use her left hand for manipulation; all left fingers extend and flex as one unit. Kendra demonstrates an even energy level across the school day. However, she demonstrates decreased writing endurance as the day progresses. Toward the end of the day, her written work is illegible. Kendra is also more likely to become frustrated with motor tasks toward the end of the school day. Her mother reports that Kendra falls asleep on the bus before she gets home and that Kendra is tired after her day at school. Figure 3-5 gives an example of the scoring on the *Coordination* item.

Environment

The physical spaces at Kendra's school facilitate her participation. She is able to access all areas and materials in her classrooms, bathroom, and cafeteria. There are also lower climbing structures, sand and grass areas, and tether balls on the playground that she can access. Physical resources inhibit Kendra's participation in activities in several settings at her school. For example, in art class she only has access to typical scissors that require bilateral coordination for success. There are many children and one teacher in her art class (two third-grade classes). The teacher is unable to provide the level of assistance needed to support Kendra before she becomes overly frustrated. Additionally, Kendra's environment only provides pencil and paper to produce written work. However, the writing demands are increasing exponentially in third grade (i.e., essays and reports). Kendra's classroom teacher is also introducing cursive writing in her class, and this is especially problematic for Kendra. The teacher wants to help Kendra, but does not want to focus all her attention on one student in a class of 20. Kendra's social environment is warm and accepting. Most of Kendra's teachers have never worked with a student that has disabilities. However, each teacher has identified that modifications/techniques are needed and have requested help to support Kendra's participation in their classrooms. Figure 3-6 provides an example of the scoring used for the *Physical Resources* item.

Occupational demands are an area of unmet needs for Kendra. Many of the activities that she is expected to do each day require motor, volitional, and/or processing skills that exceed her current abilities. In art class, examples of art activities include cutting and gluing to make collages, sculpting clay, and painting. Without modifications or assistance, Kendra is unable to meet the occupational demands, and this is negatively impacting her feelings of self-efficacy and competence. Physical education activities are primarily bilateral, and also exceed her motor abilities to meet task demands. Classroom demands to produce increasing quantities of paper/pencil activities are also beginning to limit her ability to successfully participate. Finally, Kendra and her friends enjoy playing together on the playground, but some activities require motor skills and/or problem-solving skills that exceed her current abilities. The family's routines appear to support Kendra's participation at this time. They have provided leisure activities that match Kendra's interests, engage her peers, and meet her functional skill level for participation. Many activities of daily living (ADL) tasks have been modified to ensure Kendra's participation, such as assigning chores with reduced bilateral demands, pull-on clothing, and pump bottles for soap/shampoo/toothpaste.

Questions to Consider

Goals/Treatment

1. Using the SCOPE assessment data, develop a list of strengths and challenges for Kendra.

Environment

Physical Resources

Availability of equipment, appropriate play/learning objects, transportation, and other resources (at home, community, school, and/or hospital) support the child's participation.

F	Physical resources (objects such as toys, school utensils, mobility devices) support satisfying and safe occupational participation.	***Comments:*** *Regular school materials with no modifications/adaptations (e.g. paper, pencil, scissors, clay, basketballs.) The physical properties exceed abilities, limits participation.*
A	Physical resources (objects such as toys, school utensils, mobility devices) meet the basic needs for safety and engagement in occupations, but do not fully support satisfying participation in valued occupations.	
(I)	Physical resources (objects such as toys, school utensils, mobility devices) limit opportunities for satisfying and safe engagement in occupations.	
R	Physical resources (objects such as toys, school utensils, mobility devices) are lacking, inappropriate, and/or unsafe.	

Figure 3-6. An example of the scoring used for the *Physical Resources* item. (Adapted from *A User's Manual for the Short Child Occupational Profile (SCOPE)* by P. L. Bowyer et al., 2008, Chicago: University of Illinois at Chicago, Department of Occupational Therapy, School of Applied Health Sciences. Copyright 2005 by Model of Human Occupation Clearinghouse, University of Illinois at Chicago, Department of Occupational Therapy, School of Applied Health Sciences. Adapted with permission.)

2. Review the Score Summary Table and determine which SCOPE factors need to be addressed during intervention.
3. Develop intervention goals and intervention strategies for each item listed in #2. Refer to the SCOPE School Goal Tables (Tables 3-3 and 3-4) for guidance and examples.

Intervention Plan

1. Use the *Occupational Therapy Practice Framework–2* (AOTA, 2008) terminology to determine which *intervention approach* will be used with each goal (can be more than one).
2. Compare and contrast how your approach to intervention might differ if you were providing outpatient services, instead of school-based services.
3. Evaluate how your interventions for Kendra may differ if you had not used the SCOPE, but instead relied solely on developmental assessments of motor and visual motor/perceptual skills. State your opinions about the differing interventions that may result from the two assessment approaches.
4. Do you feel that additional assessments are needed to complete Kendra's evaluation? Why or why not?
5. Assume that after 6 months of intervention, a re-administration of the SCOPE shows that Kendra's scores have improved in the area of volition. Using MOHO concepts, explain how intervention accomplished such an improvement.

References

American Occupational Therapy Association. (2008). *Occupational therapy practice framework: Domain and process* (2nd ed.). Bethesda, MD: AOTA Press.

Keller, J., Kafkes, A., Basu, S., Federico, J., & Kielhofner, G. (2005). *Child Occupational Self-Assessment (COSA)*. Chicago: University of Illinois at Chicago, Model of Human Occupation Clearinghouse, Department of Occupational Therapy, College of Applied Health Sciences.

Kielhofner, G. (2008). *Model of Human Occupation: Theory and application.* (4th ed.). Philadelphia: Lippincott, Williams, and Wilkins.

Polszaj, A. (n.d.). *SCOPE school goal chart.* Chicago: University of Illinois at Chicago, Model of Human Occupation Clearinghouse, Department of Occupational Therapy, College of Applied Health Sciences. Available at: http://www.uic.edu/depts/moho/images/assessments/SCOPE%20IL%20Schools%20Goals%20Chart.pdf

Bowyer, P., Kramer, J., Ploszaj, A., Ross, M., Schwartz, O., Kielhofner, G., & Kramer, J. (2008). *A user's manual for the short child occupational profile (SCOPE; version 2.2).* Chicago: University of Illinois at Chicago, Model of Human Occupation Clearinghouse, Department of Occupational Therapy, College of Applied Health Sciences.

Resource

Bazyk, S., & Case-Smith, J. (2010). School-based occupational therapy services. In J. Case-Smith & J. O'Brien (Eds.). *Occupational therapy for children* (6th ed.) (pp. 7173-743). St. Louis: Mosby/Elsevier.

Table 3-3

SCOPE School Goal Chart

SCOPE ITEM	SCOPE QUESTION	KEY WORDS FOR GOAL WRITING	EXAMPLE GOALS	STRATEGIES FOR INTERVENTION	THEORETICAL REASONING
VOLITION: Response to Challenge	Does student engage in new activities and/or accept the opportunity to achieve more, or perform under condition of greater demand?	• Persists • Attempts • Tries • Responds • Sustains • Accepts • Seeks • Commits	• Student will attempt to complete the first two steps of a new color/cut/paste activity. • Student will try to turn off a toy rather than throwing it. • Student will respond to a challenge by asking for help in place of throwing a tantrum. • Student will attempt to complete a difficult math activity within the allotted time.	• Structure the environment to allow the student to take risks safely and make mistakes. • Provide the appropriate level of support and/or modify tasks so that the student experiences success when attempting a new or challenging activity. • Encourage the student when he/she shows signs that a task is becoming difficult.	• To experience success in school and to progress in a curriculum, it is important for a student to engage in new and more challenging activities. • By providing support, a student's experience of doing a more challenging task is likely to be positive. This increases the student's sense of self-efficacy and competency and increases his/her willingness to engage in that activity in the future.
MOTOR SKILLS: Coordination	Does student exhibit effective gross and fine-motor movement during activities?	• Coordinates • Manipulates • Effectively moves • Completes • Grasps and releases • Handles	• With use of an adapted spoon, student will successfully scoop (manipulate) cereal into his mouth with minimal spillage. • Student will successfully grasp and move coins into piles during math lessons.	• Consult with the OT or PT for accommodations or modifications that may assist student in more effective coordination. • Adapt object and activities so that they match the students' motor skills. • Provide opportunities to practice specific motor skills	• Most school activities involve manipulation and use of tools and objects. Therefore, effective coordination supports successful performance of school activities.

Adapted from *SCOPE School Goal Chart*, by A. Polszaj, n.d., Chicago: University of Illinois at Chicago, Model of Human Occupation Clearinghouse, Department of Occupational Therapy, College of Applied Health Sciences. Adapted with permission.

Table 3-4

SCOPE School Goal Chart

SCOPE ITEM	*SCOPE QUESTION*	*ACCOMMODATIONS/ MODIFICATIONS ON IEP*	*STRATEGIES FOR INTERVENTION*	*THEORETICAL REASONING*
ENVIRONMENT: Physical Resources	Are equipment, play/learning objects, transportation, and other resources at school available and appropriate and do they support the student's participation?	Resources necessary during feeding, classroom activities, mobility, etc.: • Adaptive equipment (for seating, positioning, and mobility) • Paraprofessional • Augmentative communication • Computers • Safety precautions (helmet, etc.) • Low tech communication devices • Consult with OT, PT, SLP, Nursing, LD teacher, social worker, psychologist	• Identify and obtain an appropriate adaptive tool that will assist the student in writing activities • Be available to assist the student in using a spoon during lunch. • Consult with SLP to obtain communication device. • Connect student with a "peer buddy."	• Resources help ensure that students are able to take advantage of opportunities to participate. • The right objects, equipment, and other resources help a student meet tasks demands and perform effectively and efficiently.

Adapted from *SCOPE School Goal Chart,* by A. Polszaj, n.d., Chicago: University of Illinois at Chicago, Model of Human Occupation Clearinghouse, Department of Occupational Therapy, College of Applied Health Sciences. Adapted with permission.

Wilson: Learning Disability/ School Systems

Susan M. Cahill, PhD, OTR/L

History and Background Information

Wilson, a 9-year-old third-grader, is receiving special education and related services, specifically OT and speech and language therapy. Wilson began receiving special education and related services in kindergarten. At that time, he was found eligible for services under the Developmental Delay disability category. However, he was recently reevaluated for special education and related services and was found to be eligible under the Specific Learning Disability category. Wilson's general intellectual ability was determined to be in the average range; he received a score of 105 on an intelligence test. Despite his relatively high IQ score, Wilson demonstrated a significant discrepancy between his achievement in reading and written language as compared with his intellectual potential. His reading and written language scores fall in the high 70s/low 80s, approximately 2 standard deviations below his IQ score. As part of his reevaluation for special education and related services, he was reevaluated for OT services.

Evaluation Information

Occupational Profile

Wilson attends Jefferson Elementary School and is in Mrs. S's third grade classroom. Wilson has received OT services since kindergarten because of delayed fine-motor and handwriting skills. He reports that he enjoys math and particularly likes playing flashcard games with his classmates. He lives at home with his mom and aunt and visits his dad on the weekends. In his free time, Wilson enjoys playing driving video games and basketball. He has his own room and is responsible for making his bed every morning and folding the laundry on a weekly basis. Wilson sometimes helps to unload the dishwasher, but he would rather not. He currently does not have any pets. However, he did report that he would like to get a big dog that he could take to a dog park with his mom.

During the reevaluation for OT services, Wilson was pleasant and cooperative. He appeared to like to complete timed activities and, at one point, said, "I'm good at races." Wilson discussed his need for assistance with reading and written language. He also expressed a strong dislike for completing handwritten assignments. He stated, "I don't know why I just can't *tell* my stories. Why do I have to *write* them?"

Analysis of Occupational Performance

Wilson was observed in his classroom during several writing and drawing tasks. He is left-handed and holds his pencil with a three-fingered thumb-tuck grasp. This grasps restricts his ability to use opposition and refined distal movements. Wilson maintains a tight grasp on his pencil and shook his hand due to fatigue several times during the observation. He was also observed tilting his paper to the right, which caused him to flex his wrist and supinate his forearm to enable him to write.

During the observation, Wilson and his classmates were asked to copy 10 spelling words from the smart board. Classmates sitting near Wilson were heard saying the words out loud before starting to write. As they wrote, the classmates were often heard sounding out the words. They infrequently referred back to the smart board to check their spelling once they began writing the word. Wilson did not say the words out loud before starting to write. He was also observed not sounding out the words, and he referred back to the smart board for each letter in each word. It took Wilson approximately three times as long to copy down the spelling words as it took the three children sitting nearest him. In addition, while he was copying the words, he frequently stopped to shake his hand before getting started again.

Later, Wilson was observed working on illustrations for a book being written by his class. His job was to draw a fierce lion (Figure 3-7). After he was done with his drawing, he proudly showed it to one of his classmates. Wilson's classmates looked at the drawing and said, "It sure is a lion, but why is he smiling? He's supposed to be mean and fierce." Wilson looked at his drawing and said, "He is fierce. He's about to eat you," and then he pushed his drawing into his classmate's face. The classmate protested and then turned away from Wilson.

Nearing the end of the observation, the OT saw Wilson write down a number line from 1 to 30. Then, the OT asked Wilson to copy the sentence, "The quick brown fox jumped over the lazy hound dogs" (Figure 3-8).

Interview With Teacher

The OT interviewed Mrs. S to gain a better understanding of Wilson's performance in the classroom. Mrs. S stated that Wilson was generally able to keep up with his classmates except when it came to writing assignments. She often allowed Wilson to dictate answers to her for tests, even though this accommodation was not listed on his IEP. Mrs. S indicated that Wilson often misplaced important

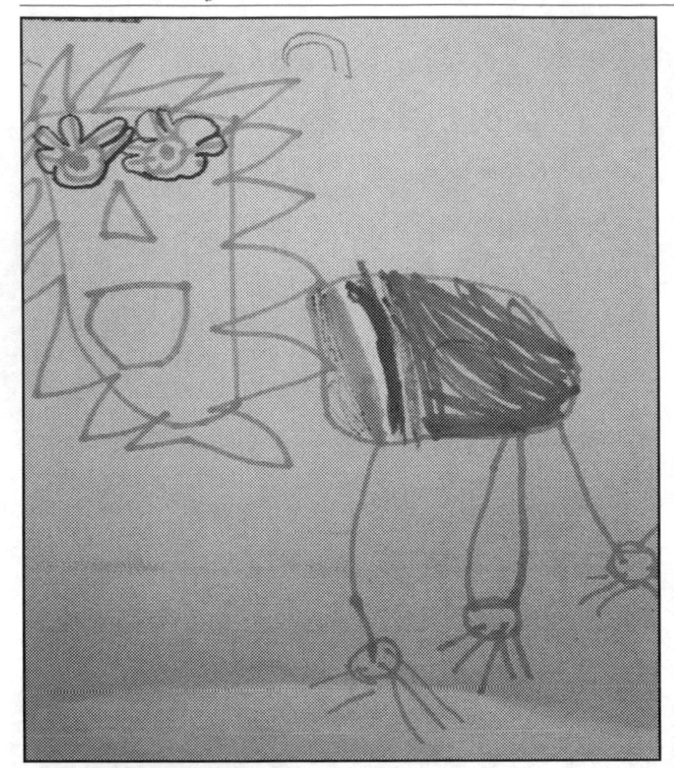

Figure 3-7. Wilson's drawing of a fierce lion.

worksheets and homework assignments and that he never volunteered to read aloud in class. Mrs. S voiced concerns about how the other students had been treating Wilson. She said, "They seem to be able to tell there is a difference between them and him now. I don't think they noticed it as much at the beginning of the year." Mrs. S also stated that on at least two occasions, Wilson stated that he was "dumber" than his friends. Mrs. S indicated that Wilson's mom is very involved in his education and is always responsive to notes home about missing assignments. Wilson's mom has told Mrs. S that it sometimes takes Wilson up to 2 hours to complete his homework. Both Mrs. S and Wilson's mom are worried that he is going to stop trying because things are becoming so difficult. Mrs. S also expressed concerns about the upcoming district-wide testing. She's worried that Wilson is not going to be able to produce his best work on the written response portion of the test. Mrs. S asked the OT if it would be appropriate to start keyboarding instruction for Wilson at this time.

Questions to Consider

1. Locate your state's board of education website. Next, find the criteria for Developmental Delay and Specific Learning Disability. Compare and contrast the criteria. Discuss why Wilson's eligibility might have been changed.

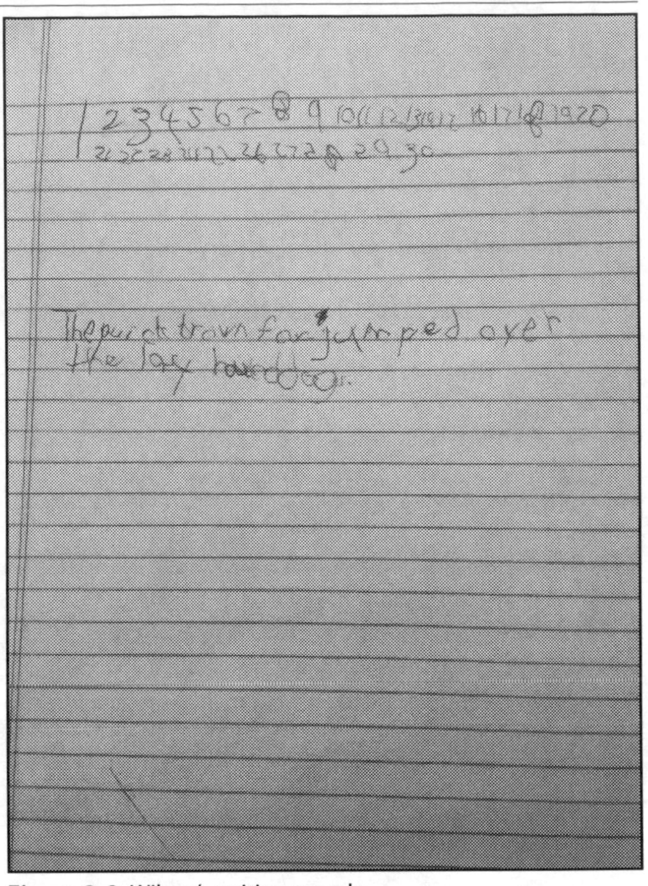

Figure 3-8. Wilson's writing sample.

2. Wilson's IQ score is within the average range. What is typically considered the average range for IQ scores?
3. Consider Wilson's pencil grasp and discuss the biomechanical factors at play that likely cause him to need to take breaks and shake out his hand.
4. Name and describe other pencil grasps that would be more functional for Wilson to use during writing.
5. Wilson flexes and supinates his wrist during writing. What is an optimal wrist position for writing? How could the environment be set up to promote Wilson's use of an optimal wrist position during writing tasks?
6. Look at the pencil grippers and supports in Figure 3-9. Would you recommend any of these for Wilson? Why or why not?
7. Discuss the pros and cons of using pencil grippers and other writing supports. Locate evidence to support the use of such equipment in practice.
8. Wilson's OT completed observations as part of the reevaluation for OT services. Identify three different assessment tools that could be used to supplement the OT's observation. Discuss the type of information that each tool would yield and discuss the pros and cons of using each tool.

9. Wilson struggles to copy from the smart board. Besides delayed handwriting skills in general, what are some other possible reasons for Wilson's difficulty?
10. Consider Wilson's drawing of a fierce lion in Figure 3-7. Does it look like the type of drawing you would expect a third-grader to produce? Why or why not?
11. Consider Wilson's writing sample in Figure 3-8. What judgments can you make about his legibility and letter production? What strategies could you use to support Wilson's handwriting production?
12. Based on Wilson's performance during the observation, what types of visual perceptual skills might he have difficulty with and why?
13. Locate the Common Core Standards for English Language Arts or your state's learning standards. Write one to two OT goals for Wilson that are aligned to these standards.
14. What other goals would you like to work on with Wilson? How would you justify your services to address such goals to Wilson's IEP team?
15. How much progress do you anticipate that Wilson will make on his goals before his next annual review?
16. Given Wilson's needs, identify and describe reasonable accommodations and modifications that could be included in his IEP. Your list should include those that can be used during typical instruction, as well as those that could be used during testing.
17. What are the pros and cons associated with introducing Wilson to typing? Do you think he is ready to use typing as his primary means for written communication? Why or why not? What prerequisite skills might Wilson need before beginning keyboarding instruction?
18. How many minutes of OT services would you recommend that Wilson get per week? Provide a justification for your answer.
19. Discuss the pros and cons of providing Wilson with integrated (i.e., in classroom) services versus pull-out services.
20. Develop an intervention plan for Wilson to address his OT goals. Discuss ways in which these goals can be carried over into the classroom.

Resources

Bazyk, S., & Case-Smith, J. (2010). School-based occupational therapy services. In J. Case-Smith & J. O'Brien (Eds.), *Occupational therapy for children* (6th ed.) (pp. 7173-743). St. Louis: Mosby/Elsevier.

Common Core Standards website: www.corestandards.org

Schneck, C., & Amundson, S. (2010). Prewriting and handwriting.. In J. Case-Smith & J. O'Brien (Eds.), *Occupational therapy for children* (6th ed.) (pp. 555-582). St. Louis: Mosby/Elsevier.

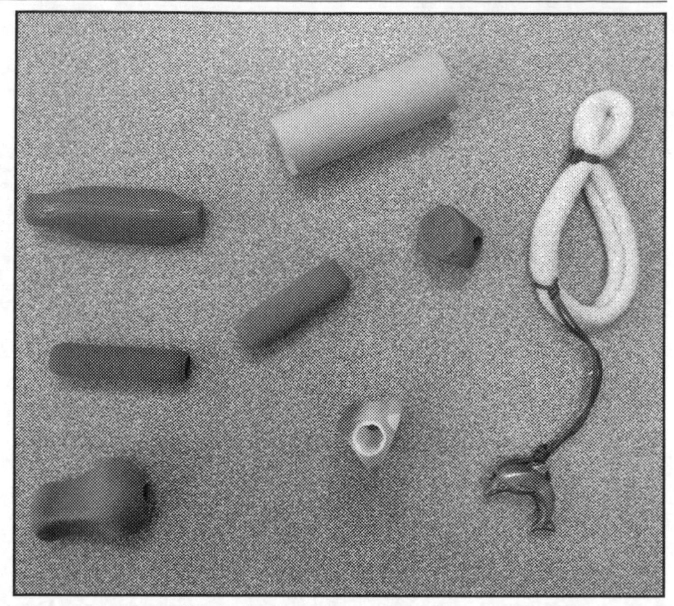

Figure 3-9. Pencil grippers and supports.

Johanna: Cerebral Palsy/ School Systems

Susan M. Cahill, PhD, OTR/L

History and Background Information

Johanna, age 6 years, attends a full-day kindergarten program. Johanna has right-sided spastic hemiplegia as a result of a left middle cerebral artery infarct. Johanna has a history of seizures, but they are currently controlled with medication. Johanna wears corrective lenses throughout the day and has a moderate case of bilateral esotropia. Johanna's functional abilities are classified at the Gross Motor Function Classification Systems (GMFCS) Level I and Manual Activities Classification System (MACS) Level III.

Johanna received early intervention services through a 0 to 3 program and was transitioned into the public school systems on her third birthday. Once she entered the school system, she received special education and related services in an early childhood special education program. During her last year in the early childhood program, Johanna was reevaluated for special education and related services. At that time, the team determined that her educational needs would be best met in general education. While in her full-day kindergarten program, Johanna currently receives special education resource services for reading and math for 300 minutes per week, speech and language therapy for 60 minutes per week, PT for 30 minutes per week, and

OT for 30 minutes per week. Johanna attends art, music, and physical education with her classmates. In addition, Johanna receives support from a special education paraprofessional who she shares with another student in her classroom. The paraprofessional assists Johanna during instructional time, sets up her lunch, and assists her in the bathroom as needed.

Johanna has been receiving OT services on a regular basis. The services usually take place in her primary classroom. Recently, the art teacher, Mr. R, has asked to meet with the OT to discuss some difficulties that Johanna is having in his class. Mr. R has never taught a student with hemiplegia before and he feels like he needs assistance to accommodate her. Mr. R thinks that Johanna would enjoy his class more if she were an active participant. He understands that Johanna can use her left hand. However, he reports that currently the paraprofessional assigned to work with Johanna ends up providing her with hand-over-hand assistance or simply completes the art projects for her. Johanna is a very pleasant and compliant student and does not challenge the paraprofessional. Mr. R feels that if he had a better understanding of Johanna's skills, he could better direct the paraprofessional.

Evaluation Information

The OT reviewed Johanna's file and found that the School Function Assessment (SFA) (Coster et al., 1998) had been completed during her reevaluation for special education and related services prior to entering kindergarten. The OT found that at the time of the evaluation, Johanna needed moderate assistance and moderate adaptations with manipulation with movement, using materials, setup and cleanup, and task behavior/completion. Given this information and Mr. R's concerns, the OT decided to reexamine Johanna's activity performance with physical and cognitive tasks using the SFA.

The OT met with Mr. R and they reviewed Part III (Activity Performance) of the SFA. Together, the OT and Mr. R determined that it would be beneficial to complete several sections related to Activity Performance to gain a better understanding of Johanna's current strengths and limitations. They decided that because they were only going to be using information from the SFA for planning purposes (versus eligibility determination), that they would not complete the entire assessment. The OT and Mr. R decided to complete the following sections: manipulation with movement, using materials, setup and cleanup, written work, and task behavior/completion.

Johanna received the following scores:

Activity Performance Sections	***Raw Scores***	***Criterion Scores***	***Standard Error***	***K-3 Criterion Cut-off Score***
Manipulation with movement	43	55	3	93
Using materials	65	55	2	83
Setup and cleanup	46	59	3	87
Written work	36	64	4	73
Task behavior/ completion	41	45	3	72

Johanna does not perform the following tasks:

- Carries objects large enough to require two hands
- Carries tray containing more than one item on top without spilling or dropping
- Removes pull-off lids from containers
- Opens cartons
- Opens sealed bags
- Copies materially accurately/legibly from a nearby source
- Recovers after failure
- Initiates work promptly after receiving directions
- Identifies materials needed for a particular task
- Lets teacher know when task information or specific assistance is needed
- Finishes project that takes several days
- Asks for help when rules or directions are not clear
- Attempts to solve a problem on own before asking for help
- Makes appropriate modifications to tasks or materials to meet his/her needs
- Has good independent work habits and makes efficient use of class time

Johanna consistently performs the following tasks:

- Carries objects small enough to be held in one hand
- Picks up materials from desk or table
- Moves objects along the floor
- Opens and closes doors
- Opens and closes a book
- Paints with brush
- Uses writing utensils to draw/write on paper
- Performs card game tasks
- Sharpens pencils with pencil sharpener (electric)
- Picks up and holds small objects with hand
- Disposes of trash in trash receptacle
- Removes food/materials from large containers
- Takes out and puts away books in desk
- Works from left to right
- Identifies appropriate starting and stopping point on a worksheet
- Listens/attends for at least 5 minutes
- Remains in designated play or work area without supervision for a specified time

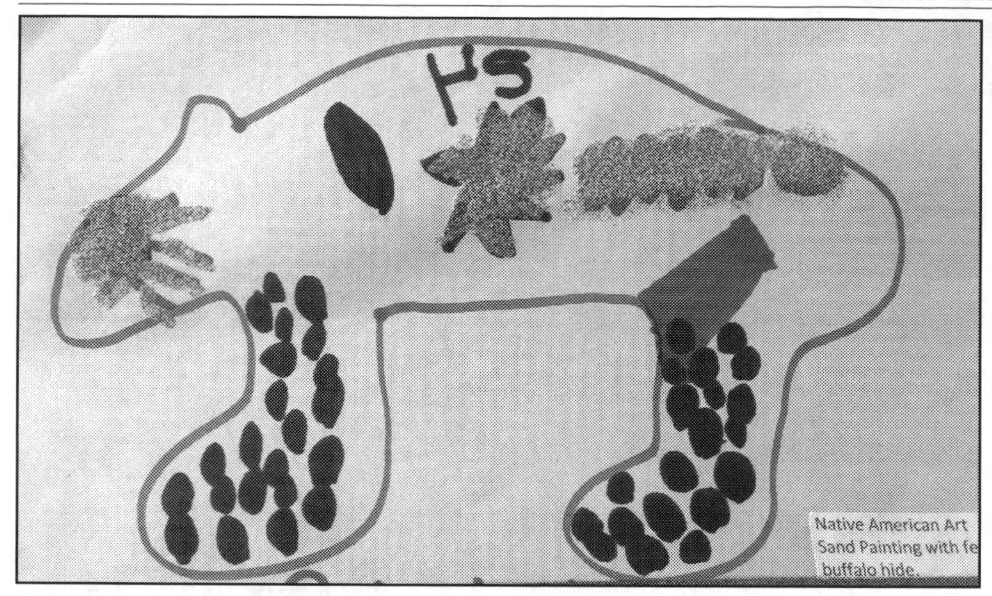

Figure 3-10. Native American–inspired sand painting on "buffalo hide."

- Attends quietly to/stays focused on audio or visual presentation for at least 20 minutes
- Attends to directions/instructions given to a small group of students
- Attends to a teacher-directed lesson for at least 15 minutes

Collaboration

After the SFA administration was complete, the OT met with Mr. R to discuss the upcoming projects that he had planned. The OT suggested that they talk about the art projects and complete a task analysis. After the task analysis was completed, the OT and Mr. R would then be able to problem solve ways that Johanna could be a more active participant in art class. Mr. R explained three different projects that the kindergarteners would be working on in the upcoming weeks and showed the OT samples of each project. Below is a description of the projects:

- Native American–inspired sand painting on "buffalo hide" (Figure 3-10). Mr. R explained that this project involves each student cutting a piece of "buffalo hide" (vinyl) off of a large roll. Next, the students select an animal shape to draw freehand or trace onto their buffalo hide with pencil. Then, students outline the shape with watercolor markers and embellish their animal shape with designs. Some of the designs are to be made with sand. The sand drawings are made by tracing over a design with glue and then sprinkling sand onto the glue. The sand is kept in a salt shaker.
- Leaf printing (Figure 3-11). Mr. R explained that this project is focused on the use of color. It involves each of the students selecting two to four leaves to print onto a white background. Students also have to select a mat color and mat their picture. In order to complete the leaf print, students have to paint tempera paint onto a leaf, turn it over, cover the leaf with wax paper, and then use a roller to roll out the leaf. In order to get the splash effect, students hit the wax paper before they begin rolling it out.
- Owl painting (Figure 3-12). Mr. R explained that this is another multistep art project. The first step involves students cutting out a piece of cardboard and painting it blue. The next step involves students tearing a section off of a brown paper bag. Once these steps are completed, the students are to finger paint a white owl body and then add black feathers. Some students will blend the paint to make gray feathers. Students then use orange for the details of the owl's face. The final step involves breaking a twig to an appropriate length and gluing it onto the piece.

Questions to Consider

1. What is esotropia? What are the functional implications associated with this condition?
2. Given Johanna's GMFCS and MACS classifications, what are functional abilities like? What are some school tasks that you think that she would have difficulty with? What are some school tasks that would be easy for her to complete on her own?
3. What aspects of the Individuals with Disabilities Education Improvement Act of 2004 (IDEA 2004; Pub. L. 108-446) are supportive of Johanna's placement in general education? Do you feel that this is the most appropriate place for her to receive her education? Why or why not? What are the pros and cons of Johanna being included in general education?

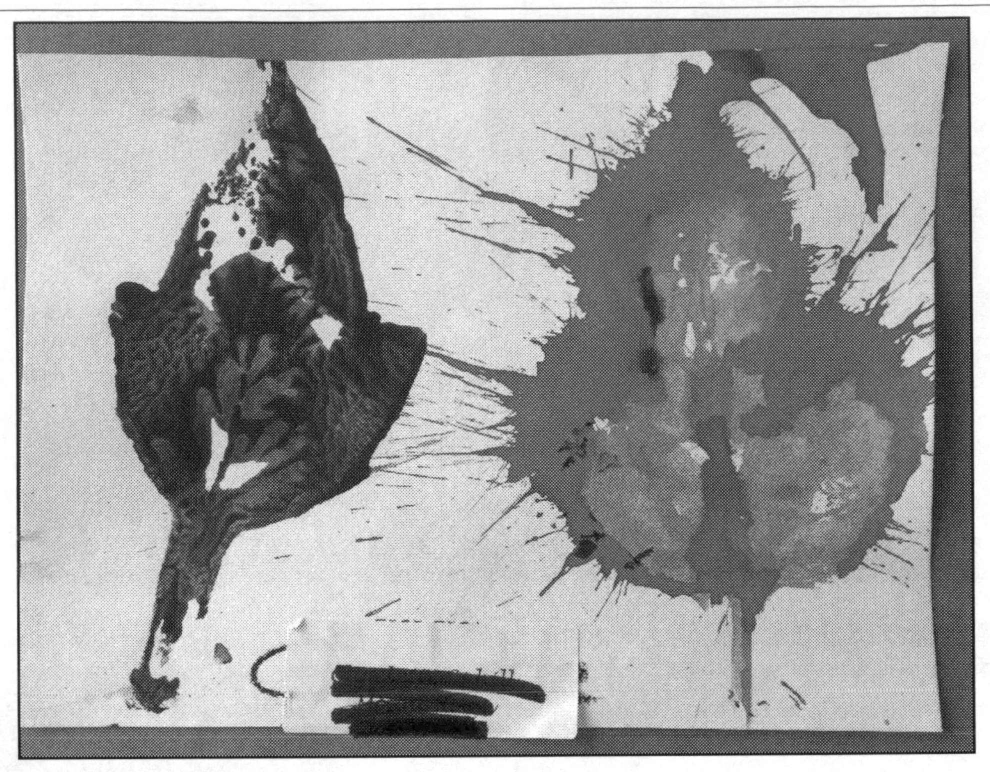

Figure 3-11. Leaf printing.

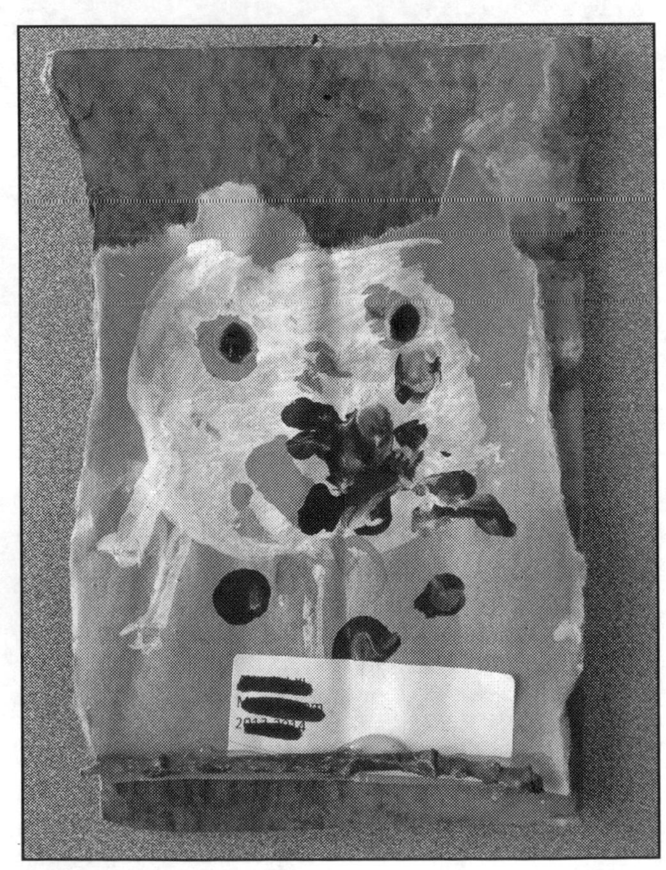

Figure 3-12. Owl painting.

4. The OT and Mr. R decided not complete the entire SFA. Given Johanna's current situation, do you think that this decision was appropriate? Why or why not? What are the limitations of completing only a portion of an assessment tool?
5. Review the SFA record form. Are there any other sections in Part III (Activity Performance) that you think might be helpful for the OT and Mr. R to complete?
6. Review the SFA to identify tasks that Johanna performed inconsistently as well as those on which Johanna demonstrated partial performance.
7. Based on the SFA, write a list of strengths and limitations for Johanna.
8. Select one of the art activities described by Mr. R and complete a detailed task analysis.
9. Once you have completed the task analysis, identify potential performance challenges for Johanna. Describe these challenges in enough detail that a substitute art teacher would have a clear understanding about what Johanna's needs are related to the specific project that you selected.
10. Describe ways that you could modify the art project and describe accommodations that may be put in place to ensure Johanna's full participation. Identify any equipment that Johanna might require.
11. Discuss how the paraprofessional could be used to support Johanna as she completes the project.

What parts of the art project would you assume that Johanna could complete independently? What parts of the art project do you anticipate she will need assistance with? How would you communicate this information to the paraprofessional?

12. Part of the OT's role to is to provide education to staff members in order to support the full participation of students with disabilities in school. What types of education could the OT provide to the paraprofessional? Describe the logistics related to providing such education (e.g., when would it be provided, what format would it take).

Resources

CanChild Gross Motor Function Classification Systems webpage: http://www.canchild.ca/en/measures/gmfcs.asp

Coster, W., Deeney, T., Haltiwanger, J., & Haley, S. (1998). *School Function Assessment*. San Antonio, TX: Therapy Skill Builders.

Eliasson, A.C., Krumlinde Sundholm, L., Rösblad, B., Beckung, E., Arner, M., Öhrvall, A., & Rosenbaum, P. (2006). The Manual Ability Classification System (MACS) for children with cerebral palsy: Scale development and evidence of validity and reliability. *Developmental Medicine and Child Neurology, 48*, 549-554.

Palisano, R., Rosenbaum, P., Bartlett, D., & Livingston, M. (2007). *Gross Motor Function Classification Systems expanded & revised*. Toronto: *CanChild* Centre for Childhood Disability Research at McMaster University. Retrieved from: http://motorgrowth.canchild.ca/en/gmfcs/resources/gmfcs-er.pdf

The Manual Ability Classification System (MACS) website: http://www.macs.nu/index.php

April: Autism/Private Separate Day School

Wanda Mahoney, PhD, OTR/L

History and Background Information

April, age 15 years, has a diagnosis of autism and severe cognitive impairment. She attends a private separate day school in a large city that contracts with her local school district. She is one of eight students with significant impairments in her classroom, which is led by one special education teacher and one paraprofessional. She has been receiving speech and OT services at school. She is nonverbal and uses a single-switch voice output communication device while in speech therapy. She receives specialized transportation between home and school.

April is an only child and lives with her father and mother in a low-income area. She has an in-home aide twice a week through state-funded developmental disability services, which will cover funding for adult services such as a day program, supported employment, and/or supportive living in the future. In last year's planning meeting, April's parents expressed that they plan for her to live at home for as long as possible as an adult but that they would like her to attend a day program.

April was referred for an OT evaluation as part of her triennial Full Individual Evaluation (FIE) for eligibility for special education services and in preparation for her upcoming IEP meeting. Because April will be turning 16 during this IEP year, the team needs to formally address her transition to adulthood (Bazyk & Case-Smith, 2010).

Occupational Therapy Evaluation

The OT evaluated April over a 1-month period during regularly scheduled treatment sessions through observation and interview with the special education teacher. The OT set up a variety of activities to determine April's interest and ability in the activities but did not administer any formal assessments. The OT knew that April required assistance for most activities. Therefore, assessment results pertaining to levels of assistance would not sufficiently describe April's current participation or the level of participation that could be developed. The OT also knew that April only engaged briefly with objects. For this reason, the OT reasoned that standardized assessments of fine-motor and visual motor skills would not be helpful in describing April's skills because they were so far below age-appropriate levels. Instead, the OT decided to complete a series of observations to assess April's participation and function with ADL, instrumental ADL (IADL), and other school-related activities. The information below is from the OT evaluation.

Self-Care

- Feeding: April feeds herself with her hands or with utensils. She sometimes puts nonfood items in her mouth and eats nonfood items. This has been a major issue for her in the past, but this behavior has decreased. April is motivated by food, seeks out food, and often can complete more complex activities (such as opening containers) when she is immediately rewarded with food. She independently operates the push bar to drink from a water fountain at school.
- Toileting: April wears pull-up diapers fulltime and inconsistently indicates the need to use the toilet. She is on a toileting schedule and consistently eliminates both bowel and bladder when seated on the toilet. She pulls her pants down consistently with gestures. April sometimes pulls her pants down independently. In a public

restroom, she usually goes directly to a stall before starting to pull down her pants. For safety and privacy, April should be in a restroom stall before pulling down her pants or getting assistance to remove/pull down clothing. She requires physical assistance with clothing fasteners, including buttons and zippers. She stands up once she is finished on the toilet and turns toward a staff member for assistance with wiping. With gestures to the toilet paper, she removes an appropriate amount, wipes her front, and puts the used toilet paper in the toilet. She needs full assistance for wiping following a bowel movement. She pulls up her pants independently or with gestures but needs physical assistance to ensure that her clothing is straightened.

- Handwashing: April independently goes to the sink following toileting and turns the water on. She performs all steps of handwashing independently or with gesture cues (pointing). She often needs repeated gestures or physical assistance for thoroughness (e.g., rubbing all surfaces of her hands with soap and rinsing all soap off her hands). She enjoys having water on her hands and usually refuses to dry her hands in order to prolong the length of time her hands are wet. April frequently puts her hands in her mouth, so it is important to encourage her to wash her hands often.
- Dressing: April takes off a jacket with gestures and physical prompts to get started. Once she understands the instruction, she independently removes the jacket. She puts on a jacket with assistance to position it correctly and needs assistance to get her second arm in the jacket. She inconsistently straightens her clothes with gestures. She needs physical assistance with all clothing fasteners, including zippers.

Home Living Skills

April has some beginning home living skills. She picks up items dropped on the floor with gestures and physical prompts. She throws trash away with gestures. She puts familiar items away with gestures and occasional physical prompts. She independently opens screw-top plastic jars. She assists another person with sweeping by holding the long-handled dustpan with cues and dumps it in the trash with physical assistance. She has started assisting with laundry tasks at school. She carries a laundry bag to the washer with someone walking with her. She loads the washer with gestures and physical redirection to return to the activity because she walks away after placing each towel in the washer. April seems to enjoy this activity because she smiles during the activity. In addition, she often chooses laundry when given a choice of tasks. Because she often has saliva on her hands, April has not had the opportunity to unload the washer or load/unload the dryer because this would involve handling clean towels.

Prevocational Skills

April has beginning prevocational skills. She completes simple one-step assembly tasks (e.g., putting two pieces together) with extended time, gestures, and minimal physical assistance for up to five objects. She has tried sorting tasks (such as separating two different types of objects) and needs physical prompting for each item to determine which container to place it in. When given sorting or assembly tasks with a comb, she often brings the comb to her hair. Although this demonstrates good recognition of the object and its typical use, her constant bringing the comb to her hair limits her participation in the assembly task. Therefore, April has limited opportunity to do prevocational tasks with combs and other familiar items.

Computer Skills

April has beginning computer use skills. She inconsistently attends to an adapted computer program (i.e., cause/effect and art activities). She seems to prefer computer activities with music. She needs simple adapted computer activities and would benefit from specialized software. She needs hand-over-hand assistance to move a regular mouse, and she is not able to double click. She is successful using a single switch connected to a power link to turn on a device such as a fan or music. She does not have a single switch for computer use. Because she frequently puts her hands in her mouth and plays with her saliva, she has had limited opportunities to use the computer. However, computer use is an area for further exploration with modifications. Computer usage may be motivating to April and it may support her skills related to item/picture identification and other prereading skills that she has been working on with her teacher. Although April used a touch screen during the evaluation, her frequently wet hands prevent this from being a viable option for regular computer use.

Motor Skills

April walks independently on a variety of surfaces, walks up and down stairs, and transitions between a variety of positions on the floor, sitting on a chair, and standing. She has delays in her fine-motor development that affect her ability to complete functional activities. She can stack blocks independently and appears to enjoy this task. She has difficulty placing puzzle pieces. She holds a writing utensil with her fingers and makes vertical lines, but she rarely engages in this task. She can turn single cardstock pages of a book.

Social Skills

April is nonverbal and communicates with simple gestures such as pulling away or pulling on someone's arm to lead him or her to a different place. She inconsistently holds out her hand to "ask for" an item. She needs time to "warm up" to a person and responds to simple turn-taking interactions (such as the OT pulling her hood up and April pulling it down) by looking up and smiling. She often withdraws from social situations by covering her head. She appears to enjoy going outdoors.

April has beginning choice-making skills. When given two objects or pictures, she usually chooses one with a physical prompt at the elbow. She has increased the variety of Boardmaker pictures that she recognizes, and she seems to understand the cause-effect relationship of choosing a picture and doing an activity. This is a skill that should continue to be developed and where she has demonstrated improvement over the past year.

April uses a voice output single switch communication device with one to four picture choices during speech therapy sessions. She most consistently uses the device to request more food during a snack and may benefit from more frequent use of the communication device.

Cognitive Skills

April often has a very short attention span, which significantly affects her ability to complete activities in school. Using motivating tasks, incorporating small amounts of food into tasks, and adding sensory components to activities has some positive effect on her attention span. She has emergent reading skills with recognizing pictures. She inconsistently matches pictures. She does not select text including her name unless given a physical prompt.

Sensory Processing Skills

April appears to process information with her senses in different ways. This is common in individuals with autism. She appears to be sensitive to fluorescent lighting because she often covers her head when sitting at her desk. This may be due to a combination of sensitivity to light and avoiding social interaction or undesirable tasks. She enjoys movement sensations such as using playground equipment or jumping. These same types of activities also give her additional sensory input to her muscles. She enjoys deep pressure sensation to her muscles and seeks this out by squeezing items, pulling objects, or moving her body so that she receives more sensory input (such as curling up on a bean bag chair). She has inconsistent responses to touch sensation. When the touch is paired with deep pressure (such as when she sucks on her finger or pulls an objects she touches), she likes the sensation and seeks it out. She frequently sucks her fingers or plays with her saliva. Deep pressure to her joints and muscles has helped calm her before starting an activity. April also enjoys strong scents, and this may be an area to further explore as a way to foster her engagement in activities.

Summary

April has significant impairments in her ability to perform activities necessary for school performance. Because she is in high school, the focus of her school program is moving toward transition to adult living, where self-care, home living, and vocational activities will take on increased importance. Her family is interested in having her attend a day program as an adult, and it would be beneficial for her to have activities that she can complete independently in that type of setting. April would benefit from OT in addition to special education services in order to increase her performance in these areas and to ensure that she is as independent as possible. April needs sensory activities throughout her day to assist with her attention and engagement in activities. These may be used as a combination of preparation prior to activities, rewards for completed work, and breaks.

Questions to Consider

Evaluation Report Language

Consider how much of the OT report information is written in parent-friendly language using a strengths-based approach. It is written in a way that is focused on what April can do rather than what she cannot do.

1. Explain why it is important to minimize the use of OT-specific jargon in an evaluation report. What are the advantages and disadvantages of doing this?
2. Consider how one of the sections of the evaluation would be quite different if written in terms of what April cannot do. How do you think the parents would respond to this type of report versus a report focused more on deficits?
3. Consider if there are ways that you can reword parts of the evaluation (or sentences within it) to focus even more on what April does well.

Self-Determination

Self-determination for individuals with significant cognitive disabilities focuses on ensuring that individuals have support and opportunities to create change in their lives. Fostering choice-making skills is one way to do this.

1. What are other ways that the OT could foster April's self-determination?
2. What could the OT recommend that the teacher and other service providers do to foster April's self-determination?
3. What questions could the OT ask the parents so that they may recognize the importance of

self-determination and figure out ways to incorporate this into April's life at home?

4. What ways could the OT work with the team to encourage April's participation in her IEP meeting? How could the team use assistive technology to encourage April's participation in her IEP meeting?

Transition to Adulthood

1. What other activities could the OT try with April at school to increase the variety of IADL and/or work tasks that April can participate in?
2. What other areas could the OT address (or encourage other team members to address) to prepare April for participation in adult settings?
3. What are potential IEP goals and objectives for April that the OT would be at least partially responsible for? Keep in mind the length of a typical IEP goal, April's current performance level, and her slow rate of progress.

Equipment and Assistive Technology

1. What are sensory activities or objects that the OT could recommend to incorporate into the classroom? Keep in mind that April has issues with putting her hands in her mouth.
2. Would you recommend technology for computer access for April? Why or why not?
3. April has been working with her teacher on cause-effect relationships and emergent literacy. Review some of the resources on adaptive computer software and emergent literacy (notice which sites have autism-specific resources) and recommend assistive technology that would address her current skill needs and be more age-appropriate than the preschool software she currently uses.
4. How might the OT approach the speech therapist and teacher about incorporating the voice-output communication device into other activities (beyond those in speech therapy)? How can the OT make such suggestions while still being respectful of the speech therapist's expertise?

Reference

Bazyk, S., & Case-Smith, J. (2010). School-based occupational therapy services. In J. Case-Smith & J. O'Brien (Eds.), *Occupational therapy for children* (6th ed., pp. 713-743). St. Louis: Mosby/Elsevier.

Resources

Strengths-Based Approach

Dunn, W., Koenig, K., Cox, J., Sabata, D., Pope, E., Foster, L., & Blackwell, A. (2013). Harnessing strengths: Daring to celebrate everyone's unique contributions, part 1. *Developmental Disabilities Special Interest Section Quarterly, 36*(1), 1-3.

Dunn, W., & Koenig, K. (2013). Harnessing strengths: Daring to celebrate everyone's unique contributions, part II. *Developmental Disabilities Special Interest Section Quarterly, 36*(2), 1-4.

Self-Determination

Abery, B. (1994). A conceptual framework for enhancing self-determination. In M. F. Hayden & B. Abery (Eds.), *Challenges for a service system in transition: Ensuring quality community experiences for persons with developmental disabilities* (pp. 345-380). Baltimore: Paul H. Brookes.

Abery, B., & Stancliffe, R. (1996). The ecology of self-determination. In D. J. Sands & M. L. Wehmeyer (Eds.), *Self-determination across the life span* (pp. 111-145). Baltimore: Paul H. Brookes.

Wehmeyer, M. (2005). Self-determination and individuals with severe disabilities: Re-examining meanings and misinterpretations. *Research and Practice for Persons with Severe Disabilities, 30,* 113-120.

Wehmeyer, M. (2007). *Promoting self-determination in students with developmental disabilities.* New York: Guilford Press.

Zager, D., Wehmeyer, M., & Simpson, R. L. (2012). *Educating students with autism.* New York: Routledge.

Assistive Technology

Ablenet: http://www.ablenetinc.com/

Attainment Company: http://www.attainmentcompany.com/

Creative Communicating (emergent literacy): http://creativecommunicating.com/

Don Johnston (emergent literacy): http://donjohnston.com/

Enabling Devices: http://enablingdevices.com/

Mayer Johnson (emergent literacy): http://www.mayer-johnson.com

Abby: Down Syndrome/ School Systems

Mickenzie Wilson, OTS; Jennifer Clone, OTS; and Agnieszka Moroni, OTS

History and Background Information

Abby, age 13 years, is attending seventh grade at her local suburban middle school. Abby is a very energetic and social girl who enjoys spending time with her friends, participating in sports like swimming and basketball, shopping with her mom, and participating in drama club at school. Abby lives with her mom, dad, older brother, and younger twin sisters. The family has one dog, and Abby is in charge of feeding the dog each day. Her stay-at-home mom helps with homework when Abby gets home from school. Abby's younger sisters walk with her each day to school. Abby's father works in the nearby metropolitan area as a civil engineer. Her older brother is very active in hockey and basketball at school, and Abby enjoys going to his games and cheering for him. Abby's family enjoys taking summer vacations at a nearby lake.

At 30 weeks, Abby's parents were informed that their baby girl had a diagnosis of Down syndrome and would probably need heart surgery after she was born. The surgery was to heal a small hole in her heart. Shortly after birth, Abby had open heart surgery to fix her atrioventricular septal defect. She continued to grow and develop at a rate slower than her typically developing peers. Abby began EI with both OT and PT at 1 year of age. The focus of EI was to encourage independent mobility for exploring her environment and to support the development of functional skills. Abby continued receiving EI services in her home until the age of 3. During this time, Abby also attended a local community Down syndrome center to participate in social and play activities with peers.

Abby began attending public school at age 3, where she received special education and related services in a cross-categorical classroom. When Abby began kindergarten, her placement remained the same, but she also attended physical education, art, and music with the general OT therapy to support the development of classroom skills and meet her IEP goals. Abby has been partially included until now. As a current seventh grader, Abby continues to be included with her peers for art, music, physical education, and lunch. Abby and her parents hope that she will continue to be included in these activities through high school.

Abby's current IEP includes goals related to the following areas:

- Independent shoe tying
- Fine-motor skill development to support dressing (e.g., zippers, buttons, jewelry)
- Independent managing of lunch time routine (including purchasing lunch from cafeteria line, as well as items from vending machines)
- Signing her name in cursive without visual supports
- Increased social participation and communication (e.g., how to properly communicate feelings and social conventions regarding specific topics of conversation)
- Following social conventions about bathroom use (i.e., redressing self before exiting bathroom, washing hands, closing the bathroom door)

The IEP team is looking forward to incorporating these goals into the transition plan that she will be following next year.

Evaluation Information

Analysis of Occupational Performance

The OT administered the COSA, an assessment based on the MOHO. The COSA allowed Abby to identify difficulties in given areas of occupational performance and indicate the importance of each task to her (Table 3-5). After administration of the COSA, the OT reviewed the following results in preparation for the next IEP meeting.

Upon reviewing the results of the COSA, the OT spoke with Abby and addressed the comments that she had indicated ("talking during class" and "taking my jewelry off") during the assessment with a series of follow-up questions. During the conversation, Abby explained the rules about wearing jewelry to physical education class. Abby stated that she had to take off all of her jewelry, including earrings, necklaces, and bracelets, to participate in physical education. Abby shared that her mother and her teacher had encouraged her not to wear jewelry to school so that she would not have to be bothered to take it off. However, Abby also said that she really wants to wear jewelry because "everyone else does" and she shared that she is frustrated because she is unable to take off and put on earrings and necklaces by herself. Abby also mentioned that she has gotten in trouble many times because she talks when she isn't supposed to during class time. She has had two visits in the past month to the principal's office to discuss talking out of turn.

As part of the evaluation, the OT also referred back to last school year's School Function Assessment (SFA). The SFA is broken down into three parts: Participation, Task Supports, and Activity Performance. The OT focused on reviewing Part III (Activity Performance). This section provided the OT with clear details of Abby's strengths and needs within the school setting (Table 3-6).

Areas of Occupation

The OT observed Abby during a part of her typical school day. In the classroom, Abby worked well with her classmates to complete a math worksheet. She was able to solve most of the math problems with some assistance from a paraprofessional. She also used manipulatives (e.g., small beads) to help her add and subtract, though she required more time than her peers. During the 30-minute math session, she was able to follow all directions and sustain attention on the task; however, when the teacher asked a question to the entire class, Abby shouted out answers without raising her hand. The teacher instructed Abby to raise her hand when she wanted to answer a question.

TABLE 3-5

CHILD OCCUPATIONAL SELF-ASSESSMENT SUMMARY RATING FORM

Myself	I have a big problem doing this	I have a little problem doing this	I do this ok	I am really good at doing this	Not really important to me	Important to me	Really important to me	Most important of all to me
Keep my body clean			X					X
Dress myself		X						X
Buy something myself		X					X	
Choose things I want to do				X				X
Do things with my friends				X			X	
Follow classroom rules		X			X			
Ask my teacher questions when I need to		X				X		
Think of ways to do things when I have a problem		X						X
Use my hands to work with things	X							X

What are 2 other things you have a big problem with that we didn't talk about today?

Talking during class.

Taking my jewelry off.

TABLE 3-6

SCHOOL FUNCTION ASSESSMENT: PART III ACTIVITY PERFORMANCE

Activity	Rating
MANIPULATION WITH MOVEMENT	
2. Picks up materials from desk or table (e.g., food, art supplies).	1 2 **3** 4
USING MATERIALS	
6. Turns pages in small book singly.	1 2 **3** 4
7. Manipulates small game pieces or toys.	1 **2** 3 4
8. Takes off and replaces caps on pens and markers.	1 2 **3** 4
10. Separates a single sheet of paper for use.	1 2 **3** 4
25. Secures paper with paper clip.	1 **2** 3 4
CLOTHING MANAGEMENT	
14. Separates and hooks zippers.	1 2 **3** 4
15. Buttons a row of buttons with one-to-one correspondence.	1 2 3 **4**
17. Buttons small buttons (less than one inch).	1 **2** 3 4
FUNCTIONAL COMMUNICATION	
3. Communicates "sick," "hurt," or "help."	1 2 **3** 4
4. Communicates need for help with a functional (non-academic task).	1 **2** 3 4
7. Communicates inquiries/requests for information.	1 2 **3** 4

1: Does not perform 2: Partial performance 3: Inconsistent performance 4: Consistent performance

During lunch in the cafeteria, Abby sat with her peer mentor (i.e., a general education student) and three other students from her special education class. Abby went through the lunch line and was able to choose what she wanted to eat and communicate her order to the lunch lady. Abby's peer mentor assisted her with finding the right amount of money to pay for her meal. Abby appeared to enjoy talking and hanging out with her friends during lunch.

After lunch, the therapist observed Abby getting ready for and participating in physical education. Abby left the cafeteria early to allow extra time to change out of her school clothes and into her gym uniform. She was independent with taking off her shirt and pants, but she needed assistance with tying her shoes and taking off her jewelry. Abby expressed frustration with trying to get her pierced earrings off, and eventually a classmate offered to assist her with this task.

After class ended, everyone went to the locker room to change. When the bell rang for the next class, Abby looked anxious because her classmates were leaving and she was still fumbling and trying to put her earrings back in. The OT asked Abby if she wanted help and she tearfully stated, "I guess, but I just want to do it myself!" After discussing this incident with the physical education teacher, the OT found that this happens often for Abby.

Questions to Consider

1. Write three measurable goals related to Abby's most prioritized concerns and her transition plan.
2. What other assessments could be used to provide more data regarding Abby's concerns?
3. Using both the COSA and SFA, identify strengths and areas of need for Abby.
4. Which of Abby's goals may be difficult to include in her IEP? Why?
5. What theories can guide intervention planning for Abby?
6. The OT will work with Abby to identify safe and socially appropriate behaviors in the context of the bathroom, as well as changing during physical education. It is also important for Abby to identify appropriate communication skills to be used in everyday conversations with her friends, including boundaries with the opposite sex.
   a. How can these outcomes be written as measurable goals?
   b. What are different strategies/tools that can be used to attain these goals?
   c. What part of learning appropriate behaviors might be the most challenging? Why?
7. In order for Abby to be more independent with dressing for physical education, Abby has identified putting on jewelry as an area on which she would like to work. Other areas of concern are tying shoes, as well as buttoning and zipping clothes.
   a. How can dressing be utilized as an intervention to help Abby with other fine-motor skills?
   b. What are some modifications that can be made to assist Abby with jewelry? Buttoning? Zipping?
   c. What social skills can be incorporated into her fine-motor tasks? (e.g., asking for assistance)
   d. How can the school environment be modified to assist Abby in being independent?
8. As Abby is transitioning into middle school, she has a larger responsibility as a student to be able to purchase her own food. It is important that she learns all the money denominations and is able to add them to get the amount needed.
   a. Consider all aspects of buying lunch in a school cafeteria. How can this activity be graded to support Abby's just-right challenge?
   b. How can the OT incorporate community outings to allow for transfer of skills?
   c. What role can the teacher and other educational personnel play in helping her achieve these outcomes?
   d. How can other goal areas (social and fine-motor skills) be incorporated into this activity?

Resources

Chapparo, C., & Lowe, S. (2012). School: Participating in more than just the classroom. In S. J. Lane & A. C. Bundy (Eds.), *Kids can be kids* (pp. 83-101). Philadelphia, PA: F.A. Davis Co.

Coster, W., Deeney, D., Haltiwanger, J., & Haley, S. (1998). *School Function Assessment.* San Antonio, TX: The Psychological Corporation.

Kielhofner, G. (2002). *A model of human occupation: Theory and application* (3rd ed.). Baltimore: Lippincott, Williams & Wilkins.

Keller, J., Kafkes, A., Basu, S., Federico, J., & Kielhofner, G. (2005). Child Occupational Self-Assessment. Chicago: MOHO Clearinghouse.

National Down Syndrome Society. (2012). *Resources.* Retrieved from http://www.ndss.org/Resources/

Shepherd, J. (2010). Activities of daily living. In J. Case-Smith & J. C. O'Brien (Eds.), *Occupational therapy for children* (pp. 474-517). Maryland Heights, MO: Mosby.

Gina: Cerebral Palsy/ School Systems

Minetta Wallingford, DrOT, OTR/L

History and Background Information

Gina is a friendly, enthusiastic, social fifth-grade student who receives special education and related services, including speech therapy, occupational therapy (OT), physical therapy (PT), and consultative assistive technology services to support her educational program. She has a medical diagnosis of cerebral palsy with spastic diplegia. She has increased tone in all extremities, which is mildly increased in her left upper extremity and moderately increased in her right upper extremity and lower extremities. Gina has diminished balance and needs support during standing. In addition, she wears bilateral AFOs. Gina's upper extremity movement is primarily demonstrated in flexion synergy pattern, but she can partially move out of the pattern to perform functional tasks. However, Gina continues to have limitations in her ability to perform voluntary, isolated controlled movements. Gina uses various grasp patterns and can grasp and hold a variety of objects. She can maintain her head in an upright position and she can sit in a classroom chair with her feet supported on the floor for short periods of time.

Gina has been receiving school-based OT services since she was 3 years old. Gina previously received direct OT services; however, she is currently receiving only consultative services to address her performance with written expression and self-help skills. Consultative services are also provided in the classroom to address Gina's positioning needs and to provide her teacher with adaptations and strategies to maximize her participation and increase her independence in the student role in her school environment.

Mobility

Gina has a customized power wheelchair and customized seating to provide support and positioning throughout her day. She uses a chest strap, lap belt, and foot supports for positioning and to support her posture for fine-motor tasks. She primarily uses the power wheelchair for mobility within the school environment. Gina uses a joystick control to drive her wheelchair through the hallway and into classrooms. Although she uses her wheelchair for mobility at school, Gina can walk short distances with a gait trainer or posterior rolling walker with pelvic support and supervision.

Gina has a one-to-one paraprofessional who assists her with transfers and setups for academic tasks. Gina is provided with opportunities for alternate positioning (e.g., sitting on the floor, prone on elbows on the floor) or supported standing at her desk throughout the day. These position changes are important for pressure relief. They also provide Gina with an opportunity to passively stretch and to participate in class in a way that is similar to her peers. For example, Gina often stands during science lab and sits on the floor during independent reading, as do her peers.

Self-Care

Gina can transfer to the toilet with minimal assistance by using the grab bar in an accessible restroom to support herself. She requires a seat back on the toilet for support during toileting. Gina is able to unbuckle and buckle the straps on her wheelchair and manage her clothing (e.g., pulling pants up and down) with moderate assistance. Gina also requires moderate assistance for toilet hygiene. Although Gina has not yet begun to menstruate, she is beginning to work on directing her toileting routine in preparation for this event. Because Gina has always had assistance with toileting, she is used to the paraprofessional directing the routine. Although Gina knows the sequence of her typical routine, she needs verbal prompts to direct the routine with substitute paraprofessionals. The team would like Gina to be able to direct this routine without prompts and to recognize that when she does begin menstruating, this routine will become more complex. Gina can feed herself with setup. Dycem (Dycem Ltd) under her tray and adapted utensils are beneficial when foods require cutting. She typically uses her own water bottle with a lid and straw for drinking liquids.

Gina requires moderate assistance with donning and doffing her jacket and her wheelchair harness. However, she can zip and unzip some zippers with the use of zipper aids once they are engaged. She requires physical assistance to retrieve and organize her school materials.

Academics

Gina is an engaged student but has limited endurance and requires some breaks in her school day. A one-to-one paraprofessional assistant provides setups for her academic tasks. There is an adapted desk in her classroom to accommodate her wheelchair. A slant board and Dycem are used to position materials on her desk. She has a wheelchair lap tray, which can be used when needed to support her laptop or other belongings when she is not in her regular classroom.

Gina can use a marker or adapted pencil to mark responses on modified worksheets, but her handwriting is not functional for most school-related written tasks. She uses a laptop and keyboarding to complete the majority of her written assignments. She predominantly uses her left hand for fine- and gross-motor activities but uses both hands while typing. Gina benefits from using an enlarged font and increased character spacing during keyboarding. She participates in a modified curriculum, and many academic activities are adapted for the computer.

Evaluation Information

The School Functional Assessment (SFA) (Coster et al., 1998) was completed by the school team. The most pertinent results are as follows.

Participation and Task Supports

Gina's scores indicate that she participates in the majority of regular education activities with some limitations in her active participation. She requires moderate to extensive assistance and adaptations in physical and a few cognitive/behavioral tasks.

Activity Performance

In physical tasks, Gina's highest scores were in the areas of computer and equipment use, eating and drinking, and maintaining and changing positions.

Gina's scores indicate that she receives significant assistance for completing most physical school tasks and activities. The scores support further exploring additional adaptations to maximize her independence and participation in school activities.

Based on the evaluation and Gina's interest in increasing her participation, she has a team goal "to independently direct others to organize and retrieve her personal belongings and school materials to achieve greater independence in her school environment."

Transition to Middle School

Gina will be attending a middle school in the district next year and is looking forward to her new courses, which include computer science, home economics, and chorus. Students at the middle school typically enter the school through a front entrance into the gym. Student lockers are located in rows near the entrance. Gina will be accessing all academic classrooms and will also be going to the gym for physical education, the computer lab, the library, and the music, art, and home economics classrooms. Classrooms are on two floors. There is one elevator, which allows access to the second floor.

Questions to Consider

1. Discuss possible explanations for why Gina's OT services have changed from direct services to consultative services.
2. Even though Gina can walk with a gait trainer, why might she opt to use her power wheelchair at school?
3. Complete a task analysis associated with what you think might be Gina's typical toileting routine. Add in steps associated with menstrual care.
4. Describe ways that you could support Gina in learning how to better direct her care. What types of supports and strategies would you provide? What would you do in a treatment session that was focused on increasing Gina's capacity to direct her toileting routine?
5. Discuss what you think a mealtime setup includes for Gina. How might Gina direct this setup in the future? Locate pictures of utensils that you might recommend for Gina based on her needs.
6. The OT and PT have been asked to conduct an accessibility assessment of the environment in the middle school that Gina will be attending. If you were conducting an accessibility assessment for Gina's transition to the middle school, what areas would you want to assess? Consider her school day from the time she arrives to school on an accessible bus to when she exits the building to the bus at the end of the day. Also consider the entrances and exits to the buildings.
7. What are the primary school tasks and activities that will constitute her student role in the middle school? Consider arrival and departure routines, academic preparation (organizing materials), academics, transitioning between periods, lunch, and self-care (toileting, changing for physical education).
8. What types of adaptations, modifications, or equipment do you need to consider for the middle school *environment* to support Gina in her student role? Consider that Gina will need to change classes between periods and that she will take elective courses like home economics.
9. Are there any adaptations or modifications you need to consider for Gina's *schedule* to support her participation in her student role in the middle school?
10. Gina was excited about middle school and expressed interest in becoming more independent in organizing her school belongings and her locker. OT is supporting this team goal. What are some ways to support Gina with this goal in her middle school environment?

Reference

Coster, W., Deeney, T., Haltiwanger, J., & Haley, S. (1998). *School function assessment.* San Antonio, TX: Therapy Skill Builders.

Resources

Schoonover, J., Grove, R., & Swinth, Y. (2010). Influencing participation through assistive technology. In J. Case-Smith & J. O'Brien (Eds.), *Occupational therapy for children* (6th ed., pp. 583-619). St. Louis: Mosby/Elsevier.

Wright-Ott, C. (2010). Mobility. In J. Case-Smith & J. O'Brien (Eds.), *Occupational therapy for children* (6th ed., pp. 620-648). St. Louis: Mosby/Elsevier.

Jefferson Union High School District: Sexuality and Dating Skills Training/ School Systems

Joanna Swanton, MS, OTR/L

History and Background Information

Jefferson Union High School District (JUHSD) is a public school district located in Daly City, California. JUHSD students receiving special education services attend classes at the district's four high schools according to their educational needs. Additionally, students ages 18 to 22 attend the transition program, which focuses on independent life skills and preparedness for adulthood. Students receive appropriate placements to accommodate for varied disabilities, including intellectual disability, cerebral palsy, autism spectrum disorders and others.

JUHSD employs one OT to provide services to students to address self-care, fine-/gross-motor, and self-regulation skills. This OT, similar to many schools-based therapists, may provide direct one-on-one services or group services to students, depending on the best context for them to reach their relevant goals. Consultation with teachers and other professionals is also a key part of the work of the OT. Many students additionally receive PT, adaptive physical education, speech therapy, and counseling services. The supervisor for this OT is an associate superintendent who is also the director of special education for the district. This administrator welcomes new programming from all staff and advises the OT to prioritize the best interest of the students.

Expanding Beyond Traditional School Services

The California Department of Education requires that all students receive HIV/AIDS prevention education. Although the state does not mandate comprehensive sexual health education, it prohibits abstinence-only education. For all HIV/AIDS prevention education and comprehensive sexual health education, the state requires that students with disabilities have access to materials and instruction that are appropriate for them. Prior to hiring this OT, JUHSD provided HIV/AIDS prevention education to students receiving special education services by inviting a speaker from a community clinic to deliver a presentation to students in a large group setting. The staff of this clinic was primarily trained to work with individuals who do not have intellectual or other disabilities.

This administrator and the teachers in the special education department are all open to expanding their understanding of the role of a school-based OT; many have previously observed interventions limited to handwriting and the development of fine-motor skills. Each of the teachers provides support to students who present with self-care and social skills concerns; the teachers are eager to collaborate with the OT on programming to address these areas of need. As the students transition through puberty to adulthood, they exhibit behaviors and ask questions related to sexual health. While all professional members of the students' IEP team offer valuable input, the OT's training is especially relevant to questions of sexual health for these students because the answers require increased body awareness, independence in self-care, practice of critical adult social skills, and development of self-advocacy skills.

Students eligible for special education services at JUHSD present with a wide range of abilities. Nearly all of the students demonstrate limited attention and processing skills. Many students require clear and literal directions with no more than two to three steps. Abstract concepts must be broken down into smaller, relatable pieces. Additionally, some students are visually impaired. Nearly all of the students exhibit decreased body and safety awareness. Most students are in the process of developing full independence in self-care; for example, all complete toileting independently but may require cues for hygiene. Social skills, particularly body positioning and impulse control, constitute a common area for skill development.

Within the category of sexual health and relevant life skills, the teachers report interest in developing the students' abilities to maintain appropriate personal space and demonstrate appropriate social touch. They express hopefulness that students will be able to develop healthy relationships as a result of the valuable socialization they gain in school. All high school-aged students and most transition-aged students at JUHSD currently require general supervision throughout each day and their teachers and parents consistently rank student safety as a high concern. All of the JUHSD are eager to prepare students to face the reality of potential sexual victimization with personal empowerment, knowledge, and self-advocacy skills because students currently defer to authority figures and follow directions in good faith. Students lack practice in determining if an authority figure should not be obeyed.

Focus of Occupational Therapy Intervention

Based on the current concerns at JUHSD, the OT, the administrator, and the teachers believe that there is a significant need for OT intervention to address sexuality and dating skills. The team decides that it would be appropriate for the OT to lead groups with the high school students to address these concerns. The team collaborates to establish the following ideal outcomes for OT intervention:

- To increase students' knowledge of sexuality and sexual health, including the ability to correctly label body parts with accurate terms and the ability to identify which types of body part contact exposes a person to pregnancy and disease
- To promote students' safety by establishing personal space boundaries and the understanding of progression of intimate touch (i.e., hugging before kissing and kissing before body/genital contact)
- To prepare students to respond to a wide range of social situations requiring the understanding of sexuality and the social rules for appropriate expression
- To instill in students the belief that their body is their own and that they are responsible for keeping themselves healthy and safe
- To develop skills for recruiting family support and reporting abuse through practiced role plays

Questions to Consider

1. Why is the OT an appropriate professional to address the area of sexual health for students at JUHSD?
2. What are the obstacles posed by the different levels of abilities in the students? How can those differences enrich the learning experience of all students?
3. What are some possible short-term goals for students at the high school level related to sexuality and dating skills? Discuss whether or not the same goals would be appropriate for older students at the transition program.
4. What legal concerns do you have about providing sexual health education for students with disabilities? Is it safer to avoid the topic of sexual health education, given the information above? Would your opinion be different in another state?
5. Investigate if there are valid curricula for the sexual health education of students with intellectual disabilities.
6. How would you communicate your plan of intervention to the IEP team, including parents?
7. How are self-care skills a component of sexual health?
8. Is it important to explain to students that they must increase independence in self-care skills in order to increase their safety from sexual abuse? Why not just promote self-care skills only? Does the intention change the intervention?
9. How can you reach out to parents to promote self-care skills as a means to improve sexual health?
10. How would you respond to parents who explain that their cultural values motivate them to care for their children with disabilities, including showering them and managing menstrual hygiene?
11. What types of visual aids would support a lesson on anatomy and identifying sexual and private parts?
12. How would you plan a group for students to learn personal space with opposite gender peers? Can you make an age-appropriate game?
13. How could you create opportunities for real-life practice recognizing the difference between private and public spaces (e.g., is a public restroom a public or private space)?
14. How would you offer consultation to teachers for ways to respond when students make inappropriate sexual comments or gestures?
15. What are two key ways students might practice expressing attraction to a peer in a socially appropriate way?
16. How would you coach parents and teachers to encourage students to question authority in a healthy way?
17. How can you create clear categories for understanding relationships for students with intellectual disabilities? What makes a friend, boyfriend, wife, and so on?
18. How can you explain how to prevent pregnancy using basic terms, simple sentences, repetition, visual aids, and opportunities for practice?
19. How would you coach parents and teachers to answer students' questions about wanting a girlfriend/boyfriend?
20. Investigate visual aids for teaching students which body parts may be touched or exposed in various private and public environments (e.g., can you put your arm around someone at school? At church? At the movies?)
21. Two students are discovered kissing in the high school hallway. Both students have intellectual disabilities. Each demonstrates a functional knowledge of appropriate social behavior and makes good use of peer models. You know that other students without disabilities sometimes hug and kiss on campus and this is not reported to their teachers. How do you coach the students in special education to understand the school rule of no public displays of affection while ignoring peer models?
22. You observe that a few of the female students have a tendency to hug any adult male who approaches them, including campus security guards and bus drivers. They do not wait for a social cue to invite these hugs and require verbal cues to let go of the person they are hugging. How can you coach the girls and the male staff to modify these exchanges and address the

social rule that young women cannot hug older men they know only as acquaintances? You want the girls to become aware of the sexual undertones of a long hug and the possibility that an older acquaintance may take advantage of their enthusiastic affection. You want the male staff members to understand that this lesson is part of sexual health education without implying that you hold a negative opinion of them or their intentions with the female students.

23. A student with an intellectual disability is highly motivated to gain attention from students in the cafeteria. He has learned that if he makes loud comments about butts that other students will laugh, so he does this repeatedly. He also attempts to hug female students whom he does not know personally and comments that they are sexy. How can you plan a group session to address inappropriate comments and offer this student a positive way to express his sexual interests?

References

American Occupational Therapy Association. (2008). Occupational therapy practice framework: Domain and process (2nd ed.). *American Journal of Occupational Therapy, 62*, 625-683.

Hattjar, B. (2012). *Sexuality and occupational therapy: Strategies for persons with disabilities*. Bethesda, MD: AOTA Publications.

MacRae, N. (2013). Sexuality and the role of occupational therapy. Retrieved from: http://www.aota.org/en/About-Occupational-Therapy/Professionals/RDP/Facts/Sexuality.aspx

Ozzy: Childhood Trauma With Neuromotor Sequelae

Kimberly Bryze, PhD, OTR/L

History and Background Information

Developmental History

Ozzy, age 9 years, was removed from his parents' care by the State's Child Welfare Agency and was placed under the care of the State to reside in a private not-for-profit residential facility for children with emotional and behavioral disorders. He lived in a group home with five other boys, ages 6 through 10 years, and attended a therapeutic day school affiliated with the not-for-profit agency.

Ozzy's early developmental history is not clear, but some basic information was obtained from his Social Work Case Manager at the facility. For the first 8 years of his life, Ozzy lived with his parents in a rural part of the state, many miles from any town. The family went largely unnoticed to school authorities until Ozzy was well into his eighth year, when a school district official pursued reports of a school-aged child living in the farmstead but not attending elementary school. Ozzy's father aggressively chased the school official from the family property, the police and the State's Child Welfare Agency were called in, and Ozzy was discovered and removed from the house. The parents were charged with felony drug charges, child abuse, and child endangerment, and they were remanded into custody. The State Child Welfare Agency arranged for thorough medical examinations for Ozzy; evidence of healed bone fractures to his humerus, tibia and fibula, and skull were identified. Ozzy was placed in a series of four foster care arrangements over the next year. The frequency of transition from one placement to another was largely due to his behaviors (i.e., fire-starting, cruelty to animals) and elopement from each foster care placement.

When Ozzy just turned 9 years old, he was placed in the residential facility, which offered greater daily supports and structure for a child with severe social and emotional disorders. He was examined by a child psychiatrist, who diagnosed Ozzy with Conduct Disorder. Ozzy had never attended school for any length of time except for his short trials in foster care and four different schools the previous year. Now at 9 years of age, with a stable living environment and therapeutic day school placement, educational testing was possible and appropriate supports initiated. It was determined that Ozzy had mild cognitive/intellectual disabilities, was performing at a first grade level in reading and mathematics, and demonstrated significant problems with focusing his attention and concentration on academic work. He avoided social interaction with children in his class, preferring to sit away from the others and, according to the psychologist, initiate opportunities to be removed from circle time.

Therapeutic Day School

Ozzy was placed in the "primary" classroom of the therapeutic day school with nine other boys, ages 6 through 10 years of age. The classroom was a large room on the first floor of an old school building. Large, high windows let in natural sunlight. Wooden, well-scuffed floors announced teachers' and students' movements during the day. The individual child desks were metal with adjustable legs and an open side closest to the child for placing books and papers inside. The children sat on hard plastic and metal chairs at their desks; the desks and chairs were arranged such that each boy sat more than an arms' length from other boys to prevent behavioral outbursts, but the desks were arranged loosely in a circular pattern facing the chalkboard at the front of the room.

Mrs. T, the classroom teacher, had taught children with SED for more than 10 years. She had a firm but warm manner, high expectations for her students, and enough energy to anticipate and manage any behavioral challenge that arose in the blink of an eye. Mrs. T welcomed Ozzy into her classroom and offered him the empty desk and chair close to her desk. She had supplied the desk with some pencils, paper, and the textbooks used by the class. The classroom aide, Mr. G, had a desk behind Ozzy's and a few other boys' desks, although he and Mrs. T rarely sat at their desks, walking around to help each boy individually.

In the far back corner was a floor mat, a shelf of books, and two large baskets filled with stuffed animals and washable quilts to create a cozy reading corner for the students. The bookshelf was secured to the wall and was filled with books ranging from preschool-level picture books to chapter books for the more advanced readers. A computer sat on a table toward the left of the classroom, and the boys could play word or math games on the computer if they had earned enough points for good behavior. While Mrs. T had a computer on her desk, the boys were not to touch her computer but could work on their computer when they earned the privilege. Children's artwork covered three large bulletin boards along the front and right sides of the classroom, and posters reminding the children of the classroom rules (e.g., "use your words, not your hands," "raise your hand to speak," etc.) were secured strategically around the room.

The classroom routine was structured in such a way that the students immediately had work to do as they arrived in the morning. Given the bus schedules, the students arrived in varying times between 8:30 and 9:00 in the morning, and tasks such as copying word riddles from the board or completing science coloring sheets were offered to provide the students with something to accomplish immediately upon their arrival. The morning was filled with 30-minute blocks of time devoted to reading, mathematics, and science, which were alternated with circle time, free time, and story-listening times. The 45 minutes for lunchtime included walking downstairs and eating lunch in the cafeteria with three other classes of students, and walking back to the classroom after lunch. The afternoon sessions were social studies, art (with an art therapist), gym time, and individual reading time.

While most of the boys had been in Mrs. T's class for more than this year, knew the routines, and were better able to control their behavioral impulses, it was not uncommon for tempers to flare up quickly and impulsive acts of aggression to occur, sometimes without warning (e.g., hitting another child while walking past the desk, sticking out a foot to trip someone, speaking an unkind word when walking past another's desk, etc.). Behavioral interventions ranged from being redirected by the teacher, losing privilege points, time-out, crisis prevention intervention, and physical restraint by the teacher(s), although the latter was the last possible approach applied to a behavioral outburst.

Ozzy had difficulty adjusting to the new routine, let alone his new living situation. Two of the boys in his class were also his group–home-mates. One of the boys sought Ozzy's friendship, while the other boy considered Ozzy to be a threat, and Ozzy seemed to need to be alert both at school and at home. Learning the routines and behavioral regulations was challenging because he had never been in a situation with rules and appropriate social behaviors and was quite unfamiliar with group norms and expectations.

The principal recognized the unique life trajectory that Ozzy had experienced up to this point and sought to build in additional supports to help him succeed at this residential/therapeutic school. He purposely touched base with Ozzy each day to inquire about his day, offer a smile, spend some informal time with him, and to provide an additional, unconditional relationship each day. When Mrs. T mentioned that Ozzy had considerable difficulty with copying, writing, and coloring tasks in the classroom, the principal took the opportunity to begin the process for an occupational therapy evaluation.

Evaluation Information

Occupational Therapy Evaluation

Evaluation Session and Results

The occupational therapy evaluation process included extended observations of Ozzy while in the classroom, lunchroom, art, and gym, and while transitioning to the van to leave for the residential center at the end of the school day. The occupational therapist also administered the Developmental Test of Visual-Motor Integration (VMI), interviewed Mrs. T, and read the information provided in his chart. The occupational therapist had previously sent a copy of the Sensory Profile Caregiver Questionnaire to be completed by Ozzy's foster parent prior to this evaluation day, and the form was completed when the therapist arrived that morning.

Mrs. T had informed Ozzy early the morning of the evaluation that the occupational therapist would be in the classroom observing him and the other boys, and would ask him to do some activities. When the OT arrived to the classroom the morning of the evaluation, the OT greeted Mrs. T, who then introduced the therapist to the class as an "observer for the day"; she situated the therapist at her desk in close proximity to Ozzy's desk so that the OT could see his schoolwork and, when the schedule permitted, work individually with him. The occupational therapist planned to blend into the routine of the classroom as much as possible and not disrupt the routines that Ozzy was slowly learning. The OT wanted to see Ozzy in the most typical or natural situation as possible to fully identify his areas of strength and need.

Ozzy sat at his desk somewhat slumped in his chair with shoulders in protraction and his arms extended in front of him on the desk. In this position, he held his book from which to read, flipped his pencil, and rearranged the inside of his desk. When it was time to write or copy from the board, Ozzy repositioned himself to sit at the edge of his chair, with his legs extended in front of him, feet on the floor, while holding his back straight and propping his wrists on the desk to write. He and the class were asked to copy five math problems from the board; he cocked his head to the left and squinted up his eyes as he looked toward the chalkboard. His right-handed grasp on the pencil was a static tripod with the middle finger anterior to his index finger, and the thumb curled over the pencil and onto his index finger. He held the pencil with a tight grasp, and used his left hand to support the paper as he wrote. However, he did not keep the paper positioned at a consistent angle, shifting it approximately 20 degrees to the left then to the right as he wrote. His letters and numerals were large and irregular. His lines were shaky and as he continued to write, he seemed to hold the pencil tighter and tighter, as if to control the shakiness of his hands. He discontinued the task after a few problems were copied and answered, and Mr. G came to his desk to help him finish the task.

As they worked on the last three problems, Ozzy would point to the board, speak with Mr. G, and occasionally put his pencil down on his desk with force as if to say, "I'm done." As Ozzy pointed toward the board, the occupational therapist noted the slowness with which he curled his fingers into a fist while pointing his index finger forward; tremors were noted as he pointed toward the problems on the board. As he retrieved the pencil to reposition it in his hand, his manipulation was awkward and he used his left hand to help position the pencil appropriately for writing.

Mr. G asked Ozzy to bring his finished work to Mrs. T's "in box" on her desk. Ozzy pushed himself off the chair away from the desk and walked the few steps over to the desk. He wore gym shoes but seemed to stamp or walk heavily with each step. When he needed to stop and turn from the desk, he seemed to turn the top half of his body at a different rate than the lower half of his body, evidence of poor trunk stability. Such awkward motor control and poor postural background movements were noted throughout the day as he navigated around obstacles in the environment or walked from one area to another. Mrs. T mentioned to the occupational therapist, "It seems like his hands and feet are loose. When he moves he seems to wiggle a lot and he doesn't mean to."

The lunchroom was located one floor down from the main classroom hallway. Ozzy and the other boys gathered up their lunches and lined up at the door (while pushing and stomping on others' feet, which delayed lunch by 10 minutes so they could practice lining up again without incident). Ozzy was originally second in line, and held his insulated lunchbox by the handle with his left hand. When Mrs. T and the first boy started to walk forward out the door, Ozzy demonstrated a delay in stepping forward and he seemed to lurch as he began walking behind his peer. When they arrived at the top of the steps, Ozzy held onto the railing with his right hand, raised his leg higher than necessary to step down to the next step, and carefully took one step at a time. The other boys ran around him to go down the stairs, not willing to wait for him and stepping out of line. Ozzy proceeded to descend the stairs, step by step, often overtly straightening his weightbearing leg as he descended to each step. He appeared to "thunk down" onto the steps while overstepping with the nonweightbearing foot. By the time Ozzy had negotiated the two flights and 16 steps to the lower level, the other boys were already unpacking their lunches at the assigned lunch table.

Ozzy unpacked his lunch of a sandwich, fruit cup, and cookies. Mr. G automatically helped him open the milk carton, but Ozzy inserted a small straw from which to drink. Ozzy's oral motor skills were effective, but his overall mealtime was somewhat slow as he had difficulty opening the fruit cup package and scooping the fruit and juice out with the small plastic spoon. He held the spoon with his right hand, palmar grasp, but used a stiff wrist movement to scoop, which limited his ability to retrieve the food from the corners of the container. He threw his trash away when reminded and slowly rezipped his lunchbox before asking to use the washroom.

Walking up the steps to return to the classroom was another laborious task for Ozzy. He demonstrated overstepping and a slow pace, and the boys arrived to the classroom before him. He was not out of breath from exertion, but his pace, facial expressions, and compensatory movements suggested that steps were difficult for him to negotiate.

The first period after lunch was a scheduled "free-time" period in which the OT chose to administer the VMI. By this time, Ozzy and the OT had communicated with each other and joked at lunch, and Ozzy seemed to be more relaxed with the therapist's presence as a stranger in his classroom. He willingly sat with the OT at a table away from where the other boys were reading in the reading corner, and he completed and received credit on the first 15 items; the raw score of 15 afforded him an age equivalency of 5 years, 6 months for visual motor integration, far below his chronological age. Given his earlier life history, it is unlikely that he was offered writing and drawing tasks, and as he had not consistently attended school, his visual motor score was not unexpected.

When he completed the VMI, he returned to the reading corner and unfortunately became involved in what seemed to be a turf war close to the bookshelf, resulting in physical redirection from Mrs. T and Mr. G. When the other boy pushed Ozzy away "because he was too close," Ozzy fell backward onto the mat, then quickly turned his body in order to kick at the boy with his feet. The occupational therapist later learned that Ozzy's style of fighting with another child, or one of the teachers, during his outbursts usually involved kicking, and that his kick was extremely powerful and seemingly well-placed. He reportedly rarely missed kicking a spot he intended to kick, creating quite an unsafe space around him when he was out of control.

Lights were turned off, boys were asked to return to their desks, and the two boys involved in the altercation were removed by Mrs. T to a quiet room to regroup. Within a short period of time, Ozzy and his now calm peer returned to the classroom for art time. The boys lined up to go downstairs to the art room where there were tables covered with colored paper. The activity for the day was cutting and gluing construction paper fall-colored leaves onto a collage for the classroom. Each boy could work on a separate section or could work together (the real goal), sharing materials and helping each other. Ozzy positioned himself at the far end of the table away from the boys, and quickly gathered his own pair of scissors and glue. The occupational therapist sat between Ozzy and another boy and hoped to encourage material sharing and assistance with cutting. Ozzy tried several times to cut the simple elm leaf pattern out using his right hand, but the tremors seemed to increase significantly. He was also unable to stabilize his wrist in order to open and close his hand appropriately without twisting and ripping the paper. The OT attempted to help him by holding the paper so that he would only have to focus on working the scissors; while that helped a bit, it was not successful. As he began to get frustrated, the OT explained to him that "scissors sure are tricky. How about if I help hold your wrist and we will cut together?" He looked at the OT seriously, and finally allowed the therapist to try helping him "only once!" Fortunately, with holding his wrist, he was able to cut the long curved line of the elm leaf, and even allowed the OT to turn the leaf to cut the other side. Ozzy and the OT then moved on to glue some leaves onto the collage.

Ozzy also demonstrated tremors with squeezing the glue bottle. He exerted increased pressure to squeeze out the glue, dropping the bottle a few times and needing to reposition his hands and squeeze again. When he briefly laid his hand down on glue on the paper, he spent considerable time searching for and using a tissue to remove all glue from his hands. After only one leaf was successfully but messily glued onto the collage, he moved himself away from the activity table until the other boys were done. He was obviously frustrated and unhappy with the activity or its difficulty, and he sat across the room glowering and tapping his feet until it was time to leave.

After art was gym time. The boys lined up in the art room to walk down the hallway to the gym area. The school did not have a physical education teacher or recreation therapist, but the teachers had arranged for several basketballs to be available, and most of the boys quickly grouped together to start an informal basketball game. Ozzy, the last one in the gym, retrieved a ball and moved to the far set of hoops away from the others. He attempted to dribble the ball (unsuccessfully, dropping it on his toe causing it to bounce away), shoot for the basket (unsuccessfully, as he could only throw the ball less than half of the distance required). He ran to retrieve the ball several times. He ran with poor coordination, his arms and legs seemingly worked against each other. As he ran toward the ball, his feet often hit the ball, requiring him to travel farther to retrieve it. He had difficulty starting to run and was unable to stop his running when he arrived at the ball. He fell frequently, and while the falls were hard enough to hear echoing through the noisy gym, he did not seem to react to the falls with pain. Regardless of the challenges, Ozzy did not give up; he attempted to dribble and shoot for approximately 15 minutes. By this time, he was breathing hard, sweating, and eventually sat on the gym floor where he slumped, leaning on the ball in fatigue. Mr. G went to Ozzy and engaged him in a game of catch with the basketball, encouraging him to use both hands to throw. Ozzy was unable to catch any of the tosses to him, although Mr. G tossed the ball directly to his midline.

After the students returned to their classroom for snack and end-of-the-day routines, the OT reviewed Ozzy's chart and scored the Sensory Profile. The results are shown in Table 3-7.

Questions to Consider for Intervention

1. In spite of his early life, Ozzy demonstrates many strengths. Identify his strengths in consideration of their possible contribution to intervention.
2. What areas of occupation are of greatest concern for Ozzy at this point? What goals should be developed to address these occupational concerns?
3. What performance skill and performance component level difficulties are of concern and may be contributing to his occupational dysfunction?
4. In what ways might his gross motor and fine motor difficulties be related?
5. What intervention strategies might be implemented to help Ozzy with his schoolwork performance? Describe your rationale for each strategy.
6. Using principles from OT theory, explain ways in which Ozzy might better participate in art and other schoolwork opportunities.

Table 3-7

Ozzy's Sensory Profile Chart Scores

	RAW SCORE	TYPICAL PERFORMANCE	PROBABLE DIFFERENCE	DEFINITE DIFFERENCE
Sensory Processing				
Auditory processing	24/40			X
Visual processing	28/45		X	
Vestibular processing	46/55		X	
Touch processing	25/90			X
Multisensory processing	23/35			X
Oral sensory processing	45/60		X	
Modulation				
Sensory processing related to endurance/tone	35/45			X
Modulation related to body position/movement	33/50			X
Modulation related to movement affecting activity level	21/35		X	
Modulation of sensory input affecting emotional responses	10/20			X
Modulation of visual input affecting emotional responses and activity level	14/20		X	
Behavior and Emotional Response				
Emotional/social responses	50/85			X
Behavioral outcomes of sensory processing	18/30			X
Items indicating thresholds for response	14/15	X		

7. Describe strategies for improving his safety and efficiency navigating the school environment, including the stairs, classroom, and hallways.
8. To what additional evaluations or professional supports might you refer Ozzy?
9. Describe at least 10 ways to facilitate Ozzy's visual-motor skill development and confidence that may further his success in completing his schoolwork.
10. Ozzy's new school and home life are so very new to him. What therapeutic approach(es) would provide him with the establishment of routines and emotional well-being?

References

Beery, K., Buktenica, N., & Beery, N. (2010). *Beery-Buktenica Developmental Test of Visual-Motor Integration* (6th ed.). San Antonio, TX: Pearson.

Dunn, W. (1999). *Sensory Profile*. San Antonio, TX: Pearson.

Resource

Bazyk, S. (2007). Addressing the mental health needs of children in schools. In L. Jackson (Ed.), *Occupational Therapy Services for Children and Youth under Idea* (3rd ed., pp. 145-166). Bethesda, MD: AOTA Press.

CHAPTER 4

Introduction to Outpatient Services

Different from hospital-based services, outpatient services are often provided to children who do not have complex medical needs. Many of the children who receive outpatient services encounter developmental challenges and require additional support to meet expected milestones and participate fully at home, school, and in the community. Others were recently discharged from the hospital and no longer need acute medical care.

Outpatient services are often provided to children and youth in private clinics. Some of these clinics cater to children with specific needs, such as sensory processing disorder. Such clinics often have large gyms with suspended equipment and climbing structures. In addition, they may also have smaller treatment rooms that provide opportunities to work on discrete skill development (e.g., cutting or handwriting).

Outpatient services might also be provided to children in their homes. The benefit of providing outpatient services in the home is that the occupational therapist (OT) can see how the child functions in his or her natural environment. Further, the OT can use materials that the child typically has access to and may be able to make recommendations that would complement the family's typical routines.

Outpatient therapy services may be billed through insurance companies and Medicaid. In addition, many outpatient clinics accept clients that self-pay.

Outpatient therapy services are generally provided when children are not attending school. Many outpatient OTs work after school hours and on the weekends. Some are self-employed while others are employed through a clinic.

Questions to Consider

1. What do you see as the pros and cons of providing outpatient services to children?
2. Besides children with sensory processing disorders, what other groups of children might benefit from this type of service?

Conrad: Sensory Processing Disorder, Fine- and Gross-Motor Delay/ Outpatient Clinic

Erin Anderson, OTR/L;
Michelle Bednarek, MS, OTR/L; and
Melissa Williamson, OTR/L

History and Background Information

Conrad is 4 years, 2 months old and has a diagnosis of an adjustment disorder with anxiety. He was brought in for an OT evaluation by his mother because he is having difficulty in his classroom environment. The teachers have concerns about his ability to participate in unstructured activities; he demonstrates immature behaviors and poor peer interactions. He is unable to sit still and generally needs one-on-one assistance. His preschool is no longer able to accommodate him at this time.

Occupational Profile

Conrad is an only child who lives with both his mother and father. His mother reports a normal pregnancy, with the only complication being maternal fibroid detection.

Cahill SM, Bowyer P, eds. *Cases in Pediatric Occupational Therapy: Assessment and Intervention (pp 89-108).*

He was born via cesarean section at 37 weeks weighing 5 pounds, 1 ounce. In regard to achieving his developmental milestones, Conrad sat up at 8 months, crawled at 11 months, walked at 14 months, and had his first words at 9 months. Conrad has not had any significant hospitalizations. He has intolerance for cow's milk but does not have any other known allergies. He has previously received OT, although he has not received any other evaluations.

Conrad's mother reports that at home he is generally mild-mannered, is able to assist with his self-care, and loves to learn. Conrad enjoys playing with trains and dinosaurs and reading books. He demonstrates adequate attention during story time and is able to discuss and remember facts in the story. He also really enjoys going to the park to climb on the equipment, swinging, jumping on the trampoline, and doing somersaults.

He follows specific routines at home and is compliant with dressing and cleaning up his toys. Conrad's mother reports that they try to keep a fairly consistent schedule at home. For the most part, Conrad is able to participate and assist in activities at home, stays regulated most of the time, and gets adequate sleep. He wakes up in a good mood, eats a large breakfast, and then attends school. If he does not attend school, mom reports that she tries to do some movement-based activity with him every day by going outside or going to the park, and she also plays with him throughout the day.

She is concerned about his impulsivity, his poor ability to shift gears, his stubbornness/inflexibility at times, and that he prefers to play with adults or older children. Conrad has difficulty playing catch with a partner and he generally does not like playing with balls. He is not always interested in participating in pretend play activities. She would like to learn some ways to help him with his anxiety and impulsivity.

Currently, Conrad is attending a therapeutic child center that addresses academic curriculum, behavior, and social development 4 days a week for 3 hours per day. He also attends a social skills group that is co-led by a speech therapist and an OT. The overall goal for Conrad is to reintegrate him into a typical kindergarten program.

Analysis of Occupational Performance

Conrad received an outpatient OT evaluation. Clinical observations were completed, as well as gross-motor testing. The Sensory Processing Measure was completed by his mother and teacher (Table 4-1). Formal fine-motor testing was not completed because he is functional and appears within age limits at this time.

Conrad presents as an inquisitive, engaging child with strong language skills and an above-average vocabulary for his age. Per his mother's report, Conrad has deficits in interacting with peers in that he has difficulty with personal space, keeping his hands to himself, and initiation during play. His mom also has observed that he appears to be rigid in his play and has difficulty adjusting his play to share with a friend or engage in cooperative play.

- Gross-motor skills: Conrad balanced on his right foot for 5 seconds and his left foot for 2 seconds, which is below average in comparison to 10 seconds by his peers. He easily hopped on two feet but cannot hop on one foot, though this skill is emerging. With a model, he completed jumping jacks moving his feet apart and together but was not able to simultaneously move his arms as well. He completed jumping side to side and front to back. Supine flexion was held for 4 seconds, although prone extension could not be assumed at this time. This suggests that Conrad demonstrates weaker core strength and postural muscles. Conrad demonstrated trouble with the balance beam with his heel to toe balance. Conrad needed moderate to maximal verbal cues to follow therapist-directed activities. He showed inflexible thinking and was frequently stuck on his own ideas.
- Fine-motor skills: Conrad is right-hand dominant and maintained a modified tripod grasp on the pencil. He required moderate assistance to complete a 12-piece puzzle. Scissor skills are emerging. He can snip with scissors, but cannot cut along a line (Figure 4-1). This is below average for a child his age.
- Activities of daily living: Conrad cannot button one-quarter–inch buttons but can snap independently. He cannot engage the zipper but can zip once it is engaged. He needs assistance with dressing.
- Upper limb coordination: Conrad caught a ball with two hands three out of five trials using a playground ball. He trapped the ball against his chest while catching.
- Academic readiness was assessed. Conrad knows his letters and sounds, which are advanced for his age. He can write the first two letters of his name.
- Sensory processing: Conrad has some difficulty interpreting vestibular information as demonstrated by decreased post rotary nystagmus after spinning. He sought out vestibular input during the evaluation by running back and forth in the hallway, spinning in circles, and jumping on the trampoline. He was seeking movement throughout the session, so much so that it interfered with his ability to complete other fine- and gross-motor tasks.
- Conrad was noted to have difficulty with modulation during the session, often seeking proprioceptive input in the pillows and Airwalker swing (eSpecial Needs) to help him focus. When another child entered the treatment space, Conrad was noted to display difficulty with body and spatial awareness in addition to needing deep pressure and verbal cues to participate in a game with another child.

TABLE 4-1

THE SENSORY PROCESSING MEASURE—HOME

	T- SCORE	TYPICAL (40T-59T)	SOME PROBLEMS (60T-69T)	DEFINITE DYSFUNCTION (70T-80T)
Social	67		X	
Visual	62		X	
Hearing	69		X	
Touch	60		X	
Body Awareness	78			X
Balance	62		X	
Planning	52	X		
TOTAL	67		X	

Per mom, Conrad has difficulty processing auditory information and seems distracted by background noises, such as lawn mowers. He always seems disturbed by or intensely interested in sounds. Conrad always bumps or pushes other children and jumps a lot. He always chews on toys, clothes, or other objects. He often falls out of his chair when changing positions.

THE SENSORY PROCESSING MEASURE—SCHOOL

	T- SCORE	TYPICAL (40T-59T)	SOME PROBLEMS (60T-69T)	DEFINITE DYSFUNCTION (70T-80T)
Social	65		X	
Visual	43	X		
Hearing	55	X		
Touch	63		X	
Body Awareness	55	X		
Balance	69		X	
Planning	62		X	
TOTAL	61		X	

In the comment section, both Conrad's mother and his teachers had concerns regarding compliance issues, such as following verbal instructions and completing familiar sequences such as dressing. His teacher noted that Conrad is always distressed or fearful of movement activities such as teeter-totters. He also shows difficulty moving his body to rhythm. Conrad also fails to complete tasks with multiple steps. He never interacts with peers during pretend play and never resolves peer conflict without teacher intervention. Per the teacher as well, he never enters play without disrupting the play that is happening. Conrad always shows distress when hands or face are dirty and he always avoids playing with messy things.

Questions to Consider

Goals and Treatment Planning

1. What long-term goals would the OT create for Conrad in order to demonstrate success with a social interaction?
2. List three short-term, age-appropriate fine-motor goals.
3. Write a long-term goal to demonstrate better sensory processing within the school environment. Describe how you would collect data on this goal in an outpatient setting.
4. How would you structure your treatment sessions with Conrad in the clinic?
5. What treatment strategies would you use with Conrad?
6. What frames of reference would you use to treat Conrad's overall deficits?

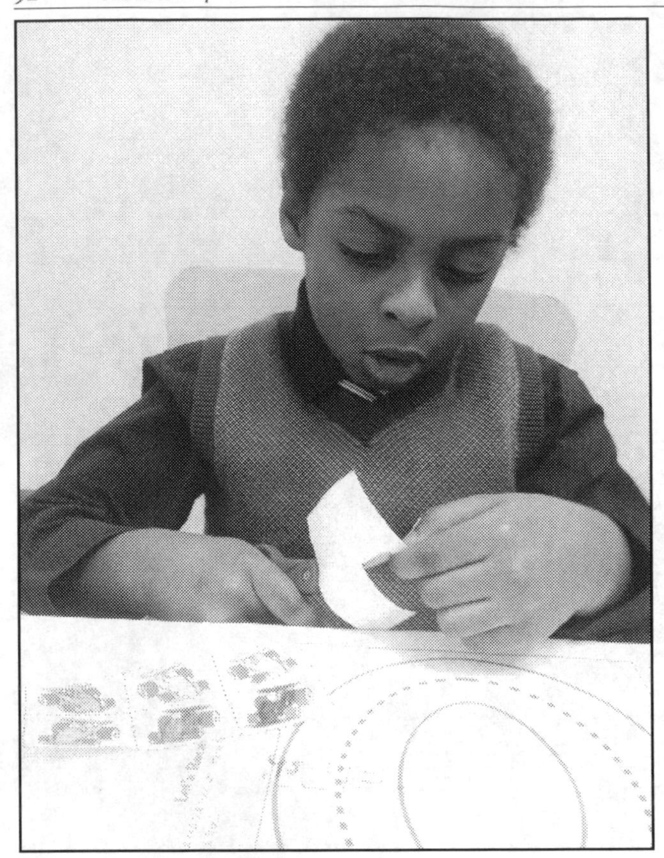

Figure 4-1. Conrad cutting.

Sensory Processing

1. How do his sensory processing skills affect his ability to interact with others and impede his ability to complete functional activities?
2. What impact does sensory processing have on behavioral outbursts, if any?
3. What impact does sensory processing play in his interaction with his family and friends at school or home?
4. What role does modulation play in Conrad's life at home and school?

Gross Motor/Fine Motor

1. What gross-motor and fine-motor tasks should a typically developing 4-year-old be able to perform?
2. What role do his delays in motor development play in his behavior?
3. What gross-motor activities would you suggest to address bilateral coordination?
4. How would you incorporate overall strengthening with gross-motor play?
5. How would you grade fine-motor tasks such as a color, cut, and paste activity with Conrad if his behavior interferes with his ability to complete the task?

School/Family Education

1. What environmental modifications would you suggest to increase his independent functioning at home and at school?
2. What equipment would you suggest to address his sensory needs at home or school?
3. Prepare a sensory diet for his mother to use at home.
4. What kind of schedule, if any, would you suggest for Conrad at home or school?
5. What other services, if any, would you suggest to address all of Conrad's and his mom's concerns?

Situations

1. Conrad has difficulty with social interactions, including play dates. He gets very dysregulated and can talk loudly, invade the friend's space, and may hit him. It is difficult for him to decide what to play and he will leave the child if he doesn't want to play what his friend wants to play. What three things would you do to make his play date successful?
2. Conrad has been receiving OT for 3 months and continues to have a difficult time transitioning into the outpatient clinic. He continues to run down the hall and disregard the therapist and his mother when coming into the clinic. This often happens when transitioning through the session as well. How would you help Conrad to have successful transitions?
3. Conrad was playing a game in the gym when a friend entered. At that time, Conrad began to run around and crash into the pillows and then got very close to the little boy, stating, "Why are you in here?" What would you do next to turn this interaction into a positive one for Conrad?
4. You've updated Conrad's treatment plan and would like others to follow through with your recommendations. Who should you follow up with to discuss the changes?
5. Conrad's mother would like assistance finding the best school placement for Conrad. What are some suggestions you can give her to help her make this important decision and enhance Conrad's success?

Discharge Planning

1. When you discharge Conrad, what do you need to have in place to ensure his success at home and school?

Resources

Bundy, A., Lane, S., & Murray, E. (2002). *Sensory integration: Theory and practice* (2nd ed.). Philadelphia: F.A. Davis Co.

Parham, L. D., Ecker, C., Kuhaneck, H. M., Henry, D. A., & Glennon, T. J. (2007). *Sensory processing measure.* Los Angeles: Western Psychological Services.

Jacob: Sensory Processing Disorder/Outpatient Clinic

Dana Pais, OTD, OTR/L

History and Background Information

Jacob, age 4 years, 3 months, was diagnosed with sensory processing disorder. Jacob was referred for an OT evaluation by his pediatrician due to concerns with neuroprocessing that are contributing to auditory and tactile hypersensitivities, decreased attention to task, and decreased eye contact. These difficulties impact his daily functioning at home and school. Jacob's parents sought an OT evaluation at a multidisciplinary private practice outpatient clinic.

The outpatient clinic is located in an urban city and houses a variety of disciplines, including neuropsychology, OT, speech therapy, PT, social work, applied behavior analysis, and dietetics. This clinic is located on a quiet street, lined with restaurants, small businesses, and homes. The one-story clinic is located on the corner of the street with the entrance at street level.

Jacob's first appointment begins with his parents filling out initial paperwork, including insurance information and a history intake questionnaire, which provides details on his developmental history, current level of functioning, current concerns, and other pertinent personal and academic information.

Evaluation Information

Upon completion of the paperwork, Jacob and his family are introduced to his OT. The OT greets the family in the lounge and walks them through a narrow hallway to the therapy gym. Jacob and his family pass the bathrooms and the therapist's office on their way to the therapy gym. The therapy gym is a large room designed for sensory equipment and gross-motor activities that take place in a large area in the middle of the space. The area is filled with a suspension system that holds a variety of equipment and swings, including the superman swing, bolster swing, rainbow swing, tire swing, and rainbow tunnel. The floor is covered by blue gymnastic mats. The space around the suspension equipment is occupied with therapy balls, a scooter board and ramp, balance beams, and three small tables and chairs. The large gym is surrounded by smaller treatment rooms, where speech therapy, mental health therapy, and behavior therapy take place. The smaller treatment rooms are also used for OT and PT, for children who may require a smaller space to help increase attention to task. In the back of the large gym is a smaller gym, with three rock-climbing walls and a 5-foot trampoline on the floor in the middle. There are two large game closets located in the smaller gym that contain board games, toys, gross-motor games, and fine-motor activities.

Jacob is quiet and reserved when he initially meets his OT, and does not make eye contact. His parents are warm and friendly, though they appear overwhelmed and apprehensive about the OT process. When Jacob walks to the back gym, his eyes light up when he sees the gym equipment and games, and he runs to the scooter ramp (Figure 4-2). The therapist instructs Jacob to dismount the scooter ramp and ushers Jacob and his parents into a small treatment room. The OT guides Jacob's parents through an unstructured interview for the first 15 minutes of the session to identify their concerns and reasons for seeking an OT evaluation. Jacob plays with the toys in the small treatment room while his parents talk to the therapist.

Occupational Profile

Birth History

Jacob was born full-term at 38 weeks gestation via vaginal delivery, weighing 7 pounds, 6 ounces. There were no complications during pregnancy or delivery, and Jacob spent no time in the neonatal nursery after delivery.

Developmental History

Jacob experienced early sleeping difficulties; he did not sleep through the night until he was 8 months old. He currently sleeps through the night and goes to sleep with ease. Jacob achieved most gross-motor milestones within typical age ranges but walked on the late side at age 16 months. Jacob has been receiving speech therapy since age 3 for concerns related to receptive and expressive language.

Medical History

No significant medical history was reported by the parents or physician. Jacob is allergic to eggs and is on an egg-free diet.

Hearing and Vision

Jacob had a formal hearing test at birth yielding normal results. No vision concerns are reported by the parents or physician.

Family Dynamic and History

Jacob lives at home with both of his parents, his older sister, Mia, age 6 years, and younger sister, Emma, age 2 years. There is no significant family medical history, but there is a history of attention deficit hyperactivity disorder and learning disability within the family. Jacob's parents describe him as quiet and clingy.

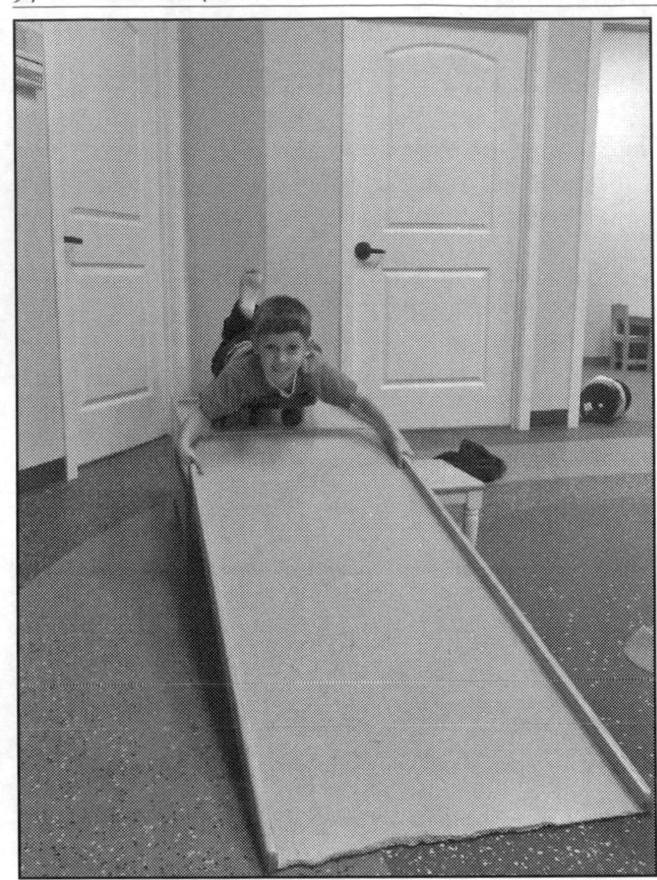

Figure 4-2. Jacob on the scooter ramp.

Educational and Extracurricular History

Jacob attends a half-day private preschool 4 days a week. Jacob's teacher has identified concerns with Jacob's ability to follow verbal directions and indicated that he frequently misses verbal directions. Jacob's teacher also noted that he has difficulty attending in the classroom and does not stay with one activity for more than 1 to 2 minutes. Jacob's teacher is also concerned with his difficulty sitting still on the carpet during circle time and the increased movement he exhibits throughout the day. Jacob also holds his hands over his ears when he enters the washroom at school. Outside of school, Jacob participates in swimming and soccer. At home, Jacob enjoys playing with trains and dinosaurs and loves listening to music. He loves going to the park to swing, climb, and go on the slide. Jacob prefers not to play with puzzles or color.

Current Functional Concerns

Jacob's parents are concerned with his hypersensitivities to sounds and touch and his lack of independence with self-care tasks, such as getting dressed. Per parent report, Jacob independently uses utensils during mealtime, is toilet trained, and has appropriate social skills. Jacob's speech language pathologist is concerned with Jacob's decreased attention, difficulty remaining seated during tabletop work, and decreased ability to follow multistep directions. These difficulties are impacting Jacob's ability to make progress in speech therapy.

Analysis of Occupational Performance

The following assessment tools were used during the evaluation:

- Sensory Profile
- Peabody Developmental Motor Scales, Second Edition (PDMS-2)
- Clinical Observations: Clinical observations were made in the areas of gross- and fine-motor skills, eye and hand usage, primitive and postural reflexes, and response to sensory stimuli, all of which affect learning, behavior and motor control.

Sensory Profile

The Sensory Profile is a judgment-based caregiver questionnaire used to measure a child's sensory processing abilities and their effect on daily performance. Scores are reported as follows: Typical Performance (corresponds to scores at or above 1 standard deviation below the mean), Probable Difference (corresponds to scores between 1 and 2 standard deviations below the mean), and Definite Difference (corresponds to scores more than 2 standard deviations below the mean) when compared with typically developing children (Dunn, 1999).

The Section Summary of the Sensory Profile provides information on Jacob's sensory processing, modulation and behavior/emotional response abilities (Table 4-2).

Jacob scored in the "Probable Difference" category for Vestibular Processing on the Sensory Profile. Clinical observations and parent report indicate that Jacob exhibits decreased vestibular/proprioceptive processing. Per parent report, Jacob frequently seeks all kinds of movement activities, twirls/spins himself frequently throughout the day, and is "on the go." During the evaluation, he moved quickly throughout the room, particularly seeking physical activities that provided vestibular input, such as jumping on the trampoline and swinging on various swings. These behaviors are correlated with inefficient processing of vestibular/proprioceptive input.

Jacob scored in the "Typical Performance" category for Touch Processing. Per parent report, Jacob never becomes irritated by socks or shoes and does not react emotionally to touch. However, Jacob's parents report that he does become irritated by certain fabrics at times.

Jacob scored in the "Typical Performance" category for Visual Processing on the Sensory Profile. However, this is an area in which he displays difficulty. Jacob had difficulty visually attending to activities due to his inability to filter out the unimportant visual stimuli around him in

TABLE 4-2

JACOB'S SENSORY PROFILE

SENSORY PROCESSING	***Typical Performance***	***Probable Difference***	***Definite Difference***
Auditory Processing	☐	☐	☒
Visual Processing	☒	☐	☐
Vestibular Processing	☐	☒	☐
Touch Processing	☒	☐	☐
Multi-Sensory Processing	☐	☒	☐
Oral Processing	☒	☐	☐
MODULATION			
Sensory Processing Related to Endurance/Tone	☐	☐	☒
Modulation Related to Body Position and Movement	☒	☐	☐
Modulation of Movement Affecting Activity Level	☒	☐	☐
Modulation of Sensory Input Affecting Emotional Responses	☐	☒	☐
Modulation of Visual Input Affecting Emotional Responses and Activity Level	☒	☐	☐
BEHAVIOR AND EMOTIONAL RESPONSES			
Emotional/Social Responses	☐	☒	☐
Behavior Outcomes of Sensory Processing	☐	☐	☒
Items Indicating Thresholds of Responses	☐	☒	☐

FACTOR SUMMARY

Factor	***Typical Performance***	***Probable Difference***	***Definite Difference***
Sensory Seeking	☐	☐	☒
Emotionally Reactive	☒	☐	☐
Low Endurance/Tone	☐	☒	☐
Oral Sensory Sensitivity	☒	☐	☐
Inattention/Distractibility	☐	☐	☒
Poor Registration	☒	☐	☐
Sensory Sensitivity	☒	☐	☐
Sedentary	☒	☐	☐
Fine Motor/Perceptual	☐	☐	☒

order to focus his attention on the important visual stimuli in front of him. His difficulty filtering out unimportant visual stimuli increased his distractibility in the gym environment.

Jacob scored in the "Definite Difference" category for Auditory Processing on the Sensory Profile. Per parent report, Jacob frequently responds negatively to unexpected or loud noises, holds his hands over his ears to protect them from sound, and has trouble completing tasks when the radio is on.

According to the Sensory Profile, Jacob obtained scores that indicate typical abilities to modulate certain sensory experiences, while scoring within the "Definite Difference" range for other modulation abilities. Jacob scored in the "Typical Performance" category for Modulation Related to Body Position and Movement, Modulation of Movement Affecting Activity Level, and Modulation of Sensory Input

Table 4-3

Jacob's Performance on the PDMS-2

SUBTEST	RAW SCORE	PERCENTILE	STANDARD SCORE
Object Manipulation	34	16th	7
*Grasping	47	25th	8
Visual-Motor Integration	118	16th	7
Fine Motor Quotient: 85	Fine Motor Percentile Rank: 16th		

**It needs to be noted that there are no items on this particular subtest between the 16 mo. and 42 mo. age range, which can inaccurately reflect in what appears to be a lower grasping subtest score.*

Affecting Emotional Responses. In these areas, Jacob is able to organize sensory input to create an appropriate adaptive response.

However, Jacob demonstrates difficulty with sensory modulation in the following areas: Modulation of Sensory Input Affecting Emotional Responses, Sensory Processing Related to Endurance/Tone, Emotional/Social Responses and Behavioral Outcomes of Sensory Processing. Per parent report, Jacob frequently has difficulty tolerating changes in plans and expectations and has difficulty with transitions.

Peabody Developmental Motor Skills-2

The PDMS-2 is a standardized, reliable, and valid norm-referenced assessment of fine- and gross-motor skills (Folio & Fewell, 2000). Results on the PDMS-2 are shown in Table 4-3.

Performance on the PDMS-2 is described by classifications of very superior, superior, above average, average, below average, poor, or very poor. Jacob scored in the *below average* range on the Object Manipulation subtest, in the low end of the *average* range on the Grasping subtest, and in the *below average* range on the Visual-Motor Integration subtest.

Clinical Observations

During the evaluation, Jacob engaged well with the therapist and was inquisitive throughout the session. Jacob had difficulty maintaining attention to therapist-directed tasks, requiring frequent verbal redirections to stay on task and complete items asked of him due to increased distractibility in the clinic gym environment. A picture schedule and reinforcement system was implemented to help Jacob remain on task. Jacob was noted to have difficulty maintaining eye contact with the evaluator.

Jacob's performance in several clinical observation tasks indicates impaired vestibular and proprioceptive processing. For example, he demonstrates difficulty maintaining single leg balance, doing so for approximately 2 to 3 seconds on each foot. A child Jacob's age is expected to balance on one foot for at least 6 seconds. During tests of antigravity positioning, Jacob had difficulty sustaining a prone extension position (lying on his belly with arms and legs extended off the ground), doing so for 9 seconds. A child Jacob's age is expected to sustain the prone extension position for 18 seconds. Additionally, Jacob had difficulty sustaining the supine flexion position (lying on his back with arms crossed over chest, legs curled into abdomen, and head lifted off ground), doing so for 6 seconds. A child Jacob's age is expected to sustain the supine flexion position for 10 seconds (Blanche, 2002).

During the evaluation, Jacob was frequently observed to walk on his toes. This observation is indicative of decreased proprioceptive processing. The increased pressure that is provided to the joints and calf muscles as a result of the toe walking may be in effort to provide him with additional sensory input that assists him to be more organized and maintain a "just right" arousal level.

Jacob also demonstrated difficulty motor planning gross- and fine-motor tasks. He had difficulty motor planning for activities when given verbal instructions, using scissors, and completing block designs. Jacob's decreased fine-motor planning has contributed to his difficulty with fine-motor tasks, such as manipulating zippers. Jacob's motor planning difficulty is complicated by decreased body awareness, decreased muscle tone, and postural control.

Jacob demonstrates an immature grasping pattern during writing activities. At times, Jacob was observed to use a dynamic tripod grasp, which is expected for a 4-year-old child. However, Jacob was also observed using a static tripod grasp, which is an appropriate grasp used by a child age 3.5 years. Jacob's tendency to alternate between grasp patterns is likely compensation for decreased hand strength and endurance.

Impressions

Jacob demonstrates age-appropriate tactile processing, oral sensory processing, and grasping patterns for fine-motor manipulation. Jacob presents with decreased sensory processing in the areas of vestibular, proprioceptive, auditory, and visual processing, as well as sensory modulation.

Jacob's difficulty with processing vestibular and proprioceptive information is impacting his behavior, attention, self-regulation, and participation in activities across environments. Because Jacob displays symptoms of reduced vestibular and proprioceptive processing, it is likely that much of the sensory seeking behavior he displays may be an effort to provide him with the additional sensory input that helps him to be more organized.

Additionally, Jacob's difficulty filtering out unimportant auditory and visual information in his environment while attending to what is important is impacting his ability to complete age-appropriate tasks. Jacob's difficulty organizing sensory input to create appropriate responses means that he may have difficulties responding appropriately to social and environmental cues, becoming inflexible or upset by situations more easily than others. These difficulties with modulation may be related to confusing information from the sensory systems, leading Jacob to feel a sense of disruption with what is going on around him. This can impact Jacob's self-regulation, self-esteem, ability to sustain attention and focus in more stimulating environments, social interaction with peers, and appropriate response to directions.

Jacob also presents with decreased gross-motor and fine-motor planning, pencil grasp, balance, postural control, low muscle tone, and attention. Jacob's decreased ability to maintain single-leg balance is associated with decreased body awareness and position in space, indicating poor vestibular and proprioceptive processing skills. Jacob's difficulty with motor planning can impact completion of age-appropriate fine- and gross-motor tasks, self-help skills such as independent dressing, and academic learning.

Overall, it appears that Jacob's nervous system is not processing sensory information efficiently, resulting in confusing information from the nervous system, difficulty attending to task, frustration and poor emotional regulation, decreased postural control, and poor motor planning. All of this is negatively affecting his participation and performance in activities throughout the day.

Recommendations

Based on review of the assessments, clinical observations, and the interview with Jacob's parents, it is recommended that Jacob receive OT services twice per week for 6 months, at which point a reevaluation would occur to assess progress and create new goals. The treatment sessions will address the areas of neuroprocessing, specifically vestibular, proprioceptive, visual, and auditory processing, and sensory modulation; body awareness; decreased muscle tone; motor planning; gross-motor and fine-motor skills; and attention. It is recommended that a school visit be completed to provide suggestions and modifications in the classroom for optimal performance. A home exercise program of activities is recommended to encourage continued progress outside of clinical therapy.

Goal Areas

- Improve vestibular and proprioceptive processing for improved body awareness, postural control, bilateral coordination, and muscle tone.
- Improve fine- and gross-motor planning skills to support effective completion of age-appropriate tasks.
- Improve visual and auditory processing to support effective completion of age-appropriate tasks.
- Reduce sensory hypersensitivities, specifically light touch, for increased participation in age-appropriate activities.

Parents' Response to Occupational Therapy Assessment

Following the completion of the OT assessment, the therapist provided a written report to Jacob's parents and set up a meeting to review the results and therapist's recommendations. During this meeting, it becomes apparent that Jacob's parents are indeed overwhelmed with Jacob's behaviors and difficulties and are very defensive regarding these issues. They are frustrated that Jacob is having difficulty in school and indicated that they do not share the same concerns related to attention as the teacher and Jacob's speech language pathologist. The therapist provided initial education around sensory processing disorder and the process of OT.

Questions to Consider

1. Discuss how Jacob's sensory processing difficulties influence his occupational performance.
2. Which OT intervention approaches from the *Occupational Therapy Practice Framework: Domain and Process,* 2nd edition (AOTA, 2014) will the OT use to address Jacob's needs?
3. What are some strengths that Jacob will bring to the treatment process? What strengths do Jacob's parents bring to the treatment process?
4. Based on Jacob's goal areas, write short-term goals for Jacob for the next 4 weeks.
5. Describe a 60-minute, clinic-based OT intervention session for Jacob. Be specific about how you would organize the clinic space, the types of equipment that you would make available, as well as any games or activities that you would introduce to Jacob.

6. What are some strategies that Jacob's parents could put into place at home to promote his occupational performance?
7. The OT would like to recommend that Jacob's parents schedule an appointment with the neuropsychologist so that further testing can be completed to identify Jacob's areas of strength and weakness related to his cognitive functioning. However, the therapist also realizes that the parents are extremely overwhelmed and may not be receptive to hearing that their child requires more testing at this time. The therapist struggles with when the referral to the neuropsychologist is most appropriate: immediately so that the therapy team can continue working toward Jacob's success or in a few weeks when the therapist has built more rapport with the parents and earns their trust. Select one option and describe why you think it is the most appropriate.
8. Imagine that the OT has the opportunity to design a treatment session for Jacob with another child on the OT caseload. What might be the focus of this treatment session?

References

American Occupational Therapy Association. (2014). Occupational therapy practice framework: Domain and process (3rd ed.). *American Journal of Occupational Therapy, 68*(S1), S1-S48.

Blanche, E. I. (2002). *Observations based on sensory integration theory.* Torrance, CA: Pediatric Therapy Network.

Dunn, W. (1999). *Sensory profile: User's manual.* San Antonio, TX: Psychological Corporation.

Folio, M., & Fewell, R. (2000). *Examiner's manual: Peabody Developmental Motor Scales (2nd ed.).* Austin, TX: Pro-Ed.

Resource

Bundy, A., Lane, S., & Murray, E. (2002). *Sensory integration: Theory and practice* (2nd ed.). Philadelphia: F.A. Davis Co.

Brad: Brain Tumor/ Outpatient

Kendall Carithers, OTR and
Lauro A. Munoz, OTR, MOT, CHC

History and Background Information

Acute Care History

Brad, age 3.5 years, was developing typically until 2 months ago, when his parents noticed a decreased activity level and vomiting. A computed tomography scan of the brain was performed, and he was found to have a right thalamic brain tumor extending into the right lateral ventricle and crossing midline with obstructive hydrocephalus. After having a seizure episode and neurological decompensation, he underwent an emergent partial resection of the tumor. Brad was transferred to a comprehensive cancer center 1200 miles away, where he was diagnosed with grade 4 glioblastoma multiforme (a type of malignant brain tumor) and underwent re-resection of the tumor. Postoperatively, he required multiple shunt placements and shunt revisions. The neuro-ophthalmologist's test were inconclusive due to difficulty with the exam, but suggested that Brad likely has dense homonymous hemianopia. Brad was seen by the pediatric OT and PT very few times during his month-long hospital stay due to medical complications and refusal.

Outpatient Rehabilitation

Brad was discharged from the hospital 1 week ago with orders to begin daily outpatient radiation therapy treatments. He was also referred to outpatient OT and PT services for impaired mobility and weakness of the left upper and lower extremity. The evaluation will take place in the outpatient gym (Figure 4-3). During your chart review, you read in numerous doctor's notes that Brad has been crying and uncooperative during visits. The outpatient PT tells you that Brad cried throughout her evaluation, and she was unable to collect much information.

Evaluation Information

1. What will you do to prepare yourself for your evaluation with Brad and his family? Is there any additional information that would be helpful prior to the evaluation?
2. What areas of occupation are developmentally appropriate for a child Brad's age to complete?
3. What theories and frames of reference will be most helpful to guide your thinking about this client?
4. What information is most important to gather during the initial evaluation?
5. How will you collect information about Brad? Which formal assessments, if any, do you feel will be appropriate to use during the initial evaluation?
6. The outpatient gym where you will evaluate Brad is set up primarily for adults, as they represent the majority of the therapists' caseload. What will you add or change to the environment to help Brad feel more comfortable in this medical setting (see Figure 4-3)?
7. What types of equipment or toys will you use during your evaluation?
8. What information can you gather from the photograph of Brad in the waiting room (Figure 4-4)?

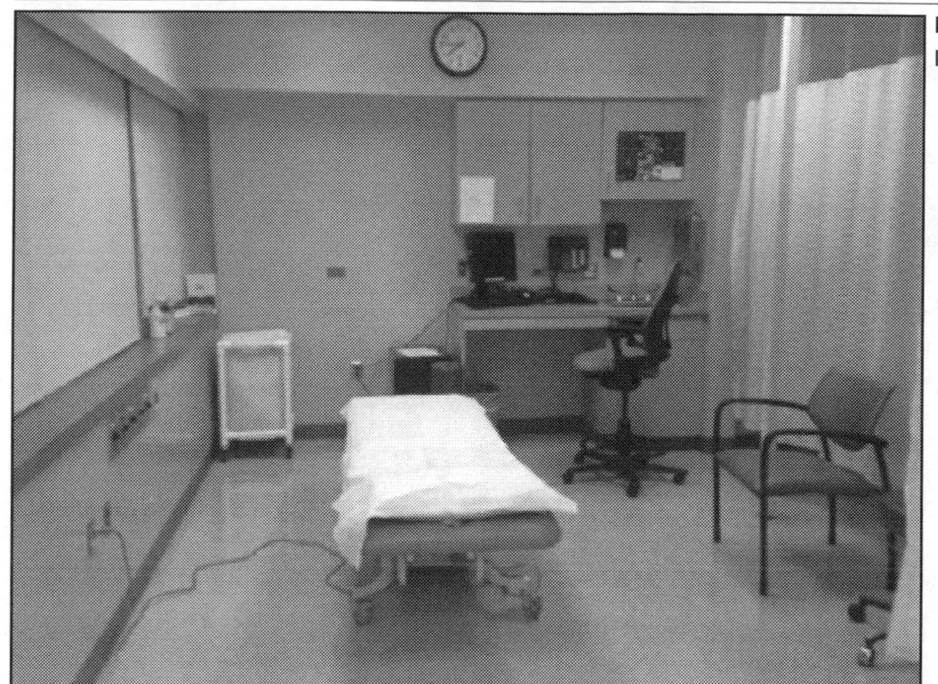

Figure 4-3. Examining room in an outpatient gym.

Occupational Profile

Brad, his mother, and his father arrive for the initial evaluation. Brad is seated in a stroller, interacting with his parents and eating a snack. In the waiting room, the OT attempts to engage Brad in conversation. Brad answers a quick "no" to all questions asked of him. The therapist continues to make attempts to engage Brad while he is seated in the stroller. Brad is not interested in answering any questions or engaging in conversation and starts to cry when spoken to. A parent interview is completed to gather an occupational profile. Brad, his parents, and two older sisters (ages 7 and 9 years) have been staying in a local apartment. His father and sisters will be returning home next week and Brad will stay with his mother during the 5 remaining weeks of radiation treatment. Brad's parents report he enjoys watching Mickey Mouse videos and playing with blocks and balls, but he is currently engaging in very little play. They report that 2 months prior, Brad was very independent and active. He was attending daycare while his parents worked and was completing typical activities of daily living for his age. At the local apartment, he interacts with his sisters, but at all times, Brad is either seated in the stroller, limiting most movements, or lying on his back. Brad's sisters or parents bring what he needs to him. Brad calms down during the parent interview after being presented with a variety of toys but cries during all movement and transition. When asked, Brad verbalizes that he is scared of falling.

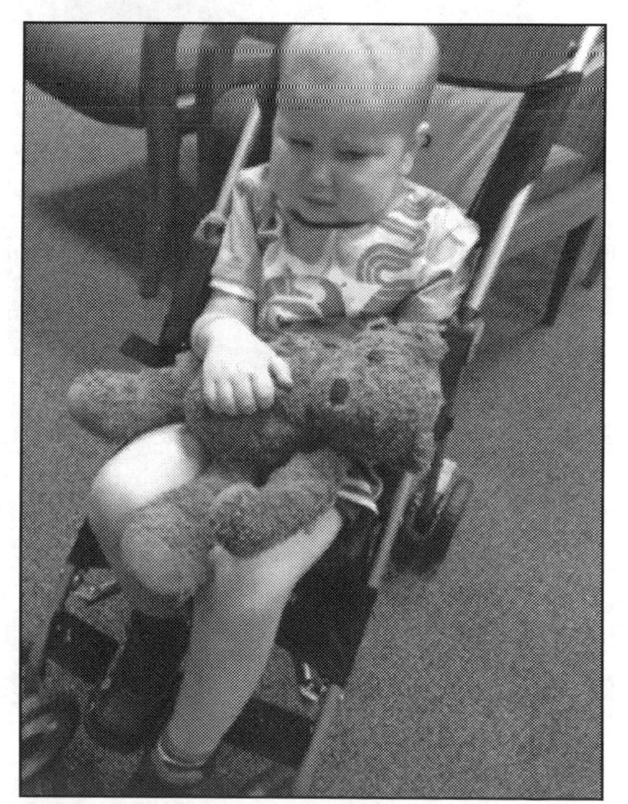

Figure 4-4. Brad in the waiting room.

Since his initial surgery, Brad has flaccid left hemiplegia. He has kyphotic posture and decreased trunk control when taken out of the stroller. He has pain with proximal left shoulder palpation and in the wrist with passive stretch, as he has developed tightness in the wrist and digits. Brad sits upright with moderate physical assistance and facilitation for approximately 30 seconds at a time. He stands with maximal physical assistance for 5 seconds. Brad's parents

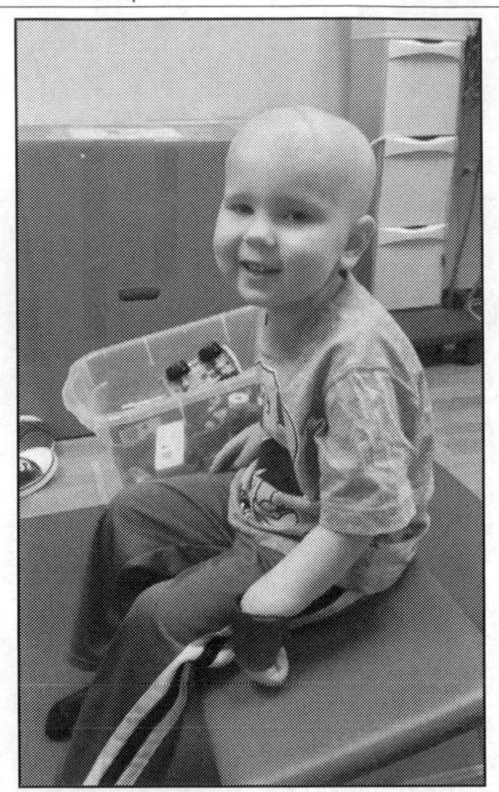

Figure 4-5. Brad during a treatment session.

report that initially after the surgery, he had significant speech impairments; however, his speech is much improved and he is able to communicate his wants and needs to his parents. Brad is able to identify three colors. He looks toward his right side throughout the evaluation, with limited scanning to the left side.

Brad currently has limited interaction with his environment, thus compromising play exploration and participation. He feeds himself, using finger feeding with his right hand. Brad's parents assist him with toileting, upper and lower body dressing, bathing, and grooming tasks. He has a difficult time sleeping and is up many times throughout the night.

Brad's Parents' Goals for Rehabilitation

- His parents report their main goal is for Brad to walk again.
- They would also like to eliminate his pain and have Brad "return to his old playful self."

Emerging Issues

The day after OT evaluation, Brad is admitted to the ICU for monitoring due to a possible shunt malfunction with symptoms of vomiting and altered mental status. While admitted, he has an additional shunt revision surgery. He is scheduled to be discharged in 2 days. The PT approaches you and asks for your opinion on discharge recommendations for Brad. She believes that Brad should go to a nearby children's inpatient rehabilitation facility, where he can be transported back and forth to his radiation therapy each day.

1. What type of rehabilitation setting would you recommend for Brad after his discharge? Explain your reasoning.
2. If Brad were to transfer to the inpatient rehabilitation facility, how well do you think Brad will tolerate 1 hour each of occupational, physical and speech therapy every day in addition to daily radiation treatments?

Occupational Therapy Intervention and Discharge

1. List 3 possible activities to use during your first treatment session and explain how each will work toward Brad's goals.
2. What changes do you see in Brad (Figure 4-5) compared to the first impression photo (Figure 4-4)?

Progress Information

After 6 weeks, Brad is finished with radiation therapy and is returning home with his mom. He has been coming to outpatient OT three times each week on days when he does not see the PT. Brad has made significant functional improvements since the initial evaluation. With Dycem (Dycem Ltd), he now completes feeding using utensils. While he continues to require assistance for ADL, he has increased participation in all ADL. He participates in daily play activities with his mother in both supported and unsupported sitting.

Questions to Consider

Goal Areas and Treatment Focus

1. What are Brad's strengths?
2. Which client factors are limiting Brad's successful participation in age-appropriate activities?
3. How have Brad's routines and roles been affected by his recent diagnosis?
4. How could Brad's vision impact his participation? How will you address this?

5. How do you explain to Brad's parents (without jargon) homonymous hemianopia and the functional implications of this visual impairment?
6. Write a list of objective, measurable goals with a time frame.
7. What obstacles might make it difficult for Brad to reach these goals?
8. In this clinic, clients are seen for 1 hour at a time. Brad's insurance has approved 90 visits combined for OT, PT, and speech therapy for the year. How often will you recommend that Brad be seen for outpatient OT? Explain your reasoning.
9. Which OT intervention approach(es) will be most beneficial to use with Brad?
10. Does Brad's prognosis impact your approach/priorities? If so, how?
11. What ideas do you have to increase Brad's engagement during OT treatment sessions? During home activities?
12. How will you establish Brad's trust and maintain rapport while encouraging him to meet therapy goals? How will you grade activities for Brad?
13. How will you incorporate Brad's family into treatment sessions?
14. What types of adaptive equipment will facilitate increased independence during activities of daily living and play?
15. What do you think is causing Brad's left shoulder pain? What are ways to alleviate this pain?

Planning for Discharge

1. What services do you recommend for Brad upon arrival home?
2. Describe the home program you will recommend to Brad and his parents.

Resources

Dudgeon, B., & Crooks, L. (2010). Hospital and rehabilitation services. In J. Case-Smith & J. O'Brien (Eds.), *Occupational therapy for children* (6th ed.). (pp. 785-811). St. Louis: Elsevier.

Longpre, S., & Newman, R. (2011). AOTA Fact sheet: The role of occupational therapy in oncology. Retrieved from: http://www.aota.org/~/media/Corporate/Files/AboutOT/Professionals/WhatIsOT/RDP/Facts/Oncology%20fact%20sheet.ashx

Nadir: Motor Disorder/ Outpatient Rehabilitation

Carly Thom, MA, OTR/L

History and Background Information

Nadir is a 6-year-old boy whose parents are seeking OT intervention in an outpatient setting. Nadir was diagnosed with a mitochondrial disorder at 6 months of age and presents with a severe motor disorder. Due to his condition, Nadir exhibits continuous uncontrolled movements in his arms, legs, head, and trunk. He also has significant reflux and recently underwent surgery for placement of a G-button in preparation for tube feedings. However, despite this, Nadir's parents refuse to use the G-tube for feeding and have continued to feed him orally.

Nadir's parents report that he was previously receiving home health services but they are now seeking services in the outpatient setting because they felt that the home health clinicians were not doing enough for their child. His parents also report that Nadir was evaluated by the school district for placement in the local school system; however, they have discontinued this process and report that they would rather keep him at home and focus on therapy right now.

Evaluation Information

Occupational Profile

Nadir is an only child living in an apartment with his mother and father. His father is employed outside the home and his mother does not work. His parents have only one vehicle and his mother does not drive. In addition to OT, Nadir is also being evaluated for speech therapy and PT services in the outpatient setting. Nadir's parents report that the speech therapy is not a priority for them and that their main goal is for Nadir to learn to walk.

Nadir arrived for his evaluation seated in a rolling car seat. The car seat has straps to support his trunk and his head extends over the top of the seat by approximately 6 inches. In addition, his feet nearly touch the ground. Nadir's parents report that this car seat was purchased about 3 years prior. They also report that Nadir has a Kimba customized seating system (Ottobock) at home that can be detached for use as a car seat; however, they feel that this is too cumbersome and prefer to use Nadir's old car seat for travel outside the home.

Client Factors/Body Functions

- Vision: Nadir is able to visually orient to music toys by turning his head/gaze toward them; however, he is unable to sustain this gaze due to lack of control over his motor movements.
- Neuromusculoskeletal and movement-related functions: When placed on the therapy mat, Nadir is unable to sit unsupported. He presents with spasticity in his lower extremities and posterior pelvic tilt, resulting in decreased tolerance for long sitting. When placed in supine, Nadir presents with an intact asymmetrical tonic neck reflex. His upper/lower extremities are in constant motion and he is unable to initiate rolling from supine to side lying. When placed in prone, Nadir is able to extend his head/neck against gravity briefly from 1 to 2 seconds at a time maximally. Nadir is also very thin—his humeral circumference measures only 3 inches. His skin color is far paler than that of his parents. Nadir's parents report that he has significant reflux and typically vomits three to four times per day. As a result, his teeth are decayed and several have been pulled. He drools continuously and does not speak, but vocalizes frequently and laughs in response to musical toys.
- Right/left upper extremity: He presents with full AROM/PROM in his upper extremities; however, because of his movement disorder, he is unable to execute voluntary movements.

Questions to Consider

Goals/Treatment Plan

1. Write out a problem list for Nadir.
2. What are Nadir's strengths? How can these be incorporated into his treatment plan?
3. What frame of reference will you use to approach treatment with Nadir? Why?
4. Write out a set of short-term goals for Nadir. What treatment modalities/approaches will you use to achieve these goals?
5. How will you address Nadir's parents' goal of him walking?
6. What obstacles to do see that might prevent Nadir from reaching his goals?

Safety Precautions

1. What safety precautions will you take during Nadir's treatment sessions?
2. Do you have any safety concerns for Nadir outside of the therapy clinic?
3. How will you address Nadir's feeding issues? How will you address his persistent reflux?

Equipment/Adaptations

1. What type of environmental adaptations or equipment recommendations would you make for Nadir? How will these address his goals/treatment plan?

Neuromotor

1. How will you approach treatment given Nadir's movement disorder?
2. How will you incorporate purposeful activity into your treatment plan?
3. Will positioning play a role in addressing Nadir's neuromotor functioning? If so, please explain why. How will you address this in Nadir's treatment plan?

Cognition/Perception

1. How will you incorporate cognitive/perceptual activities into Nadir's treatment? What functional activities would you use to address these areas?
2. How will you structure treatment to improve Nadir's visual attention?

Patient/Family Education

1. How will you approach educating Nadir's parents?
2. What do you feel are the primary areas in which Nadir's parents could benefit from parent education?
3. How will you work with other disciplines (PT, speech) on educating Nadir's parent with respect to safety and nutrition?

Situations

1. During a treatment session, you lay Nadir in a supine position and notice that he becomes agitated. He begins to vocalize more and makes facial grimaces. His parents become upset and ask that you sit him up. When you question them about whether or not Nadir is positioned supine at home they avoid the question and instead perseverate on the mats at the clinic being "too hard" and painful for Nadir. What do you do and why? How do you address Nadir's positioning in the home?
2. You discuss Nadir's feeding and potential malnutrition with his treating speech therapist. She is asking for your support in encouraging his parents to utilize tube feedings to supplement his oral intake. How do you go about approaching this issue with Nadir's parents?
3. You are recommending that Nadir utilize an alternative seating system in the car and while at home (as

he is being held most of the time). Nadir's parents are not convinced that alternative seating is necessary. How will you address this issue? What might you be able to do in your treatment sessions to illustrate your concerns?

4. How will you approach furthering Nadir's academic development? Do you feel that Nadir should be in school and receiving services through his local school district? If so, how will you communicate this to his parents?

Resource

Missiuna, C., Polatajko, H., Pollock, N., & Cameron, D. (2012). Neuromotor disorders. In S. Lane & A. Bundy (Eds.). *Kids can be kids: A childhood occupations approach*. Philadelphia: F.A. Davis Co.

Renee: CHARGE Syndrome/ Outpatient

Leon Washington, OTR, PhD, LMSW, C/NDT

History and Background

Renee, age 9 years, 8 months, was born at 31 weeks gestation. She has the primary diagnosis of CHARGE syndrome, which is a highly complex genetic condition. Renee has disturbances in communication, balance and mobility, and sensory processing deficits involving all senses (i.e., hearing, vision, smell, taste, touch, proprioception, and vestibular). In addition, Renee has multiple premature and congenital anomalies, including esophageal atresia and transesophageal fistula; ventricular septal defect; chronic lung disease; gastroesophageal reflux disease; absence of left fibula; left club deformity; dysphagia; colobomas of the optic disc, surrounding the optic nerve and involving the macula in both eyes, resulting in large scotomas, myopia, and microphthalmia; subacute bacterial endocarditis; and a gastrostomy. Renee has both hearing and visual impairment. At birth, her left leg had an absent patella, hypoplastic tibia, absent fibula to palpation, and equinovarus deformity. As a result, Renee had a left above-knee amputation prior to discharge from the hospital.

In the past, Renee has lived with several family members including her father, mother, and paternal grandmother. She currently resides with her father (who has primary custody) and they both live with his mother. Renee visits her biological mother only periodically but not consistently (once or twice yearly). Renee's father insists that she receives every opportunity in school and therapy so that she can be as independent as possible.

Renee attends a school for children with special needs and is in special education. She has an IEP based on the following disabilities categories: Deaf/Blind, Vision Impairment, Intellectual Disability, Speech Impairment, and Other Health Impairment (CHARGE syndrome). At school, Renee is followed by the special education teacher and behavior specialist, and is on a behavior intervention plan, has adapted physical education, and also has been evaluated by and had services recommended by a certified orientation and mobility specialist.

Evaluation Information

Occupational Profile

Renee was evaluated in her home. Her father and nurse were present during this evaluation. Renee was very resistant and uncooperative initially (i.e., crying and hitting out). She has no deficits in physical development in both upper extremities. She has both hearing and vision deficits and has glasses and bilateral hearing aids, which she does not wear.

Renee was not cognitively able to participate in standardized tests. The information received for the OT evaluation was through clinical observation and reports from the father and/or nurse. Renee has significant delays in all areas to include activities of daily living skills, fine-motor, bilateral hand skills, cognitive, visual-motor, visual-perception, and sensorimotor skills. Renee has a right hand preference. She enjoys scribbling with a crayon and/or marker and has an emerging ability to imitate vertical, horizontal, and circular strokes on paper; however, her attempts were very poor. Renee was also unable to cut on a half-inch line with scissors and not able to properly position the scissors in her hand. Cognitively, Renee was able to match some colors and simple shapes. She needed hand-over-hand assistance to put together a simple 2-, 4-, 6-, or 8-piece puzzle with lots of verbal cues and physical prompts (Figure 4-6). Additionally, due to visual deficits as well as visual-perceptual problems, she had difficulty distinguishing between red and orange as well as blue and green when engaged in activities requiring matching colors.

Areas of Occupation

Dressing

During the ADL portion of the evaluation, Renee had difficulty with dressing and is especially challenged with fasteners such as buttons, zippers (including catch), and tying her shoes. She will assist with all dressing such as donning and doffing a pullover shirt and pants as well as socks and shoes (Figure 4-7). She often needs demonstration and periodic hand-over-hand assistance with dressing activities. Renee wears an above-the-knee prosthesis for

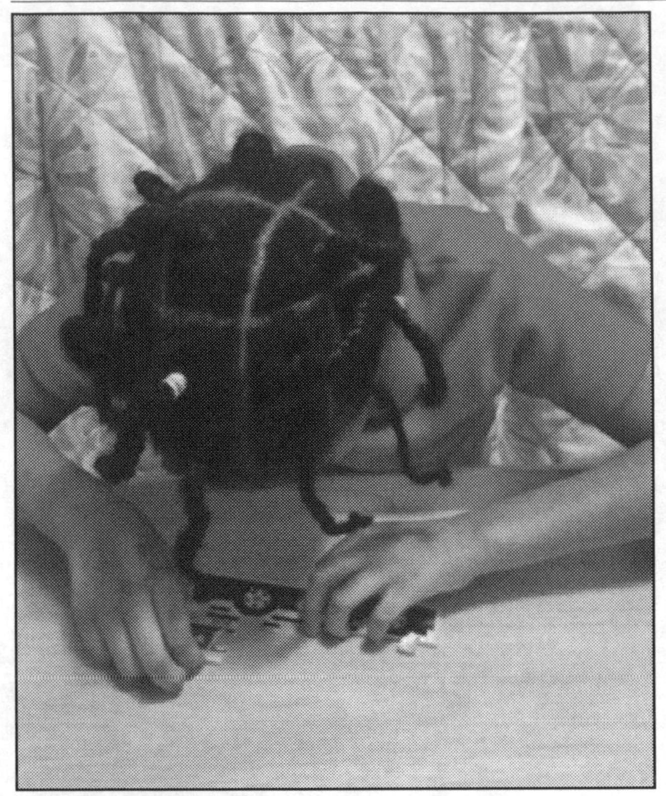

Figure 4-6. Renee requires assistance to complete a puzzle.

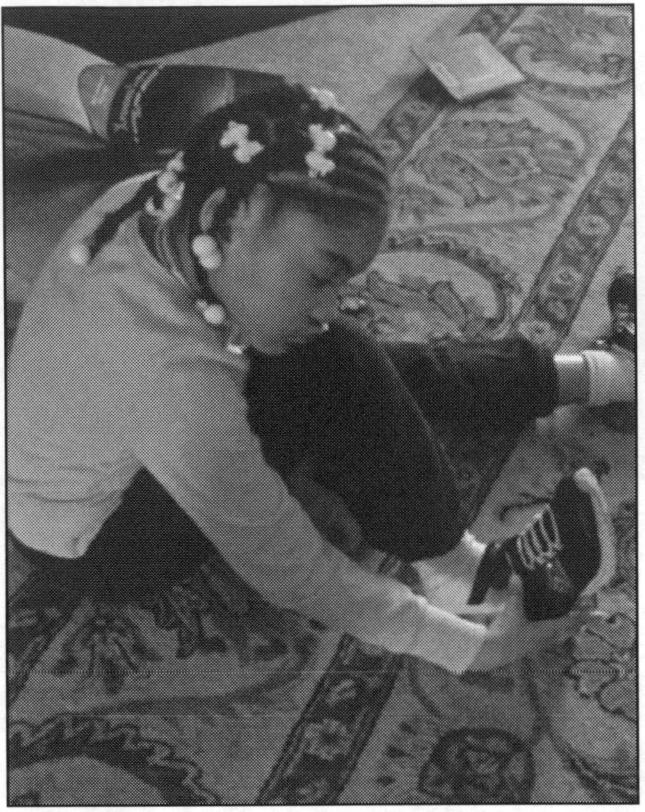

Figure 4-7. Renee assists with dressing.

the left lower extremity. She is able to don and doff her prosthetic leg but often needs help.

Feeding

Renee passed a swallow study and has been cleared to start eating. Renee eats mostly soft textured foods, often refuses to eat any foods with mixed textures, and does not chew but swallows small chunks of food. Renee is able to use a spoon or fork fairly adequately to feed herself, but prefers others to feed her.

Performance Skills

- Emotional regulation and safety: Behaviorally, Renee exhibits hyperactivity, poor attention span, poor safety awareness, poor judgment, and aggressive behavior toward other children and adults. For example: Renee hits out at others or bites her hands extremely hard and sometimes repetitiously when she gets overly excited or becomes frustrated or agitated. These behaviors are particularly noted when she encounters difficult tasks or when others do not comply with her request(s) for help. Regarding safety, Renee must be watched very closely. Some examples of safety issues include opening and walking out the door in an attempt to leave the surrounding area. Also, when Renee gets very excited or agitated, she becomes extremely rough (especially noted with children, adults, or animals).
- Sensory-processing: Renee has multisensory deficits involving all areas including hearing, vision, taste, tactile, smell, proprioceptive and vestibular. She exhibits little or no neurological responses following rotary vestibular stimulation as evidenced by post-rotary nystagmus (vestibulo-ocular reflex) in sitting or side-lying position (Figure 4-8). Renee enjoys a variety of vigorous movement in space.

Renee receives OT in her home twice weekly (45 minutes to 1 hour). She also receives speech therapy and has a full-time nurse after school and on most weekends. The father's main goals for Renee are for her to be self-sufficient and independent in all areas.

Questions to Consider

Goals/Treatment Plan

1. Write out a problem list for Renee.
2. What do you see as Renee's strengths that the therapist can capitalize on during the treatment planning process?
3. Given the father's expectations and what you know about Renee, give at least four long-term goals.
4. What short-term goals (at least six goals) would you set for Renee to help her reach the long-term goals?
5. Thinking about Contexts and Environments from the *Occupational Therapy Practice Framework*, discuss

supports and barriers to Renee's health and participation. Give examples.

6. Renee continues to make significant progress but is unable to successfully participate in standardized testing. Based on the information given about Renee's progress, what test(s) would you think she might be able to participate? Explain why you selected these tests.

Safety Precautions

1. Identify potential safety concerns other than the ones already mentioned that might occur that should be addressed and shared with the caregivers.
2. Describe in detail how you would relate/address these same safety concerns with Renee.
3. What environmental modifications would you do to address these safety concerns?
4. What specific things would you do to help Renee become more adaptable and practice safety in the areas you mentioned in the previous question?
5. Discuss how you would know that each safety concern is no longer a problem.

Intervention Plan

1. Describe a treatment session with Renee, focusing on putting on a pull-on shirt in the correct orientation (front and back).
2. Renee gets easily frustrated during dressing activities, particularly with button and zippers. What strategies would you use to facilitate the skills needed to be independent with fasteners?
3. How would you address Renee's problem with not chewing her food? Give at least three specific therapeutic strategies you might use to decrease her oral aversion to foods with various textures.
4. Thinking about the previous question, explain how you would coordinate carry-over of a home program with the family, speech-language pathologist, and nurses in this process.
5. Renee is starting to assist with very simple chores at home such as putting her clothes in a hamper or dishes in the sink (only when directed). Write out a step-by-step instruction chart of morning and after school routines for Renee. Describe in detail.

Equipment/Adaptations

1. Given what you know about Renee's history and clinical picture, what (if any) environmental modifications or equipment would you make or recommend? Your explanation must be different from question #3 in the Safety Precautions section.

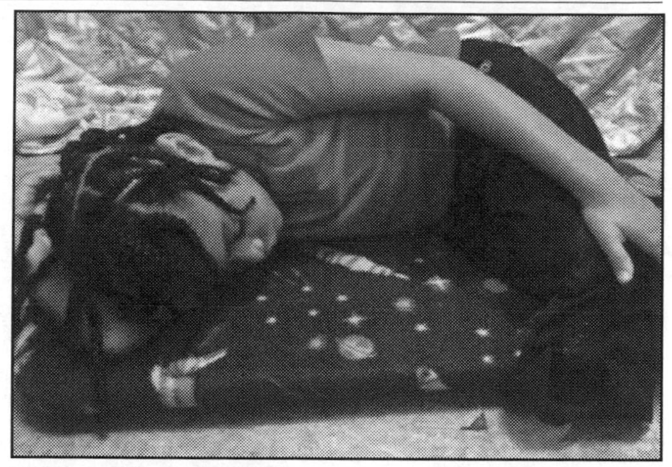

Figure 4-8. Renee in side-lying after vestibular input.

Sensorimotor

1. Renee often has unexpected falls and/or bruises as a result of constantly running and/or bumping into things. What activities might you recommend that will assist her with motor planning and coordination so that she can better understand and integrate where her body is in space?

Cognitive/Visual-Motor/Visual-Perception

1. As an OT, what types of things would you do to address Renee's cognitive deficits? In terms of role delineation and strategy intervention, how would you distinguish the difference between what you do and that of the speech-language pathologist? How would you explain this to the family?
2. What functional activities (other than the ones mentioned earlier) would you recommend to treat Renee's visual-motor and visual-perceptual deficits? Please address visual-motor activities and visual-perception activities separately.

Psychosocial

1. What behavioral issues might Renee exhibit when other children shun or do not want to be around her? Give at least two examples of each issue you identify.
2. How will you support Renee psychologically to help her adapt to others reacting negatively to her?

Neuromuscular (Fine-Motor/Bilateral Hand Coordination)

1. Renee often brings simple projects home that she has made from school that require using crayons and/

or scissors. What types of fine-motor preparation (or activities) might you do to enhance the quality of her work on these tasks?

2. What play activities can be done to enhance Renee's fine-motor and bilateral hand speed and dexterity that would make her more efficient at home and school?

Patient/Family Education

1. Would you include Renee's mother in any of the patient/family education? If not, justify your answer. If you did include the mother (given the fact that the mother rarely sees Renee), in what areas would you educate the mother?
2. How would you include the grandmother in patient/family education?
3. There are differences in opinion on how to address Renee's behavior. How would you work with the caregivers (i.e., father, grandmother, nurses, speech-language pathologist) to address these behaviors with Renee?
4. How would you relate these same behavioral concerns to school personnel?

Situations

1. You arrive at the house after school to work with Renee but she has already removed her prosthesis and clothing thinking the day is over. When she sees you, she absolutely loses it (screaming, crying, banging her head, and hitting out). What do you do? Why did you take this approach? What would you do next if this approach does not work?
2. Renee just got home from school and wants to eat. You assist her while she is sitting at the table eating from a bowl using a spoon. She puts the spoon down and starts to eat with her fingers, chew on inedible objects, such as the edge of the bowl or the table (as she typically does). You attempt to redirect her but she becomes agitated immediately, refuses to continue eating, gets up from the table, and walks away. What steps would you take to encourage her to come back to the table?
3. You have worked very diligently on assisting Renee to feed herself independently. You arrive at the home for therapy and see the nurse feeding Renee. You have repeatedly informed the nurse that the goal is to encourage Renee to be as independent as possible. The nurse agrees but continues to feed Renee when you are not present. When confronted, the nurse explains she wanted to prevent Renee from acting out and it was easier and quicker to do it for her. What would you say to the nurse? What steps would you take to prevent this from happening continuously?
4. Renee's family is very supportive of OT. In fact, Renee rarely misses an appointment (95% attendance). Unfortunately, family members are almost never around when Renee gets home from school or during therapy. Also, once the nurse arrives, the family member(s) leave almost immediately. They may observe therapy two or three times a year (even when encouraged weekly). How would you address this? How would you help the family member(s) to take ownership (or partnership) in Renee's therapy? What steps would you take to accomplish this? Who else would you include in this process? Why? How would you do this?

Planning for Discharge

1. Renee is 9 years old and has made great strides. Unfortunately, she is significantly delayed in all areas. At what point would you feel she is ready to be discharged from OT? How would you justify this knowing that she continues to make progress?
2. The father and other family members are disappointed that Renee is being discharged and do not understand why, given the fact that she continues to make progress in therapy. What do you tell them?
3. If you discharged Renee from OT, would you recommend a reevaluation at a later date? If so, why? If not, why?
4. What would you include in a home program for Renee prior to discharge?

Resources

American Occupational Therapy Association. (2014). Occupational therapy practice framework: Domain and process (3rd ed.). *American Journal of Occupational Therapy, 68*(S1), S1-S48.

CHARGE Syndrome Organization. Retrieved Jaunary 25, 2013 from http://www.chargesyndrome.org/

Hartshome, T., Hefner, M., Davenport, S., & Thelin, J. (2010). CHARGE syndrome. San Diego, CA: Plural Publishing.

Shepherd, J. (2010). Activities of daily living. In J. Case-Smith & J. O'Brien (Eds.), *Occupational therapy for children* (6th ed.) (pp. 474-517). St. Louis: Elsevier.

Finn: Autism Spectrum Disorder and Feeding Concerns

Kristin Winston, PhD, OTR/L

History and Background

Finn, age 3 years, was born at 34 weeks gestation with a birth weight of 4 pounds, 10 ounces. He was hospitalized in the NICU for 6 weeks secondary to issues with respiratory function and feeding. Finn was on a continuous positive airway pressure machine for 1 week and was fed via nasogastric tube for 5 weeks in the NICU before transitioning off of the tube to oral feedings in his last week in the NICU. He was on oral feedings when he was discharged to home at age 40 weeks chronologically. Finn has had difficulty with feeding and eating since he was born and his family has struggled to meet his nutritional needs. At 18 months of age, in addition to complex feeding concerns, Finn was diagnosed with Autism Spectrum Disorder. Finn's medical team includes a primary care physician, gastroenterologist, and dietician.

Finn lives with his parents, Joe and Maura, and his 1-year-old sister, Grace. Prior to Finn's birth, Maura was an elementary school teacher but has been a stay-at-home mom since the kids were born. Joe is an architect and works fulltime in a nearby community.

Evaluation Information

Occupational Profile

Finn was referred to outpatient OT secondary to a recent transition from home-based early intervention services to school-based services in his preschool, where there is no OT with experience in the area of feeding and eating. His primary care physician referred for an OT evaluation and intervention. This outpatient center has both individual and group services for feeding and eating concerns.

Finn was accompanied to the evaluation by his mom, Maura, and his little sister, Grace. The interview with Finn's mom revealed that there were significant concerns regarding mealtimes and Finn's inability to eat what Maura described as age-appropriate foods for a 3-year-old. Maura stated that they feed Finn in a high chair with a tray in front of the TV, which typically has a video on that is familiar to Finn. The video is used for all meals and snacks because when they try a meal without it, Finn becomes easily distressed. Maura reports that Finn will gag and frequently vomit when new foods are prepared near him or placed in front of him. He also has difficulty when other people are eating foods that are not his preferred foods. Maura reports that Finn is also very sensitive to the smell of foods. She states that the family does not eat together and she and her husband would very much like to have family meals, especially as the kids get older. Reports from the dietician indicate that Finn is at the 10th percentile for weight and is below the 5th percentile for height compared to other boys his age.

Finn's Parents' Goals

As a part of the evaluation, Finn's parents were asked to complete the Canadian Occupational Performance Measure (Law et al., 2005) to document their concerns. Their occupational performance concerns were not eating together as a family (Performance Score 1, Importance 8, Satisfaction 1), Finn gagging and vomiting with the presentation of new foods (Performance 1, Importance 10, Satisfaction 1), and Finn's limited dietary intake and variety (Performance 1, Importance 10, Satisfaction 1).

Areas of Occupation

Finn currently receives most of his calorie intake from a pureed mixture of baby foods or yogurt, high-fat oils such as olive oil, and vitamins. This mixture is fed to Finn by his parents while he is distracted by the video. In general, Finn does not tolerate puree, so this distraction is the only way they have found to get the food/calories into Finn. Maura refers to this mixture as "slop" and they feed it to Finn two to three times per day, depending on what else he eats that day. He will also drink Pediasure (Abbott) from a sippy cup.

Finn will finger-feed himself small pieces of sausage, crisp bacon broken in to bite-size pieces, goldfish crackers, saltines with nothing on them, and some thin cookies. Finn is not yet using a spoon independently to eat. As noted previously, he does drink from a sippy cup but is not yet using a straw or demonstrating the ability to drink from an open cup.

During an observation of a snack brought from home to the clinic, the following observations were noted: Finn does not visually attend to his food, he is using primarily a munching pattern when chewing, he demonstrates limited tongue lateralization, he demonstrates definite preferences for taste and texture, and he appears to have decreased strength and low oral motor tone.

Client Factors/Body Functions

The Infant and Toddler Sensory Profile was completed by Finn's parents just prior to his transition from EI, so this profile was not completed again at the time of evaluation. Table 4-4 shows the results when he was 33 months old.

Questions to Consider

Goal Areas and Treatment Focus

1. Given what you know, what additional assessment information would you gather to assist you with intervention planning?
2. Are there any formal assessments you would recommend using in addition to the Canadian Occupational Performance Measure and the Infant and Toddler Sensory Profile?
3. How do you interpret the results of the Canadian Occupational Performance Measure? How does this information help you to collaborate with Finn's family in goal writing?

Table 4-4

Finn's Infant and Toddler Sensory Profile

RESULTS OF THE ITSP	TYPICAL RANGE	PROBABLE RANGE	DEFINITE RANGE
Auditory		XX	
Visual			XX
Vestibular		XX	
Touch		XX	
Oral			XX
SENSORY PROCESSING PATTERNS	**TYPICAL RANGE**	**PROBABLE RANGE**	**DEFINITE RANGE**
Low Registration			XX
Seeking	XX		
Sensitivity			XX
Avoiding		XX	

Dunn, W. (2002). ***Infant/toddler sensory profile.*** San Antonio, TX: Pearson.

Safety Precautions

1. What are the safety issues that are important to attend to when considering intervention for Finn and his family?

Intervention Plan

1. What frame(s) of reference will guide your intervention (AOTA, 2007)? Provide support for your choices.
2. Review AOTA's *Specialized Knowledge and Skills in Feeding, Eating, and Swallowing for Occupational Therapy Practice* (2007). Entry-level practice regarding knowledge and skills in intervention is discussed within various aspects of the mealtime process. Identify one long-term goal, a short-term objective, and at least one intervention strategy aimed at addressing a contextual factor that is inhibiting mealtime participation for Finn and his family.
3. Identify one long-term goal and two short-term objectives in addition to those above that will address concerns identified in the OT evaluation.
4. Identify at least one appropriate intervention strategy for each of the short-term objectives. Include the rationale for your choice of strategy (developmental theory, frames of reference, evidence in the literature).

Planning for Discharge

1. How will you determine a discharge plan for Finn? Will you recommend transition to another model of service delivery? How might you involve his family and/or the preschool program as a part of your discharge planning?

References

American Occupational Therapy Association. (2007). Specialized knowledge and skills feeding, eating, and swallowing for occupational therapy practice. *American Journal of Occupational Therapy, 61*(6), 686-700.

Law, M., Baptiste, S., Carswell, A., McColl, M., Polatajko, H., & Pollock, N. (2005). *Canadian occupational performance measure* (4th ed.). Ottawa, Ontario: Canadian Association of Occupational Therapists.

Resources

Bundy, A., Lane, S., & Murray, E. (2002). *Sensory integration: Theory and practice* (2nd ed.). Philadelphia: F.A. Davis Co.

Rodger, S., & Ziviani, J. (2012). Autism spectrum disorders. In S. Lane & A. Bundy (Eds.), *Kids can be kids: A childhood occupations approach*. Philadelphia: F.A. Davis Co.

Schuberth, L., Amirault, L., & Case-Smith, J. (2010). Feeding intervention. In J. Case-Smith & J. O'Brien (Eds.), *Occupational therapy for children* (6th ed.) (pp. 446-473). St. Louis: Elsevier.

CHAPTER 5

Introduction to Hospital-Based Settings

When a child has a medical emergency, services may begin in the Emergency Department (ED). Once a child is stabilized in the ED, the child is moved to an acute care floor within a hospital facility. As the child becomes progressively better and stable to the point of being able to tolerate 3 hours of therapy, the child is transferred to an inpatient rehabilitation facility. All clients are medically stabilized at another facility, such as an acute care children's hospital, before being transferred or admitted to this setting. The rehabilitation facility provides 24-hour care with a full medical staff of nurses, respiratory therapy, dieticians, physicians (including physiatrists), nurse practitioners, pharmacy, social work, case management, and access to radiology and laboratory procedures. In addition to the medical staff, the therapy staff includes occupational therapy (OT), physical therapy (PT), music therapy, speech language pathology, child-life therapy, neuropsychology, and school-based services. Pediatric inpatient rehabilitation settings provide services to children from birth to 18 years, who have experienced traumatic injuries (e.g., brain injuries, spinal cord injuries, skeletal trauma), behavioral- and sensory-based feeding problems, congenital anomalies, orthopedic conditions, cerebral palsy, developmental birth disorders, and various other pediatric conditions.

A therapy treatment area or gym is located in a facility of this nature and often serves as the main treatment area for both inpatients and outpatients. Outpatient clients are able to receive therapy Monday through Friday, whereas inpatients often receive services 7 days a week. Facilities typically accept private insurance, Medicaid, and self-pay clients.

Some hospital settings also have ambulatory care clinics. Patients are seen in the clinical setting by therapists in this nontraditional outpatient model. The therapists work closely with physicians and provide assessment and intervention as the patients present in the ambulatory care clinics. The majority of the intervention that is provided by therapists in this setting is in the form of home programs.

In this chapter, you will read about a number of outpatient clients who transitioned from the inpatient unit to a rehabilitation unit. You will also read about a number of children who are referred for continuing services to outpatient clinics or other facilities.

Questions to Consider

1. How do hospital-based settings differ from other areas of pediatric practice?
2. What are the pros and cons of working with multiple medical professionals from different disciplines?
3. What do you think are the areas that OTs focus on in various hospital-based settings?

Resource

Dudgeon, B., & Crooks, L. (2010). Hospital and rehabilitation services. In J. Case-Smith & J. O'Brien (Eds.), *Occupational therapy for children* (6th ed., pp. 785-811). St. Louis, MO: Elsevier.

Cahill SM, Bowyer P, eds. *Cases in Pediatric Occupational Therapy: Assessment and Intervention (pp 109-134).*

Alexa: Pediatric Traumatic Brain Injury/ Inpatient Rehabilitation

Sara Clark, MS, OTR/L and Jennifer Schmidt, OTR/L

History and Background Information

Acute Care History

Alexa is a 6-year-old girl with no significant past medical history. She presented to Longfellow Hospital after being hit by a car while crossing the street on her way to school. In the ED, she was reported to be unresponsive to all types of sensory stimulation. Imaging of Alexa's brain showed evidence of hemorrhagic contusions in the following areas: right frontal lobe, right motor cortex, and the right temporal lobe. Alexa underwent a craniotomy with no complications. She spent a total of 3 weeks in acute care and was then transferred to the pediatric unit at Tuck Rehabilitation Hospital. At the time of the transfer, Alexa was breathing on her own, being fed continuously via a gastrostomy tube (g-tube), and started on systemic baclofen for increased tone throughout the left side of her body. She was nonverbal. Alexa's parents reported that she was intermittently following simple verbal motor commands with her right arm but not demonstrating consistent responses to any other type of sensory stimulation.

Inpatient Rehabilitation

Upon admission to the rehabilitation hospital, the Physical Medicine and Rehabilitation physician ordered the following evaluations: OT, PT, speech therapy, and psychology. Alexa received at least 3 hours of therapy a day from a combination of those therapies. Child life was also consulted for an evaluation and services were provided to Alexa throughout her inpatient rehabilitation stay.

Evaluation Information

Occupational Profile

The OT performed an informal bedside interview with Alexa's parents. Alexa's parents reported that prior to the accident, she was a healthy and happy young girl who was attending full-day kindergarten at her local public school. She excelled at writing and beginning reading skills at school. After school, Alexa was involved in dance lessons 1 day per week and basketball clinic 2 days per week at the local YMCA. On the weekends, the family loved to spend time outdoors together biking, hiking, and camping. Alexa is very social and loves being with her friends to play with her favorite toys: her bowling set and her toy pony collection. She also loves arts and crafts of any kind. Her favorite color is red.

Alexa has a 4-year-old sister. The sisters are very close and share a room. Alexa's mother was a real estate agent before having her children. Now she is home full time with the girls. Alexa's father is a firefighter who works three 24-hour shifts a week and then is home with his family the other 4 days of the week. The family lives in a two-story home with four steps to enter and no hand rails. The first floor has a half bathroom. Alexa's bedroom and the only full bathroom, with a tub shower, are on the second floor.

Alexa's parents also report that Alexa loves to be as independent as possible with her self-care tasks. She is able to dress herself, brush her teeth, and go to the bathroom on her own. She needs some help with washing, drying, and brushing her hair. She also needs help with small fasteners on clothing and tying her shoes.

Alexa's Parents' Goals for Her Rehabilitation Stay

- Alexa will walk soon.
- Alexa will be able to play with her sister soon.
- Alexa will be strong enough to be able to go back to school with her friends this year.

Alexa was unable to verbalize her goals for therapy at the time of the initial evaluation because of cognitive and expressive language impairments.

Analysis of Occupational Performance

Tuck Rehabilitation Hospital uses a specific set of outcome measures for pediatric traumatic brain injury admissions, based on the recommendations of the *Common Data Elements—Pediatric TBI Outcomes Work Group* (McCauley et al., 2012). The required outcome measure at Tuck Rehabilitation Hospital, for all therapy disciplines, is the Functional Independence Measure for Children (WeeFIM). Scores must be submitted to the electronic medical record within 72 hours from admission. Alexa was assessed bedside, by all therapy disciplines on day 2 of admission (Table 5-1).

Client Factors/Body Functions

- Vision: No consistent fixation on objects and no consistent tracking.

Table 5-1

Alexa's WeeFIM Admission Scores

Physical therapy	Score of 1 in all areas of mobility
Speech therapy	Score of 1 in all areas of cognition
Occupational therapy	Score of 1 in all areas of self care

- Right upper extremity: Alexa was right hand dominant prior to admission. Movement noted in minimal ranges, inconsistent purposeful use, full passive range of motion, normal tone.
- Left upper extremity: No active movement noted, significant increased flexor tone in synergy pattern: shoulder internal rotation, elbow flexion, wrist and digit flexion, and thumb adduction. The Modified Ashworth Scale = 2 in all joints.

Progress Information (2 Weeks After Admission)

The OT is required to complete a weekly summary of progress to submit to the insurance company, in order to continue to justify intensive inpatient rehabilitation.

New precautions (listed in chart by the Physical Medicine and Rehabilitation physician) were modified diet (soft and nectar liquids), aspiration precautions, fall precautions, direct hand offs, use of four side rails, and bed exit alarm.

Client Factors/Body Functions

- Pain: Unable to formally rate pain using a facial or numeric scale due to cognitive impairments. Alexa shows signs of discomfort in her left arm as evident by facial expressions during movement and positioning of her left arm (Figure 5-1).
- Expressive language: Alexa is responding to simple questions with delayed, one- to two-word answers. Her speech intelligibility is poor, especially to an unfamiliar listener. She rarely initiates verbalizations.
- Global mental functions: Currently, Alexa is very impulsive with her movements and use of her right upper extremity for functional tasks. She needs tactile and verbal cues for pacing during activities. She demonstrates significant neglect of her left environment and left upper extremity. Alexa is inconsistent with following one-step motor commands for functional tasks.
- Specific mental functions: The speech therapist completed the Children's Orientation and Amnesia Test (COAT) each day with Alexa. This week, Alexa met age-appropriate norms for 2 consecutive days on the COAT, demonstrating learning potential for new skills. The COAT is also a recommended outcome measure by the *Pediatric TBI Outcomes Workgroup* (McCauley et al, 2012). Alexa does continue to demonstrate challenges with executive functions such as problem solving through novel tasks, due to damage of her prefrontal cortex.
- Vision: The OT was unable to formally assess vision using formal assessments due to cognitive impairments and challenges with accurately verbally expressing what she is seeing. During functional tasks, Alexa is fixating more on objects and tracking from her right side toward midline, but continues to be inconsistent with tracking past midline to the left and demonstrates inconsistent visual attention to her left environment. Alexa's eyes are misaligned. She tends to keep her neck flexed to the left side, and when reading appears to use only one eye (indicative of possible diplopia). When the OT attempts to cover one eye to relieve the diplopia, Alexa becomes very agitated, pulling the therapist's hand away in frustration.

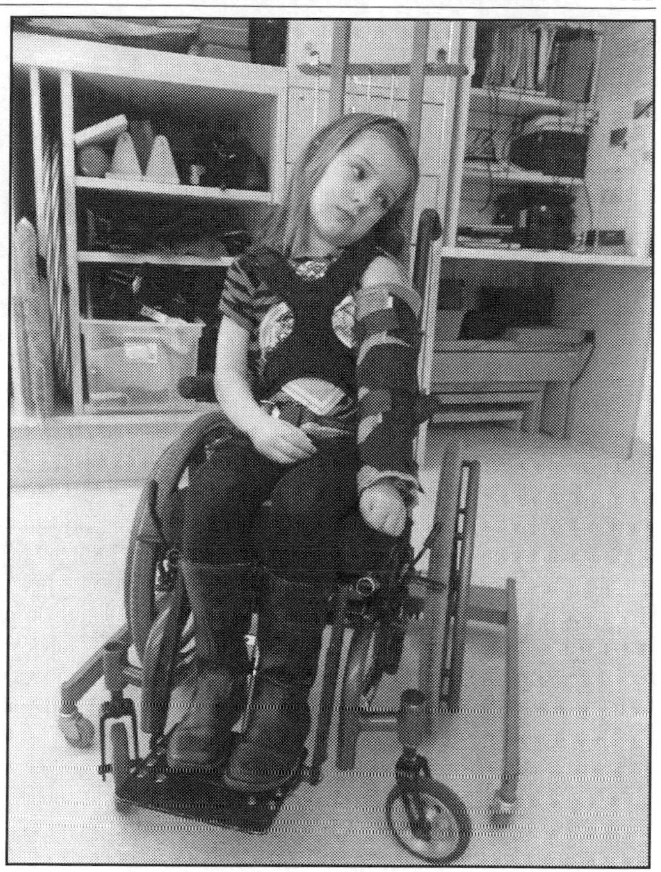

Figure 5-1. Alexa shows signs of discomfort in her left arm.

Table 5-2

Alexa's Modified Ashworth Scale Ratings

JOINT	*MUSCLE*	*MUSCLE GRADE*	*MUSCLE ACTION*
Shoulder	Anterior deltoid	2+	Forward flexion
	Middle deltoid	2+	Abduction
Elbow	Biceps	2+	Flexion
	Triceps	1	Extension (trace palpation)
Forearm	Supinator	2+	Supination
	Pronator quadratus	1	Difficult to accurately assess active pronation from gravity assisted pronation and tone
Wrist	Extensor carpi radialis and Extensor carpi ulnaris	2+	Extension
	Flexor carpi radialis and Extensor carpi ulnaris	1	Difficult to accurately assess active wrist flexion from gravity assisted flexion and tone
Digits	Extensor digitorum	2+	Digit extension
Thumb	Abductor pollicis longus	2+	Thumb abduction

Neuromusculoskeletal and Movement-Related Functions

Muscle Endurance and Balance

- Unsupported static sitting edge of bed or mat: Moderate assistance, leans to left, poor neck extension endurance (neck rests in left lateral flexion)
- Unsupported static standing: Maximal assistance with right upper extremity support, leans to the left
- Right upper extremity current function: No motor concerns. She initiates purposeful use of the right upper extremity for functional tasks, but continues to be impulsive with movement.
- Left upper extremity current function: Difficult to accurately assess formal manual muscle test scores due to age and cognitive impairments. All scores listed in Table 5-2 are estimates of the *least* muscle grade demonstrated by Alexa this week. Significant flexor tone is present in the left elbow, wrist and digits, and thumb when Alexa attempts to use her left hand. She presents with a Modified Ashworth Scale rating of 1+ in her shoulder, and 2 in her elbow flexors, wrist flexors, finger flexors, and pronators (see Table 5-2).

Areas of Occupation

Current Occupational Therapy WeeFIM Scores

The occupational therapist uses constant activity analysis of all Alexa's self-care tasks, during interventions sessions, in order to provide the team with a weekly update on functional performance improvements (Table 5-3).

Functional Mobility

Alexa requires total assistance for manual wheelchair mobility due to hemiparesis, and moderate assistance with power wheelchair mobility with right hand joystick (assistance needed for safety due to left neglect).

Contexts and Environment

The *Common Data Elements—Pediatric TBI Outcomes Workgroup* encourages assessment of psychosocial risk and protective factors when working with any family impacted by a child with a traumatic brain injury (TBI) (Gerring & Wade, 2012).

Alexa is cooperative, loves coming to therapy when therapy is not focused on self-care skills, and loves being around other kids in the gym and common room. When Alexa is presented with more challenging tasks that involve use of her left arm or standing, she tends to request going back to her room.

When Alexa's dad is able to be present for sessions, he actively participates and assists with all of Alexa's care and transfers. He is eager to learn her hands-on care and acts as a great coach by encouraging Alexa to participate and try challenging tasks. He has a great deal of experience moving and assisting people who are critically ill because of his job as a firefighter.

Alexa's mom is more hesitant to participate in hands-on care or with transfers. This week, Alexa's mom vocalized a fear of doing something wrong, guilt for Alexa's injury, and hope that Alexa will be back to normal in a few weeks.

Table 5-3

Alexa's WeeFIM Scores

SELF CARE TASK	WEEFIM SCORE	DESCRIPTION
Feeding	4	Needs set up and supervision for pacing due to being impulsive with her right upper extremity as well as minimal assistance for accuracy in getting food onto utensil and bringing to mouth
Grooming	2	Performed from wheelchair level, needs maximal assistance with brushing her teeth, washing her face, and combing her hair
Dressing (upper and lower body)	2	Supportive long sitting in bed, cries and demonstrates signs of frustration when attempting dressing skills
Toileting	2	Continues to need to wear a pad due to inconsistent continence with bladder, full continence with bowel movements; also does need maximal assistance for clothing management and hygiene
Toilet transfer	2	Squat pivot with use of grab bar with right hand
Bathing	1	Very poor sitting balance with wet surfaces, leans to the left, currently using a fully supportive rolling shower chair with lateral, arm, head, and leg supports and chest and pelvis straps (Figure 5-2); also needs total assist for completion of bathing tasks
Shower transfer	1	Squat pivot from bed to/from rolling shower chair, poor balance with wet surfaces and bare feet, leans to the left

Questions to Consider

Goal Areas and Treatment Focus This Week

1. Which OT intervention approaches from the *Occupational Practice Framework* (AOTA, 2014) will you use when working with Alexa and her parents?
2. What strengths will Alexa bring to the treatment process? What strengths do Alexa's parents bring to the treatment process? How do Alexa's parents enrich the hospital's social environment and how does this support Alexa?
3. Write short-term goals for Alexa for this week.
4. How will your goals and approach to feeding differ from the speech and language pathologist's goals and approach for feeding?
5. Outline a 60-minute treatment session for Alexa. Indicate whether your intervention activities are occupation-based, purposeful activities, or preparatory methods.
6. What are some strategies that may be helpful for addressing Alexa's challenges with executive function during functional tasks?
7. What are some evidence-based intervention strategies that you can use to support Alexa?

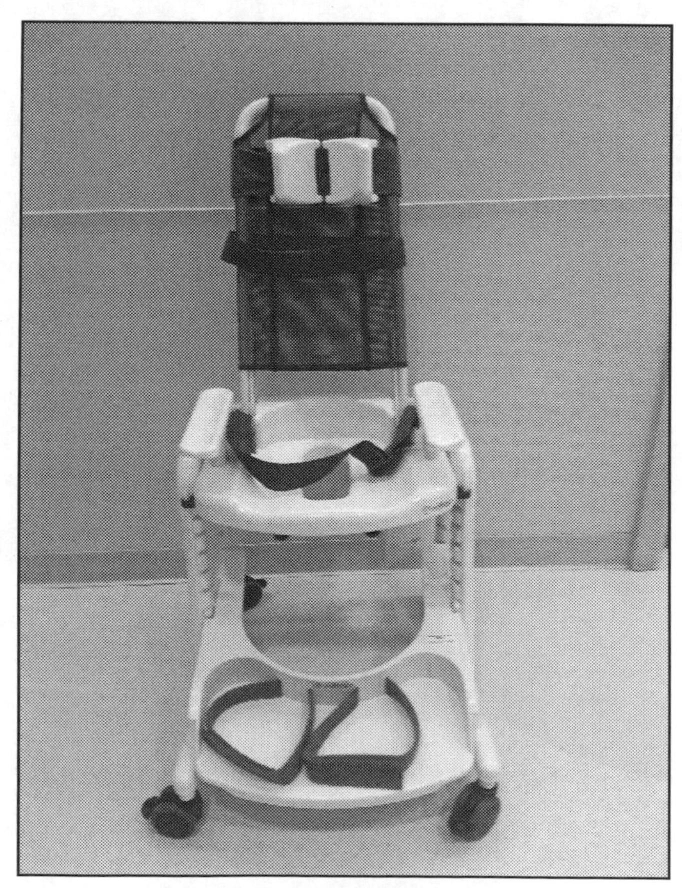

Figure 5-2. Pediatric rolling shower chair.

Safety Precautions

1. What are the main safety issues to consider when working with Alexa?
2. How will these safety issues influence your intervention?

Planning for Discharge to Home

1. Describe OT's role in the following factors when planning for discharge to home:
   - Obtaining a wheelchair for Alexa to use at home
   - Ensuring that Alexa has physical access into the home and to the second floor
   - Addressing bathroom equipment needs
2. Given Alexa's progress to date, what do you anticipate Alexa's long term WeeFIM goals would be by discharge in 8 weeks? Consider the following self-care skills: feeding, grooming, bathing, dressing, toileting, toilet transfer, and shower transfer.
3. What type of therapy will Alexa receive when she is discharged to home?
4. When is Alexa able to receive education services from her public school district? What do you anticipate these services will look like?

References

American Occupational Therapy Association. (2014). Occupational therapy practice framework: Domain and process (3rd ed.). *American Journal of Occupational Therapy, 68*(Suppl 1), S1-S48.

Gerring, J. P., & Wade, S. (2012). The essential role of psychosocial risk and protective factors in pediatric traumatic brain injury research. *Journal of Neurotrauma, 29*, 621-628.

McCauley, S. R., Wilde, E. A., Anderson, V. A., Bedell, G., Beers,S.R., Campbell, T. F., ... Yeates, K.O. (2012). Recommendations for the use of common outcome measures in pediatric traumatic brain injury research. *Journal of Neurotrauma, 29*, 678-705.

Resources

Uniform Data System for Medical Rehabilitation. (2006). *The WeeFIM II® Clinical Guide, Version 6.0*. Buffalo, NY: UDSMR. http://www.udsmr.org/WebModules/WeeFIM/Wee_About.aspx

Bohannon, R., & Smith, M. (1987). Interrater reliability of a Modified Ashworth Scale of Muscle Spasticity. *Physical Therapy, 67*, 206-207.

Ewing-Cobbs, L., Levin, H., Fletcher, J., Miner, M., & Eisenberg, H. (1990). The children's orientation and amnesia test: Relationship to severity of acute head injury and to recovery of memory. *Neurosurgery, 27*(5), 683-691.

Jenna: Complex Regional Pain Syndrome/ Hand Therapy

Susanne Higgins, MHS, OTR/L, CHT and Jennifer Bobo, MOT, OTR/L, CHT

History and Background Information

Jenna is a 14-year-old girl with a history of complex regional pain syndrome (CRPS) in her right foot and ankle. Jenna acquired CRPS in her right lower extremity after she tripped while running for a soccer ball approximately 2 years ago. Jenna received physical therapy for 3.5 months to treat the pain and dysfunction in her lower extremity, during which time her symptoms resolved. Jenna's most recent injury occurred 4 weeks prior to her first OT visit. While attempting to close her locker door at school, she accidentally banged it on her right, dominant arm. Jenna developed severe burning pain in her hand, wrist, and forearm that increased over the course of the next few days. During that time, Jenna was seen by a pediatric orthopedic surgeon, who diagnosed her with a contusion and CRPS.

Lately, Jenna has been missing school and avoiding many social events due to the problem with her upper extremity. Her mom reports that Jenna has been cranky and irritable. Jenna's mom expressed frustration of not knowing what to do and how to help her. Her friends seem to have a hard time understanding what is wrong with her because her arm looks the same as it did prior to her injury. In the past, she often got together with a large group of friends and connected through frequent texting and social media. Recently, she has only been seeing her two closest friends.

Evaluation Information

Occupational Profile

Jenna was seen at an outpatient OT clinic that primarily services clients with orthopedic conditions. The OT who evaluated and worked with Jenna is also a certified hand therapist with many years of experience. Jenna's mom accompanied her to the first therapy visit and noted that she has been assisting Jenna with her self-care routine, typing her homework, and driving her to school so she doesn't have to take the bus. Jenna lives in a suburban community in a single family home with her parents, a younger sister, and a brother. Jenna has her own room.

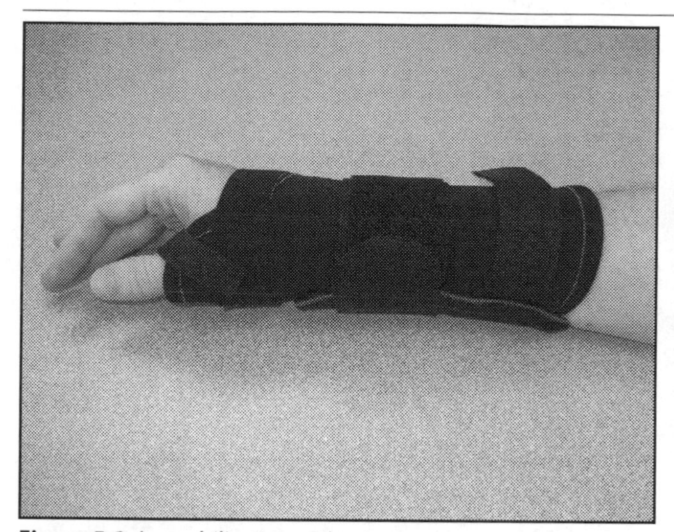

Figure 5-3. Immobilization orthosis.

Table 5-4	
Patient-Rated Wrist/Hand Evaluation	
PAIN SUBSCALE	
0 = NO PAIN, 10 = WORST EVER	
Pain at rest	6/10
Fasten shirt buttons	6/10
When lifting a heavy object	10/10
FUNCTION SUBSCALE	
0 = NO DIFFICULTY, 10 = UNABLE TO DO	
Turning a doorknob	9/10
Using bathroom tissue with affected hand	8/10
Performing recreational activities	10/10

As a freshman in high school, Jenna takes honors classes and gets mostly A's. She runs on the high school junior varsity track team and plays junior varsity volleyball. She enjoys hanging out with her large group of friends. Her only other hobbies include using multiple forms of social media.

Jenna and her mother recently returned to see her doctor at the pain clinic of a large urban children's hospital. Her doctor prescribed pregabalin and amitriptyline for pain management. Jenna refused treatment with a stellate ganglion injection, stating that even the thought of a needle going into her neck was intolerable. As part of usual care by the pain clinic, she was also given a referral to see a psychologist. Jenna's mom reports that they think they misplaced the paper with the information and haven't "gotten around to doing anything about it."

Jenna stated her current goals for therapy include a desire for her "arm to get better and to be back to normal." When prompted to identify what she meant by "back to normal," Jenna identified eliminating pain, using the computer, styling her hair, and playing volleyball as activities that she would like to perform without difficulty.

Analysis of Occupational Performance

During the past month, Jenna reports that she has had pain that she rates at 10/10 when it is at its worst. She experiences this level of pain intensity on a daily basis. Using a pain diagram, Jenna indicates that she has severe, burning pain in the area of her volar and ulnar hand, wrist, and distal forearm. Her pain is aggravated by any movement of her hand/wrist/forearm or attempts at functional usage such as using a fork, keyboard, or turning a doorknob. Jenna carries her hand and arm in a "guarded" position against her body, demonstrating little spontaneous usage. She avoids resting the volar side of her hand or distal forearm on hard or soft surfaces, such as a tabletop or the armrest of a chair. Sleeves or bedding that touch her arm trigger burning pain. Jenna has been using a prefabricated wrist extension, thumb palmar abduction immobilization orthosis (Figure 5-3) that was issued by her orthopedic surgeon. She has worn the orthosis nearly continuously for the past 4 weeks because she is fearful of any unexpected touch, movement, or bumping of her hand/wrist. The OT encouraged Jenna to gradually decrease her use of the orthosis by wearing it just at night and when she is out of the house.

Even though she is right hand–dominant, Jenna has been eating, brushing her teeth and hair, and writing with her left hand. She lifts her backpack with her left upper extremity. She is frustrated because it is slow and difficult to perform these tasks with her nondominant upper extremity. No obvious edema or color changes are seen.

Jenna completed the Patient Rated Wrist/Hand Evaluation (PRWHE) (MacDermid, 1996). Her overall score was 76 (out of a possible 100). Her scores for some of the items on the PRWHE are shown in Table 5-4.

During the initial assessment, Jenna wore her right sleeve pushed up above her elbow. She avoided resting her forearm on the table. Active range of motion (AROM) at the shoulder and elbow were not impaired. Forearm and wrist AROM are shown in Table 5-5. With extra time and encouragement, Jenna was able to make a nearly complete fist with her fingertips about a half inch from her palm. She was able to fully extend her finger and thumb and oppose her thumb to the tips of her index, middle, and ring fingers, but not her small finger. The motion of the digits was slow and labored. She reported increased pain with motion of the forearm, wrist, and hand. When attempting to manipulate a small object (such as a coin) in her hand, she

TABLE 5-5	
AROM RIGHT UPPER EXTREMITY	
FOREARM	
Supination	0 to 30 degrees
Pronation	0 to 20 degrees
WRIST	
Extension	0 to 30 degrees
Flexion	0 to 7 degrees
Radial deviation	0 to 4 degrees
Ulnar deviation	0 to 10 degrees

dropped it three times and had difficulty moving it to a tip pinch between her thumb and tip of her index finger. With the therapist supporting the weight of the dynamometer and pinch gauge, Jenna did not apply enough pressure to produce a measurable score. During her time in the clinic, Jenna was not observed using her right upper extremity and avoided resting it on the table. She drank a small glass of water using her left hand. She handed paperwork to her mom, who completed it for her.

Treatment Parameters

Jenna is scheduled to attend OT 2 times per week for the next 6 weeks. She plans to return to see her orthopedic physician in 4 weeks, at which time she will be reevaluated. If it fits into her schedule, the therapist will accompany Jenna to her visit with the doctor, whose office is in the same building as the OT clinic. Her insurance allows a total of 60 OT visits per calendar year.

Questions to Consider

Goals/Treatment Plan

1. Create a problem list for Jenna.
2. Which of Jenna's strengths do you think may help her in her rehabilitation?
3. Identify potential obstacles that Jenna may encounter.
4. Describe Jenna's roles and how they are impacted by this injury.
5. List the short-term goals for Jenna for the first 4 weeks of treatment.
6. How will you prioritize the focus of your treatment initially?
7. Indicate which other team members (health professionals and others) might be involved with Jenna and what each team member's role might be.
8. Create a home program for Jenna. Be sure that it is in a format accessible to a 14 year old.

Safety Precautions

1. In light of her current medications, are there any side effects or precautions to be aware of?
2. If Jenna continues to avoid using her upper extremity, what are possible consequences?

Self-Care/Work/Leisure

1. Jenna's mom is helping her with styling her hair and dressing. Describe a series of two to three treatment sessions that are designed to increase Jenna's independence in self-care.
2. Jenna reports that she is tired during the day and has difficulty falling asleep at night because she can't find a comfortable position for her hand and arm. If she attempts to sleep without her orthosis, the weight of the sheets and blanket are painful. What strategies could you explore with Jenna to help her to get a good night's sleep?

Equipment/Adaptations

1. In order to complete her school work, Jenna needs to write and/or use the computer extensively. What adaptations could you incorporate to enable her to independently and efficiently complete her school work? What strategies could you teach her to promote the increased use and function of her right upper extremity?
2. Jenna is fearful of people bumping into her during the passing periods at school in the crowded hallways. She is also worried about her performance on exams because she has difficulty writing with her left hand. Describe accommodations and modifications that you can recommend to Jenna's school team to address these concerns and difficulties.

Neuromusculoskeletal

1. How would you address Jenna's nonuse of her affected, dominant upper extremity?
2. Jenna has been hesitant to decrease the usage of her orthosis. How would you explain to Jenna why you want her to wear it less?

Psychosocial

1. Jenna previously had CRPS in her lower extremity. In what ways might this impact her coping abilities and her current OT program?
2. What do you think is the psychological impact of having chronic pain? Describe pain management techniques that Jenna could use.

3. Jenna and her mom have not followed through with the referral to the counselor/psychologist at the pain clinic. Do you think it is the role of the OT to initiate a conversation about this? If so, what would you say? What would be your goal of the conversation?

Patient/Family Education

1. How would you explain CRPS to Jenna and her parents?
2. Imagine that Jenna and her parents had done some research on the Internet and read some frightening stories about people who had CRPS. How would you address these concerns?

Situations

1. After the first OT treatment session, Jenna's mom dropped her off and ran errands while Jenna attended therapy. Describe how you could include Jenna's parents in her OT (to ensure carryover with her home program) while encouraging Jenna to take responsibility for her rehabilitation.
2. The precipitating event for this injury appeared to be a minor one. Jenna's hand and arm do not appear discolored. Some of Jenna's friends and teachers at school do not seem to believe that her condition is "real." How do you think this affects Jenna and what can she do about it?
3. Jenna's OT includes Graded Motor Imagery and use of a "mirror box" as part of her treatment program. Briefly describe what this is and how it could be beneficial.
4. After several weeks of involvement in OT, Jenna begins to use her hand more spontaneously. She is now using her right hand for eating, writing, and using the computer. She is only using her orthosis occasionally and is having less frequent and less intense pain. Jenna asks the OT if she will be able to try out for the volleyball team with all her friends in 2 months. How do you answer her question and help her work toward this goal?

Discharge Planning

1. When it is time for discharge from OT services, what would you tell Jenna about the possibility of further reoccurrences and how to respond if this happens?

Reference

MacDermid, J. C. (1996). Development of a scale for patient rating of wrist pain and disability. *Journal of Hand Therapy*, 178-183.

Resources

Kachko, L., Efrat, E., Ben Ami, S., Mukamel, M., & Katz, J., (2008). Pediatric complex regional pain syndrome. *Pediatrics International, 50*(5), 567-752.

Logan, D. E., Carpino, E. A., Chiang, G., Condon, M., Firn, E., Gaughan, V. J., . . . Berde C. B. (2012). A day-hospital approach to treatment of pediatric complex regional pain syndrome. *Clinical Journal Pain, 28*(9), 766-774.

McCabe, C. (2011). Mirror visual feedback therapy. A practical approach. *Journal of Hand Therapy, 23*, 170-179.

Priganc, V. W., & Stralka, S. W. (2011). Graded motor imagery. *Journal of Hand Therapy, 24*,164-169.

Jonathon: Pediatric Spinal Cord Injury/Rehabilitation

Gail A. Poskey, PhD, OTR

History and Background

Jonathon was injured at age 2 years during a motor vehicle collision. He was restrained in a car seat and sustained a cervical spinal cord injury (SCI) from the collision. He lived with his teenage mother and her immediate family and would also stay at his teenage father's home periodically, who lived with his maternal grandparents. Jonathon's primary caregivers were his maternal grandparents, his mother, and his father. At the time of the injury, both of his parents were still in high school but not married.

Jonathon sustained a complete fracture of the C7 vertebra, which was classified as an American Spinal Injury Association's (ASIA) A injury. Although this was his level of injury, he later presented with functional return of T1 on his left side and C8 on the right. Following the motor vehicle collision, he was transported from the scene by ambulance to a large metropolitan children's hospital, where the workup revealed the SCI. Jonathon's fracture was stabilized and he was placed in a halo jacket and vest. Following an extensive 6-week stay in the acute care facility, he was transferred to the pediatric rehabilitation facility, where he received comprehensive rehabilitation services. Once he was medically stable and his caregivers were independent with all levels of his care, he was discharged to his home with his mother and maternal grandparents, who lived in a suburban area. Jonathon returned to the same pediatric rehabilitation facility to receive outpatient OT and PT. The case study now focuses on Jonathan's recovery process as an outpatient. Although he received therapy for over 2 years as an outpatient, the current scenario is Jonathon at 4 years of age.

Evaluation Information

Jonathon is a typically developing 4 year old and is in the lower percentile for his height and weight but still within the normal range. He is shy around strangers but very interactive and curious with his family and those whom he knows. He has a port-wine stain (or nevus flammeus) on his face, which is unrelated to his injury. His primary caregivers must travel approximately 1 hour to attend outpatient therapy from the suburb where he resides. Often, it is a different caregiver who brings Jonathon in for his outpatient therapy. Jonathon may be accompanied by his mother, father, maternal grandmother, or maternal aunt. His grandmother and mother will sometimes attend the therapy sessions together. All of his caregivers are independent with Jonathon's basic care and in assisting with his mobility. What is not typical is his age in regard to his injury, as Jonathon was traumatically injured at the age of 2 with a complete cervical injury and resulting tetraplegia (Vogel, Hickey, Klaas, & Anderson, 2004). The resulting SCI posed specific and unique problems related to his early development, the maturity of his body and systems, and ongoing changes to his general physical growth and development (Young, 2003).

Jonathon was initially assessed using manual muscle testing and dermatome testing to reveal his muscle strength, functional level, and his sensory level. In addition to manual muscle testing and sensory testing, his self-help skills were assessed in conjunction with age-appropriate developmental scales, the Hawaii Early Learning Profile (HELP) for 0 to 3 years, and the HELP for Preschoolers for 3 to 6 years.

Intervention strategies include developmentally based treatment congruent with Jonathon's functional spinal cord level and family-centered care. This is paramount because the important role the family and caregivers play in the child's life and the need for the care to be developmentally based and responsive to the ongoing dynamic changes that will occur naturally as a result of growth and development (Vogel, Betz, & Mulchahey, 2010). Intervention strategies for Jonathon includes self-feeding, manipulation of feeding and writing utensils, mobility (bed, mat, and wheelchair), age-appropriate dressing activities, grooming, gross- and fine-motor activities, awareness of protection of skin, and play skills.

Jonathon's injury was classified as a C7 ASIA A, being a complete injury. However, clinically he presented with a T1 functional level on the left side and C8 on the right side. He demonstrated full head and neck movements with good muscle strength and had paralysis of his lower extremity and trunk from T1 and down. On the right side, he demonstrated full elbow flexion and extension, full wrist flexion and extension, and partial finger movement/flexion, showing extrinsic finger muscles and thumb flexors but absence of the intrinsic thumb and finger muscles. On the left side, he demonstrated full elbow flexion and extension, full wrist flexion and extension, and finger flexion and partial finger extension and finger adduction on the ulnar side.

In regard to self-care and self-help skills, Jonathon required setup and occasional assistance with self-feeding. He often used his fingers from his left hand with his right hand stabilizing to pick up food and preferred to use a spoon as his utensil. His parents or caregivers would prepare his food and also cut the food for him or in some situations might help hold the food. He was able to pick up lightweight plastic cups and drink directly from them, and he was also able to drink from a lightweight cup with a straw.

His family provided intermittent catheterization every 4 hours and total care for his daily bowel program. Additionally, they provided diligent monitoring and care of his skin. Jonathon initially had occasional bowel accidents and wore a diaper after the injury. However, around 4 years of age he had a more regimented and consistent bowel program and wore regular underwear. Therefore, occasional accidents were more the exception. Jonathon assisted with bathing by helping to wash his face and upper body. He had overall minimal assistance with grooming (mainly for thoroughness), brushing his teeth, and brushing his hair. Upper extremity dressing was typically accomplished in a long sitting position from the bed level. Lower extremity dressing was usually completed on the floor.

At the time of discharge from outpatient services, Jonathon received minimal assistance with donning and doffing socks, setup with upper extremity dressing of a pullover top from wheelchair level, and set-up to minimal assistance with upper extremity dressing from bed level; setup to minimal assistance with donning and doffing long pants/slacks and minimal assistance to don/doff underwear. He required moderate assistance to don his shoes and minimal assistance to doff shoes. It is important to note his self-care routine did take more time than that of a typically developing 4-year-old, as would be expected for any client who has an SCI. Although Jonathon had achieved a high level of age-appropriate independence with his self-care, on various occasions and usually due to time constraints, his caregivers would perform a significant portion of his dressing and grooming routine for him.

Jonathon was able to self-propel his custom wheelchair (Figure 5-4) short distances on level surfaces. He was fitted in a wheelchair with a custom seating system including a custom back with lateral supports that still allowed him freedom of movement from his upper extremities and provided appropriate support to his back and trunk. At the time of discharge, level transfers from the wheelchair required moderate assistance and transfers to higher or lower surfaces from the wheelchair required moderate to maximum assistance. For bed and/or mat mobility, he required supervision to minimal assistance (Figure 5-5).

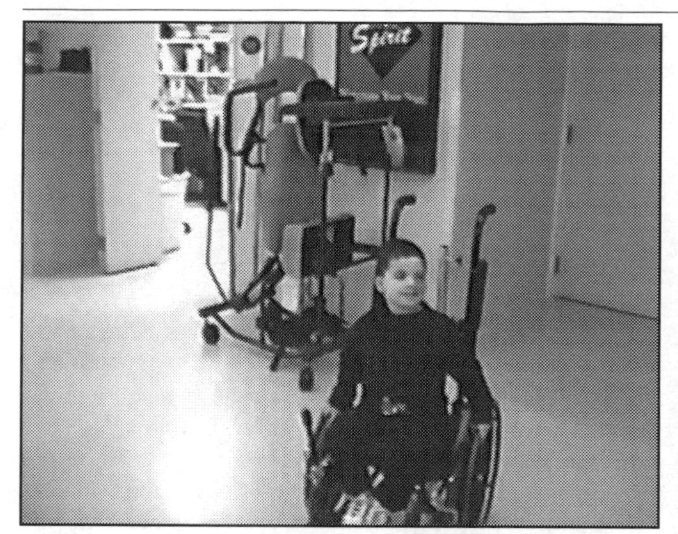

Figure 5-4. Jonathon propelling his wheelchair.

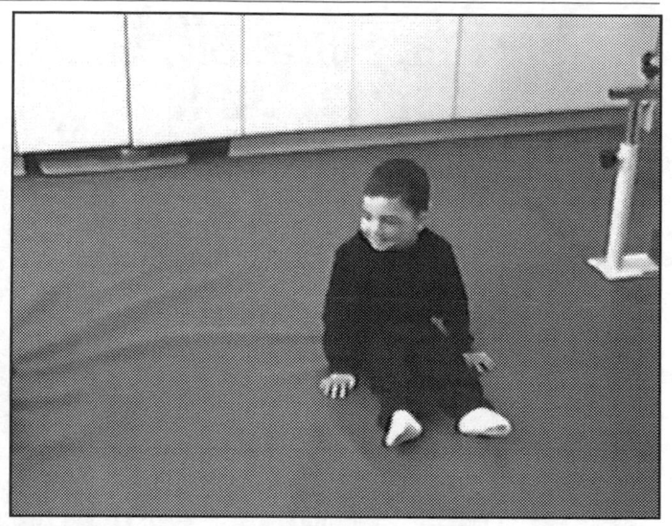

Figure 5-5. Jonathon performing mat mobility.

Jonathon received outpatient OT services 2 times a week for over 2 years. He also was followed by the facility's pediatric physiatrist and received PT services once a week for 1 year. Child life worked consistently with Jonathon as an inpatient and continued to work with him in conjunction with therapy during his 2-year outpatient program. Social work services and case management continued to be involved with his case to ensure appropriate resources for funding and to provide ongoing emotional support and resources for the parents and maternal grandparents. Additionally, neuropsychological services worked with the family as an inpatient and continued to provide intermittent support on an outpatient basis.

Questions to Consider

1. What were Jonathon's strengths before his accident? What are his strengths now?
2. What does ASIA A level mean?
3. Discuss the challenges and benefits of so many caregivers being involved in Jonathon's case.
4. What are some developmental skills that children Jonathon's age without disabilities are working on?
5. Jonathon's OT used two versions of the HELP. Why do you think that this decision was made? What sort of information did the OT expect to gain?
6. Locate pictures of adaptive equipment that might be helpful for Jonathon to use during eating. Discuss why you selected each piece of equipment.
7. Write a goal for Jonathon to be independent with skin checks.
8. Design a 30-minute treatment session to address the goal that you wrote for question 7. Specify the set-up of the environment, as well as the materials that you would need for this treatment.
9. What other types of equipment might Jonathon benefit from?
10. What is a child life specialist? How does the role of the child life specialist differ from that of the OT?

References

Vogel, L. C., Hickey, K. J., Klaas, S. J., & Anderson, C. J. (2004). Unique issues in pediatric spinal cord injury. *Orthopaedic Nursing, 23*(5), 300-308.

Vogel, L. C., Betz, R. R., & Mulcahey, M. R. (2010). Spinal cord disorders in children and adolescents. In L. Vernon (Ed.), *Spinal cord medicine: Principles and practice* (2nd ed.) (pp. 595-623). New York: Demos Medical Publishing.

Young, W. (2003). CareCure community: Pediatric spinal cord injury. Retrieved from http://sci.rutgers.edu/dynarticles/PediatricSCI.pdf

Resources

American Occupational Therapy Association. (2008). Occupational therapy practice framework: Domain and process (2nd ed.). *American Journal of Occupational Therapy, 62*, 625-683.

American Spinal Injury Association website: http://www.asia-spinalinjury.org/pediatrics/mobility_guidelines.php

National Spinal Cord Injury Association (NSCIA) website: http://www.spinalcord.org/resource-center/askus/index.php?pg=kb.book&id=23

Shiner's Hospital for Children website: http://www.shrinershospitalsforchildren.org/en/CareAndTreatment/SpinalCord.aspx

Vogel, L. C., & Anderson, C. J. (2003). Spinal cord injuries in children and adolescents: A review. *The Journal of Spinal Cord Medicine, 26*(3), 193-203.

Martha: Spina Bifida/ Hospital Clinic

Rachel Galant, MS, OTR/L

History and Background Information

Martha began coming to the myelomeningocele clinic when she was just 2 months old. This clinic is led by an orthopedic surgeon but involves an interdisciplinary team that includes a urologist, neurosurgeon, nurse(s), resident, nurse practitioner, social worker, psychologist, dietician, orthotist, recreation therapist, PT, and OT. Often, the team will all enter the clinic room together for a new exam so the family does not have to repeat the child's medical history multiple times. Otherwise, each discipline can assess the family's needs separately on a case-by-case basis. Unfortunately, these clinic services are not billable from a therapy standpoint, but they are viewed as a very important and viable service. These clinics see children with spina bifida (SB) as early as shortly after birth to age 21. Luckily, this population is living longer and longer into adulthood and enjoying satisfying, fulfilling lives. On the other hand, adult SB clinics are not as common and are desperately needed to address the specific needs of this patient population into adulthood.

Martha was born at 37 weeks gestation via cesarean section because the family was aware of her diagnosis before she was born. She had her sac closure hours after her birth, and she had a ventriculoperitoneal (VP) shunt placed for her hydrocephalus several days later. She has had no other surgeries and was an otherwise healthy girl. She was soon connected with early intervention (EI) services (birth to 3 program). Martha was initially getting PT weekly and developmental therapy monthly. She did not have any specialized equipment yet.

Evaluation Information

When she first came to the myelomeningocele clinic, the orthopedic doctor looked at her back closure and checked if her spine was fairly straight, which it was. He also looked at her general range of motion. The PT and OT worked together to do a gross developmental screen. Martha was able to tolerate the prone position for up to 20 seconds before fussing. She was able to bring her hands to midline and hold onto age-appropriate toys. At the time, Martha's mother was nursing her but also supplementing her nutrition with formula and bottle feeding. Martha had a 5-year-old sister who was very interested in helping her mother and father care for her sister. Martha's father was in school to become an electrician and also worked a part-time job. Martha's mother stayed home with her, while her sister had just recently started kindergarten. Martha's funding source was through All Kids, the public aid program set up for children in Illinois.

The PT and OT both reviewed their roles to the parents and stressed the importance of independence as Martha gets older. Martha's parents were very anxious to know if she would ever walk, and the doctor discussed that it was too early to tell. However, the doctor did review the likelihood of needing foot bracing and some type of ambulatory device as she gets older, as well as the probable need for a wheelchair to some extent. The therapists addressed the importance of tummy time for Martha and different methods in which to promote this, especially if Martha has a hard time tolerating lying prone on a flat surface or the floor at home. They discussed how tummy time leads to posterior neck strengthening and arm strengthening, which supports sitting, crawling, and upright play. The family was grateful for all of the education and the idea of being hopeful about Martha's future without making any promises. They were quite overwhelmed by the team experience, even though they reported that they appreciated it. Martha's parents were also issued a book about living with a child with SB and a home teaching folder, including educational materials on latex allergies, tethered cord, shunt malfunction symptoms, and the business cards of all the team members. They were advised to come back in 4 months for follow-up.

Progress Information

Martha and her family returned to the clinic when Martha was 6 months old. Martha seemed to be more interactive and smiled frequently. Martha was not sitting yet; however, she was tolerating tummy time better than she was before. She was just starting to eat baby food and rice cereal and gaining weight appropriately. An issue that Martha's EI PT was concerned about her not showing any active movement in her lower extremities. In addition, Martha was starting to develop some plantarflexion contractures. The orthopedic doctor requested that the OT fabricate bilateral ankle foot orthoses (AFOs) for Martha, to be worn at night and periodically during the day. Definitive AFOs were not yet indicated, as they were meant to be only positional at this time and not for assisting with standing. Also, at this age, a child is growing so much that by the time definitive AFOs were ready, Martha may have outgrown them. Therefore, the OT fabricated AFOs for Martha with splinting materials in the clinic. Great attention was given to the bony prominences in her feet to prevent pressure ulcers. This population is at high risk for pressure ulcers due to their impaired sensation.

Wounds can lead to a long road of healing and intervention, especially as they become more severe. Precautions around wearing the AFOs and the likelihood of skin breakdown were reviewed with the parents. Martha's parents were encouraged to check her feet and lower legs often in the beginning to make sure the splints were not creating any red spots. Martha's mother redemonstrated donning and doffing of the splints and summarized the written instructions that were issued. These instructions included the wearing schedule, precautions, and care of the splints. The doctor requested that they return to the clinic in another 3 to 4 months.

Martha returned to the clinic when she was 9 months old. She was still not sitting independently, but she did hold her head up well in supported sitting. She had started to feed herself finger foods, but her mother said that she often shoveled many baby puffs into her mouth instead of one at a time. She was able to put weight on her legs when supported in standing. Her AFOs had worked out well; however, there were some pressure points as she was growing. The OT made modifications on this date for better fit. Based on her urodynamics testing, the urologist recommended beginning catheterization every 3 to 4 hours. She was demonstrating kidney reflux and not emptying her bladder completely into her diaper. The family was instructed in clinic how to do this, and they were issued some samples to get them through until they could get their own supplies from their medical supply company. They were to return when Martha was 1 year old.

At the 1-year appointment, the OT observed Martha and discussed with the family how she was using her hands to manipulate toys and food. She had not yet mastered grasping items with her thumb and index finger and usually just used a gross grasp. Her parents were encouraged to practice this type of grasp with Martha, but they were also assured that it was typical for children with SB to be delayed in this development. Martha was using both hands equally and not demonstrating a preference. The OT recommended EI evaluation for OT services. At this time, Martha was finally sleeping through the night and continued to tolerate the AFOs; however, new ones were fabricated because she had outgrown the old ones. Her ankles remained tight but maintained range of motion well with the braces.

Martha returned to the clinic 6 months later when she was 18 months old. Martha had begun receiving OT every other week through EI, and continued to receive weekly PT and monthly developmental therapy. She had proved herself to be a determined young lady. At this visit, Martha was sitting independently and beginning to commando crawl. The PT and the orthopedic doctor felt confident that she would benefit from a parapodium standing frame, which allows the child to stand upright without any support from others. Martha would be able to play at the couch or toddler-sized activity table using her hands functionally for fine-motor tasks. The stander also supports social participation because Martha would be able to be at the same level as her peers. Standing programs are recommended for children with SB for multiple reasons. Standing promotes bone density from weight bearing, stretches the hip/knee/ankle joints, and uses gravity to assist with bowel and bladder emptying. At this time, it was also recommended that Martha be fitted for definitive AFOs by the orthotist. She had outgrown the AFOs that the OT fabricated, and she was ready to have a sturdier brace, especially if she was going to be weightbearing in the parapodium. Before the family left, Martha was measured for a parapodium in clinic and molded for AFOs, and she was scheduled to return in 1 month for brace fitting and training with the PT on how to don/doff the brace, as well as wearing schedules and other recommendations.

After her parapodium was issued, Martha's mother was advised to continue coming to the clinic every 6 months to monitor Martha's development and orthopedic issues. The parapodium and AFOs were effective in keeping her ankle joints supple. At home, she was commando crawling to get around or scooting on her bottom. The clinic OT continued to assess her upper extremity function and strength through the years as well as her development with her ADL. Martha was evaluated and assessed for a manual wheelchair, which she received around the same time that she started preschool at age 3. The wheelchair also had a pressure-relieving cushion, which was key to her skin integrity. Martha continued to have fine-motor deficits and was mostly dependent with her ADL until she was 5 years old. Martha continued to get catheterized by her parents, although she was involved in gathering her supplies and washing her hands. At age 5, Martha was able to don/doff her shirt and wash her hands and face with a rag, but not at the sink because it was not accessible at home. Martha did have enough strength in her arms and trunk and desire to walk and was subsequently fitted and issued with a reciprocating gait orthosis and walker to begin upright mobility. The clinic PT and her community PT were in close contact regarding this training and recommendations. The clinic OT recommended ways for Martha to increase her independence with her self-dressing techniques, including sitting against the wall or in a corner on the floor for better support with dynamic sitting. She also trialed a pediatric sock aid to don her socks after her parents set up the socks on the sock aid for her. All of this practice was recommended for the weekends and weeknights, as the parents were often in a rush in the mornings trying to get the girls ready for school. The clinic OT also issued them a dressing achievement chart (Figure 5-6) to track Martha's progress and post stickers every time she was able to do the tasks in order to motivate her.

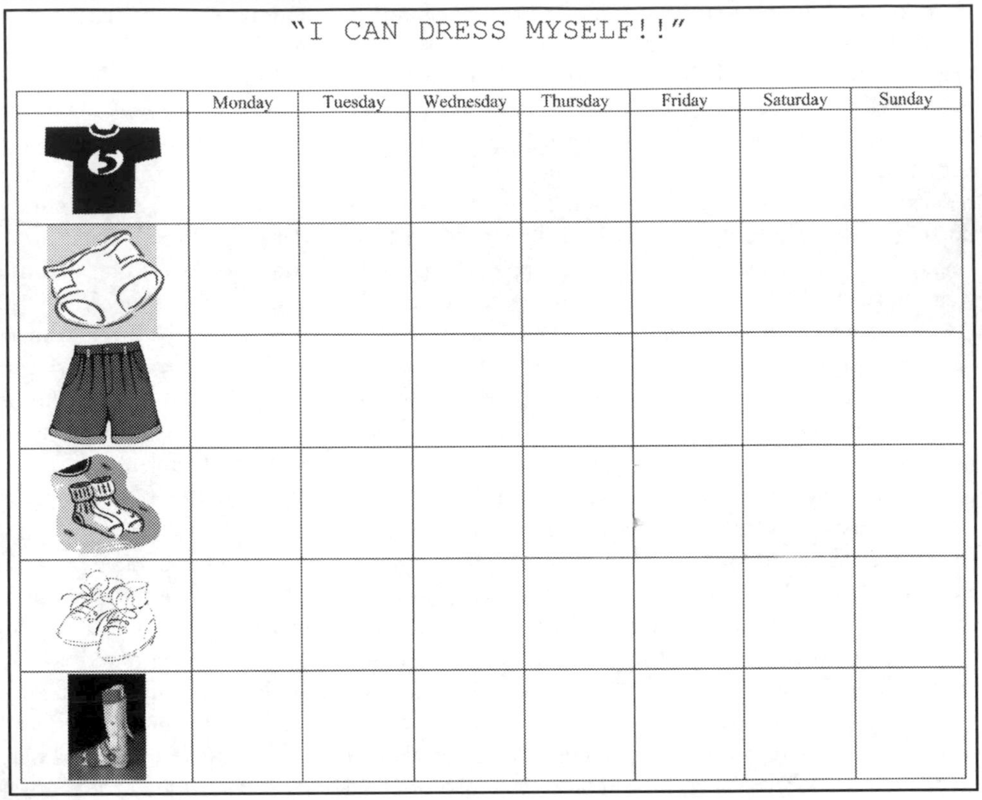

Figure 5-6. Dressing chart for Martha.

"I CAN DRESS MYSELF!!"

	Monday	Tuesday	Wednesday	Thursday	Friday	Saturday	Sunday

Occupational Therapy Intervention

When Martha was 9 years old, her mother reported to the clinic staff that she was beginning to feel very stressed and anxious. Martha's mother was performing catheterization on Martha and even going to the school to do it. The school nurse was willing to catheterize Martha, but Martha's mother did not feel comfortable with anyone else doing it. Therefore, Martha's mother was going to school two to three times per day in order to do it. Martha's mother was trying to get a part-time job and would not be able to continue with this schedule. She was wondering if there was any chance that Martha could learn to catheterize herself. The OT did an updated screen on skills related to self-catheterization. She assessed sitting balance in different positions (i.e., long sitting, short sitting, and ring sitting), as well as ADL status, fine-motor coordination, visual perception, and grip and tip/lateral pinch strength. Martha was finally independent in all her ADL, except for getting her pants over her bottom, donning her shoes over her AFOs, and perineal cleansing for bathing.

Despite the strengths listed above, Martha has some cognitive learning issues as well as mild deficits in fine-motor coordination and visual perception. However, the OT thought that Martha could be a good candidate for self-catheterization.

An intensive outpatient OT program was set up that involved Martha coming to the hospital for several hours each day to work with the OT and a nurse in order to learn catheter insertion as well as all the pre- or post-activities that are related to this. Martha's mother agreed to the plan. The OT and nurse worked closely with Martha when she came in for intensive therapy for self-catheterization training. The treatment plan centered on improving the skills stated previously as well as actual trials for catheter insertion. Before this was trialed, Martha was instructed to remove the catheter and get familiar with the anatomy of where the tube was located. Adaptive tools were used, such as a mirror that sat on the bed so that she could watch the nurse and see what she was doing when she tried herself. The ultimate goal was to get Martha to be able to do this without any mirror, as it is not always convenient or realistic to use one.

Questions to Consider

1. Develop a time line that outlines Martha's developmental progress. Compare this time line to typical development. Include motor development, as well as self-care skills.
2. Describe strategies that the EI OT and the clinic OT could use to share information about Martha. What would need to be in place before they could communicate?

3. How is the role of the clinic OT different from the role of OTs in other pediatric settings?
4. What are the steps involved in self-catheterization?
5. Write two to three short-term goals for Martha that lead to independence with self-catheterization.
6. How many visits do you think Martha will have to attend before she is independent with self-catheterization?
7. What are some assessment tools that could be used to assess Martha's readiness for self-catheterization?
8. What are some informal ways that Martha could be evaluated for readiness skills? Provide specific examples.
9. Describe a 60-minute treatment session that addresses at least one of the goals you developed above.
10. Imagine Martha is ready to try self-catheterization at school. Design a self-catheterization kit that Martha will take with her into the bathroom. Be specific about what is included in the kit.
11. What do you think is the next developmental challenge that Martha will encounter related to self-care?
12. How could OT address Martha's next self-care developmental challenge?

Resources

Liptak, G. (2013). Neural tube defect. In M. Batshaw, N. Roizen, & G. Lotrecchiano (Eds.), *Children with disabilities* (7th ed., pp. 451-472). Baltimore: Paul H. Brookes Publishing.

The Ohio State University Wexner Medical Center. (2012). Female self-catheterization. Retrieved from: https://patienteducation.osumc.edu/Documents/fem-sf-c.pdf

Shepherd, J. (2010). Activities of daily living. In J. Case-Smith & J. O'Brien (Eds.). *Occupational therapy for children* (6th ed.) (pp. 474-517). St. Louis: Elsevier/Mosby.

Liam: Acute Myeloid Leukemia, Septic Shock, Cardiac Myopathy/ Oncology

Lisa Robken, OTR

History and Background Information

At 35 months old, Liam was an energetic boy and had achieved all of his milestones. He lives with his mother and grandmother and is the only biological child of his mother. The father is estranged from the family. Liam loves to do crafts, run, and watch the Disney Channel. For 1 month, Liam sought treatment for low-grade fever, mouth sores, and lethargy, which did not improve despite multiple antibiotics. He then presented to the local ED with a fever of 104°F. Blood work revealed pancytopenia. Liam was immediately transferred to a specialized oncology hospital for diagnostic workup and treatment.

At the oncology hospital, Liam received the diagnosis of Acute Myeloid Leukemia (AML). The 5-year survival rate for pediatric AML is 60% to 70% (cancer.org). A central port was placed and Liam immediately began treatment, consisting of five cycles of cytarabine, tobramycin, and etoposide. His last chemotherapy cycle was an intrathecal combination of cytarabine and mitoxantrone. His cancer treatment was unremarkable for complications, and Liam remained playful with high energy. Peer and public interactions were limited due to a compromised immune system. Functional mobility and hand skills remained normal. Plans were also in place for him to attend preschool in the fall with doctor approval.

Seven months after the completion of his treatment, when Liam was 47 months old, he developed a cough, runny nose, and fever despite a round of amoxicillin. He was admitted to the inpatient pediatric unit for management and found to have relapsed. Within hours of his admission, he experienced septic shock and respiratory failure requiring intubation and sedation. He required the use of vasopressors to manage his blood pressure. At week 1 of intubation, his ejection fraction dropped to 30%. An OT order was received 2 weeks after Liam's admittance, during which time he remained sedated and intubated.

Evaluation Information

Occupational Profile

Prior to entering the room, the therapist speaks to the bedside nurse and advanced practice nurse, who report the patient is stable for therapy. Liam's immediate environment included an abundance of stuffed animals and blankets. He lies supine and is buried so deep in blankets that only his face is visible. He appears to be very anxious. Liam whimpers when the OT introduces herself. His mother is present and agrees to the evaluation. The OT gently engages Liam in conversation, and he allows her to borrow his favorite owl puppet. According to mom, Liam loves his stuffed animals. The OT uses the puppet to coax Liam into a rapport-building activity, and Liam smiles and participates. Upon request from the therapist and owl puppet, Liam sits up with her on the edge of the bed, then he immediately withdraws and becomes silent.

Mom reports that he has become increasingly fussy when he is taken out of his "cocoon."

Liam's Parents' Goals for Rehabilitation

The OT discusses goals and the role of OT with the mom. Mom reports that she would like Liam to return to the skills he had before the intensive care unit (ICU), which include walking, toileting, dressing, and performing all transfers independently. She hopes to see these improvements in 1 week if not sooner.

Analysis of Occupational Performance

With encouragement, Liam reluctantly agrees to leave his cocoon as long as he can keep his blanket on his lap. As Liam moves, the therapist notes a stage II pressure sore behind his ears and muscle atrophy throughout his entire body. When he grasps for his stuffed animal, he must slide it along the bed because he says it feels "too big."

Client Factors/Body Functions

- Bilateral upper extremities: Passive range of motion (PROM) is within functional limits, and active range of motion (AROM) in shoulder flexion and abduction is 90 degrees against gravity.
- Bilateral lower extremities: Liam's lower extremities' PROM and AROM knee flexion are -20 degrees.

Neuromusculoskeletal and Movement-Related Functions

- Sitting: Maximal assistance is required to bring Liam from supine to sitting for the first time since intubation, and he is in a diaper despite being potty trained. He requires moderate assistance throughout sitting because of his weakened core. His abdomen is distended from fluid overload. There are no arches in the left hand and minimal arches in the right. Liam cries the entire 7 minutes he sits. There is an arterial line in his left hand in addition to a peripherally inserted central catheter, pulse oximeter, and heart monitor. His resting heart rate of 100 beats per minute increases to 120 and his oxygen saturations drop from 99% to 94%.
- Standing: Mom is encouraging the therapist to move Liam to a standing position because she feels it is important for him to move immediately.

Questions to Consider

1. As a therapist working with a very anxious little boy, what can you say to make him feel more comfortable?
2. What could you change in the ICU room environment to reduce Liam's anxiety?
3. What other activities can you do to establish rapport?
4. With multiple patients to see, how much time would you spend building rapport before physically cueing Liam to task?

Goal Areas and Treatment

1. What are Liam's strengths?
2. Develop a problem list for Liam.
3. What short-term goals should you address first given Mom's broad list? Write a list of four short-term goals and four long-term goals.
4. Do you think Mom's expectations match the time frame you are expecting in Liam's recovery? If no, how would you address this?
5. What are some of the obstacles that could prevent Liam from achieving the goals?
6. Which frame of reference would be appropriate to consider when developing treatments?
7. What would be a good frequency to see Liam?

Safety Precautions

1. Would you stand Liam as mom requests? If not, what would you tell mom?
2. Should mom's eagerness be discussed with the medical team?
3. What other precautions should be taken while Liam sits up for the first time? Would you consider having another discipline present?
4. What physical signs of intolerance would you look for in Liam during treatment?
5. How could you communicate to Liam, on a level he would understand, to be mindful of the arterial line in his left hand? Why does the arterial line require specific caution compared with his peripherally inserted central catheter and monitors?

Areas of Occupation

1. What is appropriate for a boy 47 months old in terms of his ADL?
2. Would you consider Liam's ADL impaired? Which ones?
3. What other ADL not mentioned might also be impaired?
4. Would you discuss with mom the importance of regaining his achieved ADL at the evaluation? Why or why not?
5. Because of Liam's problem list, is it likely that he will be attending preschool as planned?
6. Based on what the therapist observed in his hand skills, do you think he has become delayed in expected hand grasps that precede functional handwriting?

7. At this time, would you consider this delay a priority? Why or why not?
8. Do you think Liam feels like playing right now?
9. What could you do to help incorporate play into the evaluation and treatment sessions?
10. Do you think he is capable at this time to engage in play the way he used to? Do you think this might frustrate Liam, and if so, how can you ease his frustrations?

Client Factors

1. Which of Liam's body functions are most impaired?
2. Do your goals incorporate these body functions?

Habits, Roles, Routines, Rituals

1. What are some of Liam's routines that have been impacted?
2. Have any of his routines remained the same? If not, how could you establish them in your treatment plan?
3. What are the typical roles of boys Liam's age? Have any of these roles been impacted?

Occupational Therapy Intervention

Session 3

Liam improves in sitting tolerance requiring minimal assistance-supervision. He is officially weaned from his vasopressors but continues to have an elevated heart rate at 130 beats per minute. Would you consider standing Liam? Whom might you consult on the pediatric ICU team prior to doing this? How could you incorporate an occupation-based activity into standing?

Session 5

After 1 additional week in the ICU, Liam improves medically and transfers to the inpatient pediatric unit. Liam is exhausted and only gets out of bed with help from OT and PT. He also continues to cry and fuss, which inhibits his participation. The mom verbalizes to the therapist that he is fussy as a means to delay treatment. The therapist believes this to be accurate because Liam always asks her to come back later or will take 10 minutes to chew one chicken nugget when he takes 2 minutes with mom. The OT decides to use the Model of Human Occupation (MOHO) to better understand Liam's volition. With this model, the therapist learns that Liam will do anything for a hug from his mom, his favorite candy, going on wheelchair rides, and coloring.

1. What are some ways to incorporate these aspects into his treatment?
2. What else can you do to help Liam enjoy his therapy sessions?
3. How can you grade these activities to progress with his goals?
4. Would you consider it a poor outcome if, despite these efforts, Liam continues to cry and be fussy?
5. Could you use this discovery to build his sense of competence? How?

Session 6

The therapist's discoveries from the MOHO framework have helped to move the sessions along, although Liam continues to cry whenever the therapist and any medical staff enter his room. The crying becomes louder when the therapist/staff touch anything on his bed or tell him to do something. The therapist believes that Liam might be acting out during the little opportunity he has to exercise control and decision making in the hospital environment.

1. What other context and environment could be influencing his behavior besides the hospital? Consider the cultural, personal, temporal, virtual, physical, and social aspects.
2. What are the positive influences in his environment and what are the negative? Create a list.
3. Out of the above list, can the therapist address any of these in his treatments?

Other Treatment Situations

Session 7

Two weeks have passed since Liam left the ICU. He sits with supervision while engaging in craft activities, and AROM shoulder flexion is within normal limits as evidenced in reaching for toys and assisting mom in donning his shirt. Because of decreased extension in his lower extremities, he has great difficulty standing. You suspect that standing is the biggest factor inhibiting his mobility.

1. Why would mobility be a concern for OT?
2. What occupation-based interventions could you develop to incorporate mobility?
3. Due to the nature of leukemia and chronic low blood counts, fatigue is an important factor in Liam's therapy. How could you tell if this is a contributing factor to his limited mobility in addition to decreased extension?
4. What treatments could you provide to help increase his activity tolerance?

Session 10

Liam's white blood cell count becomes increasingly low, reading 0.1 per L. The normal range is 3.0 to 5.0 per L. As a result, all visiting staff and friends must wear a mask when interacting with Liam. The mask covers the wearer's face from the nose to the neck, leaving the eyes visible and muffling the voice. The OT notices that the mask increases Liam's anxiety. Subsequently, the OT decides to bring markers that have been used with other patients so that Liam can draw a nose and mouth on the therapist's mask.

1. What should the therapist do to the markers prior to taking them into Liam's room due to Liam's critically low white blood cell count?
2. How can the therapist set up Liam's treatment in order to address his decreased standing and out of bed activity?
3. What if Liam is nervous to do the task with the therapist? Who else in his personal environment would you consider involving to make the activity less daunting?
4. What adaptations may need to be considered in order for Liam to utilize the markers?

Session 16

Unfortunately, it seems that Liam has plateaued during the past six treatment sessions. The therapist believes it is because mom does not consistently follow up with therapist recommendations for increasing out-of-bed activity. She does not want to be perceived as the "bad guy" when Liam has been so sick.

1. What practice framework would you consider to better understand this situation?
2. Why is this important to address with Liam's mom?
3. What are some considerations when discussing your concerns with mom?
4. If mom does not agree to increase out-of-bed activity outside of therapy treatment, would you consider discharging Liam?
5. How could you support mom during this time?
6. What other disciplines might be helpful in providing insight into this situation? Would you consider making a referral to another discipline?

Session 18

Liam is having a particularly fussy day. When the therapist walks in, Liam states, "Doing therapy today is not possible." There are no medical reasons that would prevent therapy, and Liam's mom is encouraging therapy. What should the therapist do?

Session 19

Over the past few sessions, the OT has implemented a routine with Liam, where she comes 15 minutes before therapy is to start to let him know what time therapy will begin. The therapist also asks Liam what he would like to do today, and she incorporates this as a reward at the end of the session. What other behavioral approaches would you consider?

Session 20

Liam considers himself well enough to attempt to get out of bed without help. When the therapist walks in, mom is in the bathroom and Liam is climbing over the bed rails. What should the therapist do?

Session 21

The therapist decides that Liam would benefit from an obstacle course. He fatigues more quickly than in previous sessions and his abdomen appears distended. Should the therapist be concerned? Who should be alerted of the therapist's observations?

Planning for Discharge

Liam is medically stable and preparing for discharge. The therapist assesses his progress and realizes he has not achieved his long-term goals, despite demonstrating increased sitting tolerance and out-of-bed activity. The therapist considers recommending home health therapy and outpatient therapy.

1. Would Liam do better in home health or outpatient care?
2. How might Liam's low blood counts influence his therapy setting?
3. Would the expected outcome change depending on his setting? Why or why not?

Reference

Surivival rates for childhood leukemia. (2013). Retrieved August 20, 2014, from http://www.cancer.org/cancer/leukemiainchildren/overviewguide/childhood-leukemia-overview-survival-rates

Resources

Dudgeon, B., & Crooks, L. (2010). Hospital and rehabilitation services. In J. Case-Smith & J. O'Brien (Eds.), *Occupational therapy for children* (6th ed.) (pp. 785-811). St. Louis: Elsevier.

Longpre, S., & Newman, R. (2011). AOTA Fact sheet: The role of occupational therapy in oncology. Retrieved from: http://www.aota.org/~/media/Corporate/Files/AboutOT/Professionals/WhatIsOT/RDP/Facts/Oncology%20fact%20sheet.ashx

Robby: Feeding Disorder/ Hospital-Based Feeding Clinic

Patricia W. Ideran, OTR/L, CEIM and Jennifer L. Zieman, MOTR/L, CEIM

History and Background Information

Robby, age 4 years, has a diagnosis of feeding disorder and was recently diagnosed with autism. He lives with his mother, father, and 2-year-old typically developing sister. He is being raised in a middle-class household with both parents, who are employed full time. He is currently attending an early childhood program 3 days per week and receives speech therapy and OT as a part of his programming. He was not receiving any additional outpatient services at the time of assessment. He attends a home daycare when he is not in school.

Medical History

Robby was born at 38 weeks gestation with no prenatal or postnatal complications. He had respiratory syncytial virus, bronchiolitis, and ear infections as a baby. Robby has a history of constipation. He is under the care of a pediatric gastroenterologist and developmental pediatrician. Robby is also followed by ophthalmology and wears glasses. He is currently on the following medications: gummy vitamins and Miralax (polyethylene glycol). His mother reports he currently holds his bowel movements and spends one-quarter of the day in the corner trying to not go to the bathroom. He is potty trained. His weight was slightly below the 50th percentile and his height was in the 25th percentile.

Robby was breastfed for the first 6 months of life with no difficulties and then transitioned to the bottle without difficulty. He was introduced to baby cereal at 4 months of age, pureed stage I at 5 months, and pureed stage II at 6 months, all without difficulty. When Robby's mother introduced pureed stage III foods, he started to display gagging and head turning upon presentation of the spoon. Robby's parents went back to stage II foods, which were successful. At 7 months, the parents began to introduce table foods such as smashed banana and puffs (meltable solids) with gagging, choking, and refusals observed. Because of Robby's negative response to stage III and table foods, his parents continued with stage II until 1 year of age. At this time, his parents brought the child in for his well exam and voiced concerns regarding Robby's feeding difficulties. The pediatrician advised Robby's parents to switch him from formula to whole milk, continue with purees, and continue offering table foods. Robby was accepting adult purees (e.g., pudding, yogurt, applesauce) but was still not accepting foods with texture. At 19 months of age, Robby had a choking incident on a chicken nugget and has refused them since then. There were no concerns with liquids.

At 3.5 years of age, the parents continued to voice concerns regarding Robby's inability to accept more food groups and textures. At that time, Robby's pediatrician made a referral to the pediatric feeding team at the local children's hospital. The pediatric feeding team consisted of a pediatric gastroenterologist, behavioral psychologist, nutritionist, speech therapist, and OT. They evaluated Robby and concluded that he continued to have problems with constipation; he had appropriate height and weight for his age on the pediatric growth chart and had no oral motor concerns. Feeding concerns were primarily behavioral and sensory-based, which generated a referral to OT.

Evaluation Information

Robby was evaluated by an OT specializing in feeding therapy. He was 3.5 years old and was accompanied by his mother. Robby was evaluated for feeding only. Developmental delays and sensory processing deficits were evident, though these were not formally evaluated. At this time, Robby would eat only the following foods: small white powdered donuts, Goldfish crackers (Pepperidge Farms), cheese crackers, plain white bread, McDonald's french fries, Gerber fruit strips, green grapes, yogurt (strawberry and blueberry), apples, cherries, oranges, soft-serve vanilla ice cream, applesauce, pretzels, Quaker Oats Life cinnamon cereal dry (no milk), Lucky Charms cereal dry (General Mills), Nilla wafers (Nabisco), potato chips, crispy rice treats (homemade only), peanut butter and honey on toast, Hershey's chocolate (plain only), M&M's (Mars), Oreos (inside frosting only; Nabisco), and blue-flavored suckers. Liquids included water, orange juice, apple juice, and berry juice. The parents, therapist, and Robby were seated at a kid-sized table for the evaluation. His parents brought some preferred foods and some nonpreferred foods to the evaluation. His mother set out foods for him to eat and modeled eating. The observation revealed conflict when any nonpreferred food was offered. Robby turned away, said no, and pushed his mother's hand away. Robby eagerly ate his preferred foods.

Based on the parent interview, Robby does not have regular scheduled meals or snacks; he grazes on food and liquids throughout the day. Robby eats either at the kitchen table or child-sized table and chair. Robby needs encouragement to stay seated for all meals and frequently fidgets when seated. He independently feeds himself finger foods, uses a spoon with a palmar grasp, and drinks from an open cup. He was able to use a fork, though had difficulty piercing foods successfully.

Sensory processing as it relates to feeding includes gagging at the sight of nonpreferred foods. His preferred texture is crisp and crunchy. He smells all food, including preferred and nonpreferred. He chews on ice cubes. He does not like to touch certain foods or get his hands messy, resulting in frequent requests for a napkin to wipe his hands during meals.

Behavioral outcomes with feeding and the introduction of new foods include verbal refusal, gagging, spitting, verbal negotiation/bribing, and a history of vomiting when a new food is presented.

Robby presented with mild gross-motor and motor planning deficits. He also exhibited decreased muscle tone globally.

Questions to Consider

Goals/Treatment Plan

1. Write out a problem list for Robby.
2. What strengths do you see with the child?
3. What are positive details about his diet?
4. What deficit areas does this child exhibit?
5. What short-term goals and long-term goals would you establish?
6. What OT frames of reference would you use?

Safety Precautions

1. What are the primary safety concerns with Robby?

Neuromusculoskeletal

1. Identify how deficits in this area affect feeding.

Psychosocial/Behavioral

1. What impact do his behaviors have on the family at mealtime?
2. How are his feeding problems impacting his ability to participate in social outings?
3. How are his feeding problems affecting participation at school and daycare?

Family Education/Home Programming

1. Describe important topics that should be discussed with the family.
2. What are some specific activities and/or structures you would recommend to the family?
3. Identify long-term consequences of these feeding problems if they are not addressed in feeding therapy.

Discharge Planning

1. When do you discharge from feeding therapy?
2. What home program would you provide to the family upon discharge?
3. What kind of follow-up would you recommend?

Resources

Arvedson, J., & Brodsky, L. (2002). *Pediatric swallowing and feeding: Assessment and management* (2nd ed.). San Diego, CA: Singular Publishing Group.

Chatoor, I. (2009). *Diagnosis and treatment of feeding disorders in infants, toddlers, and young children.* Washington, DC: Zero to Three.

Ernsperger, L., & Stegen-Hanson, T. (2004). *Just take a bite: Easy, effective answers to food aversions and eating challenges.* Arlington, TX: Future Horizons, Inc.

Fishbein, M., Fraker, C., Cox, S., & Walbert, L. (2007). *Food chaining: The proven 6-step plan to stop picky eating, solve feeding problems and expand your child's diet.* New York: Marlowe & Company.

Kedesdy, J., & Budd, K. (1998). *Childhood feeding disorders: Biobehavioral assessment and intervention.* Baltimore: Paul H. Brookes Publishing Co.

Morris, S., & Klein, M. (2000). *Pre-feeding skills* (2nd ed.). Austin, TX: Pro-ed.

Lyrik: Amyoplasia Multiplex Congenita/Outpatient

Angela R. Shierk, PhD, OTR

History and Background Information

Lyrik is a 5-year, 3-month-old female with amyoplasia multiplex congenita. Her past medical history includes a right elbow release, triceps plasty, and carpal wedge osteotomy at age 3. She has also used wrist and elbow splints in the past to promote wrist extension and elbow flexion. Lyrik's parents and the physician attribute increased use of her right upper extremity during functional tasks to improved positioning of her elbow and wrist postoperatively.

Lyrik and her parents presented to an ambulatory care clinic and were seen by a hand surgeon. The hand surgeon recommended a carpal wedge osteotomy and possible thenar release on the left upper extremity. The family was going to consider this surgical option and would contact the hand team when they were ready to proceed. At the end of the visit, the physician wrote an order for an OT to fabricate elbow splints and address independence with ADL. Prior to seeing Lyrik, the OT reviewed her medical record and obtained the following information.

Evaluation Information

Orthopedic Surgeon Note

Lyrik was seen by an orthopedic surgeon at age 5 years, 2 months. During that visit, Lyrik's mother reported that her outpatient PT wanted to try some long-leg bracing to see if it would provide Lyrik with some stability to stand independently. At the time of the visit, Lyrik was not able to pull to stand independently or stand without support. The physician reported that Lyrik had good trunk control and that her spine appeared straight. She had good abduction of both hips during the clinical exam, and her knee range of motion was from 0 to 30 degrees of flexion. The physician recommended trying plastic knee-ankle-foot orthoses (KAFOs) to see if they would provide some stability at her knees and enable her to stand independently. She will follow up with the orthopedic surgeon in 1 year for repeat evaluation. A referral was made to orthotics to initiate making the KAFOs.

Orthotics Note

Lyrik was provided with solid gutter splint-style KAFOs with heel wedges at age 5 years, 3 months (Figure 5-7). She was also provided with a size medium KAFO sock. Lyrik and her parents were educated on donning and doffing techniques, skin care, and brace wear and care schedule.

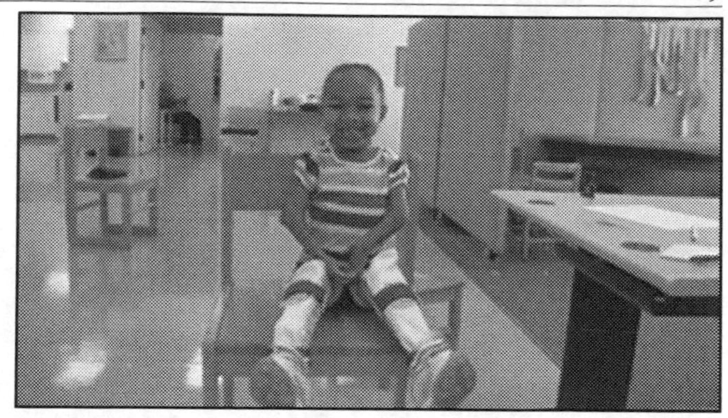

Figure 5-7. Lyrik sitting in chair wearing KAFOs.

Previous Hand Surgeon Note

Lyrik was last seen by the hand surgeon at age 4 years, 8 months. The physician reported that Lyrik had not been seen in quite some time due to the family having difficulty making it to follow-up appointments. As a result, the mother stated that she had not been doing much in terms of stretching for Lyrik and noticed some loss of motion in the elbows. The hand surgeon emphasized the need to continue range of motion exercises and wrote a referral for OT to review passive range of motion exercises.

Previous Occupational Therapy Note

Lyrik was seen by an OT at the same time as her last appointment with the hand surgeon at age 4 years, 8 months. The previous evaluation and home program focused on improving passive range of motion for bilateral elbow flexion and passive range of motion for left wrist extension. Lyrik's passive range of motion measurements were 95 degrees for right elbow flexion and 105 degrees for left elbow flexion. Her right wrist has been in a neutral position since surgical intervention, and her left wrist was lacking 25 degrees to neutral passively. The family was also provided with lightweight utensils and cylindrical foam to increase independence with feeding at home. The family was encouraged to continue daily passive range of motion exercises to improve elbow flexion bilaterally and left wrist extension.

Occupational Therapy Evaluation

1. Based on the information that you have, what additional information would you want to collect during an OT evaluation?
   a. Areas of occupation
   b. Client factors
   c. Performance skills
   d. Performance patterns
   e. Context and environment
   f. Activity demands
2. Which evaluation tools would you use to guide your assessment?
3. Review Lyrik's diagnosis and write a brief paragraph explaining amyoplasia multiplex congenita.
4. Review developmental milestones and make a list of activities that are age-appropriate for a 5 year old (cognitive, social, gross motor, fine motor, self-care).
5. After reviewing the diagnosis and developmental milestones, make a list of activities that you think Lyrik may have difficulty completing independently.

Occupational Profile

The OT completes an evaluation including patient and parent interview, observation, range of motion measurements, and the Canadian Occupational Performance Measure. Lyrik is a bright and pleasant young lady. She is very articulate, socially appropriate, and easy to communicate with during the OT evaluation. Based on conversation and observation, Lyrik's cognitive ability is average or above average compared with peers her age. She is able to answer the therapist's questions, voluntarily asks questions, and helps with problem solving throughout the therapy session. She is able to verbalize an appropriate motor plan to complete an action, but due to limitations in active and passive range of motion in her upper and lower extremities, she has difficulty completing motor tasks. She has some fear with trying new tasks that involve standing due to a fear of falling, but she is able to verbalize her concerns and will try a new task after specific instructions are given and she knows that she will be safe. Her vision and hearing are within normal limits, and she is otherwise healthy.

Lyrik's and Her Parents' Goals

- Increase independence with toileting
- Increase independence with dressing
- Increase independence with self-feeding
- Strategies for writing/coloring using her hands
- Increasing upper extremity passive range of motion

Areas of Occupation

Lyrik is dependent or requires maximum assistance for most activities of daily living including bathing, toileting, and self-feeding with utensils. She can independently drink from a straw if the cup is sitting on the table, and she can eat finger foods independently with her right hand. The family tried using the utensils and cylindrical foam provided at the previous OT session, but they report that the foam and utensils are too heavy for Lyrik to use independently. She can independently take off her jacket if it is already unzipped, and she is able to remove a pair of boots and her socks independently. She is dependent for putting her shirt on and taking it off and for donning her pants. She requires moderate assistance to doff her pants. She is dependent for fasteners, including buttons, zippers, snaps, and shoelaces. She brushes her teeth with setup and supervision. She can color using her feet and is starting to write letters. She can loosely hold a pencil in her hand, but has difficulty putting enough pressure on the paper, making her writing very light.

Client Factors

Lyrik presents with the diagnosis of amyoplasia multiplex congenital, a condition that is associated with multiple congenital joint contractures.

Neuromusculoskeletal and Movement-Related Functions

- Bilateral upper extremities: At rest, Lyrik's bilateral upper extremities are positioned in an internally rotated, adducted position with her elbows extended, wrists in flexion on left and in neutral on the right, and fingers extended. She has 30 degrees of active shoulder flexion and 110 degrees of passive shoulder flexion. She does not have any active shoulder abduction, extension, or external rotation. She has 90 degrees of passive elbow flexion bilaterally and no active elbow flexion. Her left wrist lacks 25 degrees to neutral passively, and her right wrist is in a neutral position.
- Bilateral upper extremity function: Lyrik uses her right hand, demonstrating a weak grasp, and is able to release objects independently. She uses her hands together at midline to move and hold objects, and she also uses her feet to manipulate objects and for functional activities. She can bring her hand to her mouth or face by propping her right arm on a surface or her leg and passively bend her elbow using her leg or her trunk to bring her hand toward her face.
- Bilateral lower extremities: Lyrik has good active and passive range of motion at the hips. She has 30 degrees of knee flexion, and her feet are in a plantarflexed position. She has good dexterity using her first and second toes bilaterally.
- Sitting and standing: She has good head control, rolls independently, transitions from supine to sitting independently, sits independently and scoots on her bottom independently. She uses KAFOs for standing with support and is working on independent standing.
- Mobility: Lyrik uses a stroller for community mobility. She uses a power wheelchair in the home but is unable to use it in the community because she is not able to transport the wheelchair in the family's vehicle. The family is working with a vendor for vehicle modifications so that the wheelchair can be transported.

Contexts and Environment

Lyrik's parents are supportive of her desire to gain independence and meet her goals. She currently stays at home during the day and will attend kindergarten in the fall. She receives outpatient OT and PT two times per week. Her daily routines are typical for a 5-year-old child and include getting up, getting dressed, eating breakfast, playing, eating lunch and dinner, taking a bath, and spending time with family.

Questions to Consider

Goals/Treatment

1. Create a list of Lyrik's strengths and challenges.
2. Based on the information presented, where would you start with intervention (think about physician referral and what is important to the family)?
3. Write out short-term and long-term goals for Lyrik.
4. What are the activity demands of each goal that you are planning to address?

5. List strategies that you would use to assist Lyrik in meeting her short- and long-term goals.
   a. What remedial strategies would you recommend?
   b. How would you adapt tasks to increase independence?
   c. How would you adapt the environment to increase independence?
   d. What education would you provide to the patient and parents?
   e. Are there any additional referrals that you would make? If so, to whom?
   f. Is there anyone that you would collaborate with regarding Lyrik's plan of care?

Intervention Plan

1. Describe the treatment session that you would provide in conjunction with the physician visit.
2. Write out a home program for the family to work on until their return to clinic.
3. How would you assess the outcome of intervention?
4. When would it be appropriate to discharge the patient?

Situations

1. During the OT session following the evaluation, custom elbow splints were fabricated and a prefabricated wrist cock-up splint was provided for her left wrist to be worn at night time to increase passive range of motion. At the follow-up visit, Lyrik had gained 10 degrees of passive range of motion at each joint. What would be the next step in the plan of care to continue to increase range of motion?
2. Lyrik and her parents were educated on the use of a toilet aid to assist with toilet hygiene. The parents report that the toilet aid is too heavy and is difficult for Lyrik to use. What other strategies could you recommend to increase independence?
3. Lyrik and her parents were educated on the use of a sock aid to don socks, and Lyrik is now independent with donning her socks using the sock aid. She would now like to be more independent with donning her shirt and pants. How could you adapt the environment to promote independence?

Resource

Shepherd, J. (2010). Activities of daily living. In J. Case-Smith & J. O'Brien (Eds.), *Occupational therapy for children* (6th ed., pp. 474-517). St. Louis: Elsevier.

Jane: Pediatric Spinal Cord Injury/Inpatient Rehabilitation

Elizabeth Kohler-Rausch, OTR/L

History and Background Information

Acute Care History

Jane is a 17 year old diagnosed with an incomplete C6 SCI due to a diving accident. Jane had been drinking during a graduation party at a friend's lake house prior to the incident. She assisted her friends in pulling herself out of the pool and reported that she hit the back of her head and could not move her legs. Her friends immediately called 911. Upon arrival to a local hospital, her blood alcohol level measured 0.155. The following day, Jane was transferred to a Chicago-based hospital for further care. She was sedated, paralyzed, and intubated for airway protection before being moved. Upon arrival at the medical center, Jane underwent an emergency tracheostomy due to respiratory arrest. While on a ventilator, Jane was able to answer yes/no questions by nodding. Additional medical procedures included a C5 corpectomy, anterior and posterior spinal fusion with allograft and instrumentation, and gastrostomy. Her acute stay lasted 6 weeks.

Additional evaluation information can be found in Table 5-6.

Inpatient Rehabilitation

Jane was admitted for inpatient rehabilitation at a Chicago-based facility. She remained in the PICU for 3 days and then was moved to the inpatient unit. At present, she is being weaned off g-tube feedings with daily monitoring of her caloric intake. Jane has one wound located at the tracheostomy site. Respiratory considerations include plans to place a smaller tracheostomy tube, introducing a passy-muir valve, and capping schedule. Precautions for OT treatment include wearing a cervical collar when out of bed for the duration of the rehabilitation stay. The current plan for discharge is 3 months from her admittance to this facility.

TABLE 5-6

STRENGTH

MUSCLE	RIGHT	LEFT
Elbow flexion	3+	3
Wrist extension	2	2
Elbow extension	1	1
Finger flexion	0	0
Hand intrinsics	0	0
Lower extremity	0	0
Sensory level measured at approximately T4 for light touch.		

Evaluation Information

Occupational Profile

Upon Jane's admission to the Chicago hospital, the OT completed a chart review of her acute care stay and consulted nursing for any spinal precautions. Then the OT completed a bedside interview in order to obtain an occupational history, goals, and concerns with Jane and her father.

Prior to the SCI, Jane was independent in all of her daily activities. Jane had just recently graduated from high school and planned to attend community college in the fall. Her interests include basketball, swimming, and spending time with her family and friends. She often will play board games with her family or paint her nails with her sisters. They chose this specific rehabilitation facility due to the availability of aquatic therapy. Her main goals include walking and texting on her smart phone.

Analysis of Occupational Performance

A standard protocol was created for the inpatient SCI unit. However, it is up to the therapist's clinical reasoning to find and analyze the most relevant information in regard to the client's home environment and her body functions and structures. It is also up to the therapist's clinical reasoning to select additional assessment tools for the evaluation process. Jane's plan of care includes OT and PT services two times per day, with a total of 900 minutes of therapy per week. Jane's ASIA testing placed her at a B level.

Client Factors/Body Functions

- Mental functions: Jane demonstrates age-appropriate cognitive function, safety, and judgment.

TABLE 5-7

RANGE OF MOTION

	AROM	PROM
Neck	WFL	WFL
Upper extremity	Limited	WFL
Lower extremity	Limited	WFL

- Pain: During the evaluation, Jane complained of pain in her right hand due to the IV insertion.

Neuromusculoskeletal and Movement-Related Functions:

- Height: 175 cm
- Weight: 105 kg
- Hand dominance: Right
- Range of motion (Table 5-7)

During the ROM evaluation, the therapist noted compensatory shoulder movements to achieve a greater end range. Jane demonstrated no active grasp; however, tenodesis was noted in both hands. She also demonstrates decreased balance and fine motor skills consistent with her level of injury (Table 5-8).

- Sensory function:
  - Light touch sensation
  - C2-C6, C8, T2, T3 normal
  - C7, L5, S1, and S2 impaired
  - Remaining spinal segments absent

Areas of Occupation

Currently, Jane is dependent for catheterization and bowel management. Maximum assistance is required for feeding, grooming, bathing, and dressing activities. She is dependent for all functional mobility tasks and transfers. She plans to complete an evaluation for a manual wheelchair and home evaluation for potential modifications.

Social Environment

Jane grew up in the south side of Chicago and lives with her mother, father, and two sisters. Pets include one dog. A brother and additional sister live in a nearby suburb. Jane is the youngest child. Many of her friends live near her neighborhood or in neighboring suburbs. Jane made most of her friends from being on the high school basketball and swim teams.

Physical Environment

Jane currently lives in a bilevel home. Seven steps lead to the bathroom and bedrooms. Two steps lead to the home entrance. Jane has her own room and shares a

Table 5-8

STRENGTH

JOINT MOTION	RIGHT	LEFT
Elbow flexion	5	5
Elbow extension	1	2-
Wrist extension	3+	4
Finger flexion	0	0
Hand intrinsics	0	0
Lower extremity	0	0

bathroom with her sister. The bathroom has a tub shower (Figure 5-8).

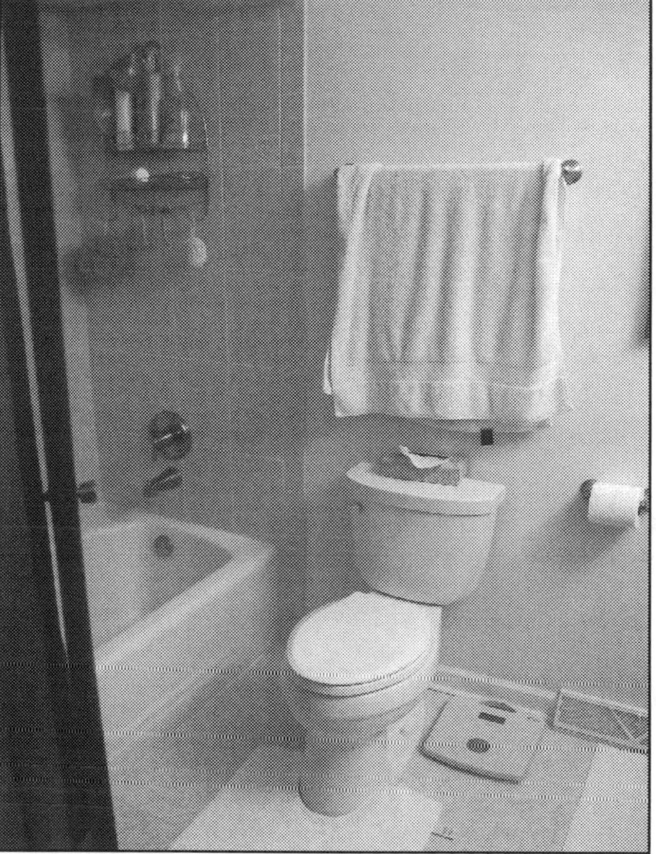

Figure 5-8. Jane's bathroom at home.

Progress Information

Jane has made gains in OT. She is able to tolerate ring sitting without back support for approximately 5 minutes. Positive protective responses have been noted when practicing mobility tasks in therapy sessions with OT and PT. She has increased her participation in grooming, feeding, and upper extremity dressing. Jane has demonstrated problem solving by independently texting a four-word sentence on her smart phone following several attempts. The OT and speech therapist conducted a co-treatment session for evaluation of computer needs and provided Jane with a typing cuff. She continues to show good potential for rehabilitation by demonstrating improved motor planning by completing strategies for ADL tasks following minimal therapist demonstrations and verbal cues. ADL assessment and level of assistance is provided in Table 5-9.

Social Environment

Jane is always accompanied by her father during OT sessions. He has participated in learning safe transfers for home use. Jane's mother is unable to attend the therapy sessions due to her distress of seeing Jane in this situation. Social work and psychiatry are addressing these concerns. In the evening and on the weekends, Jane is often visited by her siblings and friends.

Jane's mood fluctuates between sessions. Jane often requires encouragement that she is progressing in therapy. She is often focused on tasks that aim to strengthen her upper extremities and functional mobility. She is hesitant to attend any trips into the community because she does not want to be seen wearing the cervical collar in public.

Questions to Consider

Goal Areas and Treatment Focus

1. What strengths does Jane have that will enhance the treatment process?
2. What are some areas of weakness that may impact the intervention sessions?
3. Write three short-term and two long-term goals.
4. How will your goals and treatment differ from PT?
5. How will Jane's culture impact intervention and her functional outcomes?

Safety

1. What are some strategies that will increase Jane's safety when completing transfers?
2. What are signs for autonomic dysreflexia and how is it treated?
3. Does Jane have other safety concerns and how will these be addressed in your treatment sessions?

TABLE 5-9

JANE'S ACTIVITIES OF DAILY LIVING ASSESSMENT AND LEVEL OF ASSISTANCE

SELF-CARE TASK	DESCRIPTION
Grooming	Following set up of materials, Jane completes her oral care routine with minimal assistance. Currently, she completes this task in bed with back support. She utilizes a built up toothbrush and bilateral hands to align and move the toothbrush. She is dependent for hair care.
Upper extremity dressing	Jane requires moderate assistance to dress into t-shirts and her sports bra. She completes this task in bed with back support. She is unable to reach behind to pull the shirt down her back due to decreased balance.
Lower extremity dressing	Jane requires maximum assistance to complete this task in bed. She participates in threading her feet into athletic shorts and pulling them over her knees with assistance. She requires maximum assistance to pull her shorts over her backside in side lying position. She is dependent for donning and doffing socks and shoes.
Bed to wheelchair transfers	Jane completes this task with maximum assistance x 2 and with a slide board.
Self-feeding	Jane feeds herself 75% of her meal independently with a universal cuff. She requires assistance to don and doff the cuff. She is dependent for set up of the meal items.
Bed mobility	Jane requires moderate assistance to initiate momentum for rolling into sidelining when in bed. She requires a three count for task initiation and is dependent for leg management. She participates in this task by pulling herself into side lying with use of the bed rails.

Interventions

1. Describe three methods for addressing decreased fine-motor coordination and dexterity.
2. What occupation-based interventions will be included in her plan?
3. What preparatory methods may be used in the intervention process?

Discharge Planning

1. What will you recommend to Jane and her family in regard to the accessibility of their home?
2. How would you address IADL tasks such as continuing education and driving?
3. What services will you recommend postdischarge?

Resource

Shepherd, J. (2010). Activities of daily living. In J. Case-Smith & J. O'Brien (Eds.), *Occupational therapy for children* (6th ed., pp. 474-517). St. Louis: Elsevier.

Chapter 6

Introduction to Mental Health Settings

The roots of occupational therapy (OT) lie in providing mental health services. In fact, at the beginning of the 20th century, the principles of moral treatment were being applied to individuals who were chronically mentally ill, and the first meeting of the National Association for the Promotion of Occupational Therapy was convened (Kielhofner, 2004). Early occupational therapists (OTs) were physicians, nurses, architects, and artisans who shared a common vision that was guided by five constructs:

1. Humans need to be occupied.
2. An individual's health is dependent on and reflected in the habits that he or she uses to organize how time is spent on a daily basis.
3. The mind and body are connected.
4. Disruption in an individual's participation in daily activities could be a result of poor health *or* could cause poor health.
5. Participation in everyday activities (or occupations) could be applied therapeutically to enhance a person's mental health (Kielhofner, 2004).

In 1926, Bryant, as cited in Bryden and McColl (2003), spoke of the power of OT for children:

> We know we are helping these misfit children to self-possession in the broadest sense of the word, to realize that they are responsible little folks with real things to do. We help them to form good habits, to be observant, attentive, cooperative, honest, well-behaved children. We know that their salvation lies in handwork, and so we are encouraged to try again and again. (p. 30)

Today, despite an ever-changing reimbursement system, OTs are continuing to provide mental health services to children in various settings, from inpatient psychiatry units to therapeutic day schools to community organizations. Contemporary pediatric mental health services are provided within the context of a tiered public health framework and include prevention, promotion, and direct intervention (Bayzk, 2011). Occupational therapists are involved in minimizing the risks associated with certain mental health conditions, reducing symptoms, and supporting children and youth to build capacity to function independently within their given roles (Bayzk, 2011).

Occupational therapists collaborate with various professionals to meet the mental health needs of children and youth across practice settings. These professionals include psychiatrists, psychologists, social workers, counselors, mental health providers, and nurses. In addition, OTs also collaborate with their clients and their families to ensure that their services are relevant and meaningful.

Questions to Consider

1. What are some examples of the ways that OTs can be involved in providing services that target mental health prevention and promotion?
2. What is unique about the type of services that OTs can provide to children and youth with mental health needs compared to other providers?
3. What are some examples of theories and frames of reference that may be used when working with children and youth with mental health needs?

References

Bazyk, S. (2011). *Mental health promotion, prevention, and intervention with children and youth.* Bethesda, MD: AOTA Press.

Cahill SM, Bowyer P, eds. *Cases in Pediatric Occupational Therapy: Assessment and Intervention (pp 135-154).*

Bryden, P., & McColl, M. (2003). The concept of occupation 1900 to 1974. In M. McColl, M. Law, D. Stewart, L. Doubt, N. Pollock, & T. Krupa (Eds.), *Theoretical basis of occupational therapy* (pp. 27-37). Thorofare, NJ: SLACK Incorporated.

Kielhofner, G. (2004). *Conceptual foundations of occupational therapy practice* (3rd ed.). Philadelphia, PA: F. A. Davis Co.

Abigail: Aggression/ Inpatient Psychiatric Unit

Lisa Mahaffey, MS, OTR/L, FAOTA

History and Background Information

Abigail, age 9 years, has a history of aggression and a diagnosis of Disruptive Mood Dysregulation Disorder. She and her brother were adopted from eastern Europe when Abigail was 2 years old and her brother was 5 years old. At the time of the adoption, Abigail weighed approximately 13 pounds. Her brother was also severely underweight. After coming to the United States, both Abigail and her brother were evaluated and received early intervention (EI) services to support the development of cognitive and social emotional skills. Since being adopted, Abigail has endured multiple medical problems, including whooping cough, severe flu-like illnesses, and multiple ear infections.

History of Hospitalization

Abigail was admitted to the inpatient psychiatric unit at the local hospital because of extreme aggression toward her family, especially her mother and brother. In addition, Abigail has a history of demonstrating aggression toward her teacher and other students in her third-grade classroom. On the unit, it was noted that Abigail was extremely verbally aggressive when she became angry. She often used foul language directed at the individuals who were near her or the source of her anger. On occasion, Abigail would also become very physically aggressive when angry. Abigail continues to be underweight and, despite her small stature, would strike out and injure staff that tried to contain her during bouts of anger. Abigail's bouts of anger often lasted upward of 20 minutes and typically included physical aggression, yelling, and screaming. The psychiatric unit's social worker contacted Abigail's teacher after she received consent to do so from Abigail's mother. Abigail's teacher reported that Abigail is making progress academically, but she believes Abigail could achieve more if she could manage her behavior in the classroom. The teacher stated that Abigail cannot sit still, is unable to tolerate the presence of other children in close proximity to her, and is often observed screaming at them if she thinks they are too close or too loud. When the classroom gets too loud, Abigail responds by screaming at people to be quiet. Because of her outbursts, the teacher has not sent her to physical education or music class for the past month. Just before Abigail was hospitalized, she became very aggressive with a classroom teacher and a teacher's assistant. In addition, she physically attacked another student. The school asked the parents to have her evaluated for mental health problems.

Evaluation Information

Occupational Profile

Abigail's day includes school and homework during the week. She is currently taking swimming lessons on Saturday mornings, which she likes. Abigail's mom said they have tried to sign her up for dance as well as soccer and t-ball, but she had trouble listening to the coach and got in trouble. They have been thinking about trying lacrosse because the park district has a program for kids with special needs. On Sundays, the family goes to church in the morning and then Abigail usually plays with a neighborhood friend, plays video games, or does homework. Mom states that Abigail does better if her time is structured. Abigail identifies many interests, including drawing and simple craftwork, reading books and magazines about nature, video games, games on her mom's iPad like Fruit Ninja and Bike Race, playing with her friends at school, swimming, and playing with her Barbie dolls. Abigail stated several times that she would like to ride a bike but can't. She also stated that she has two chores during the week: she has to help clear the table and run the vacuum in the bedrooms. Abigail is responsible for cleaning her room and making her bed in the morning. She really wants a cat, but her mom said they couldn't have one until she learned to be nicer to her brother, whom she doesn't get along with because "he bothers me." Abigail has two friends near home, but her mom says sometimes they won't play with her if she gets mad at them. Abigail prefers playing with one friend at a time and, according to mom, she has trouble with being bossy and not letting her friends choose the activities or take the lead in their games or play activities. Abigail had several friends from school, but she has gotten angry and verbally aggressive when she has gone to their homes, so they no longer invite her to play after school or on the weekends.

Abigail's parents are both professionals. Abigail's father works in business and her mother worked as a teacher prior to adopting Abigail and her brother. When it became apparent that Abigail would not be able to stay in day care due to her behavior, Abigail's mother quit teaching to stay home and be with the children. Abigail's mother has a physical disability, resulting in limited use of one arm and a slower gait. She feels this has contributed to her difficulty in physically controlling some of Abigail's behavior. Abigail's parents' goals for her inpatient stay are that she become more tolerant of other people in her family and school classroom, that she be able to remain attentive and listen during groups and school time, and that she find alternative ways to cope when she doesn't get her way.

Analysis of Occupational Performance

Abigail's inpatient evaluation included an observation of her during a group held on the unit. The OT group runs on Friday afternoons after lunch, which is sometimes a difficult time for the children on the unit. On this day, the group activity was a sensory motor activity designed to provide sensory input but also to work on cooperation, listening, and turn taking. Some of the activities required the children to help each other. All of the activities required group cooperation to be successful. Interventions included pointing out when a member is not working with the group and the outcome of that action. The parachute and several balls were used for the group on this day. The group started with introductions and a discussion about the participants' favorite games. The activities started with simple raising and lowering of the parachute to help the kids learn to work together and get a feel for the chute. Balls were added and the children worked together to bounce them 10 consecutive times and roll them around the edge of the parachute. During the last activity, each child took a turn sitting in the center of the parachute and the group wrapped the child up like a flower bud and then spun him or her out. The group ended with a discussion of sensation and the participants' levels of alertness, how the parachute activity made them feel, how each member supported the group activity and what they learned about working together, as well as what happened when they did not work together. When the children were able to understand the metaphor, the discussion was applied to other areas of their lives. In this group, there were seven children, the OT, and a student OT. Abigail joined the group without hesitation and was attentive. She tended to be very directive with her peers and frustrated when they didn't listen to her. Two children had difficulty calming themselves in order to listen to instructions. Three children were actively engaged and able to follow directions. One child began with the group but appeared to lose interest after 10 minutes and required consistent redirection throughout the remainder of the activity. The OT student worked closely with this child, redirecting him and demonstrating what he needed to do. He was eventually able to do all of the activities but showed minimal interest in other children in the group.

During this activity, the OT noted that Abigail had a distinctive response to auditory input. In fact, Abigail appeared to be very sensitive to the chatter that took place and when other children raised their voices. When the room got louder, Abigail would initially ask people to quiet down, using a very high-pitched tone of voice. If the people in the room didn't respond, she would escalate by asking louder until she was eventually screaming. At one point, she was asked to leave the space. Once she calmed herself, she was able to return to the group and continue the activity. Abigail refused to be wrapped up during the final activity. She did agree to try sitting in the parachute with the OT student while the group walked around very slowly, turning her in the parachute for one full circle. She enjoyed this activity and asked to do it again.

In addition to group, Abigail was observed on the inpatient unit during the school hour. During this hour, patients work on grade-appropriate school work with a teacher. Abigail worked on her school work with minimal support. Abigail wore glasses throughout the day, yet when working on her school work, she still sat hunched over with her head approximately 4 inches from the paper. She held her pencil with a thumb wrap grip. Her grip was tight and she pushed on the paper hard enough to occasionally cause small rips in the paper. When asked to use a ruler to mark a line, Abigail was able to position the ruler correctly and follow the edge with her pencil, though it was noted twice that she was pushing so hard on the ruler that it moved. She attempted to put the ruler back but struggled with lining it up. She eventually became frustrated, completing the line without lining up the ruler. Abigail complained several times to the teacher that she couldn't find her vocabulary words in an assignment where the words were hidden in a puzzle. Once she was helped to locate the first or last letter, she was able to pick the word out and circle it. She also complained that the light in the room (fluorescent lighting) was bothering her and giving her a headache. At one point during the school period, a peer became frustrated and loud. Abigail's response was to tell her peer to be quiet. When her peer continued to escalate, Abigail's response was to yell louder for him to be quiet. When redirected, she complained that her peer was not listening to her and it was too loud for her to concentrate. Once the peer was removed from the situation, Abigail was able to settle back down to her school task.

The OT made the following observations of Abigail:

- Her muscle tone was generally low.
- She had poor muscle co-contraction and at times her joints were hyperextended.
- She had poor balance in standing and kneeling.
- She used a thumb wrap grasp for gripping a pencil and her grip was extremely tight.
- She had decreased body awareness and was not able to draw a recognizable person.
- She "slapped" her feet on the ground when walking.

Progress Information

One week after her initial evaluation, Abigail was seen by the OT in a group that was focused on exploring self-regulation during new challenges. During this meeting, the participants imagined that they were characters from Star Wars and were attending the "Jedi Academy." The children were taught a choreographed Jedi sparring routine that required them to repeat a series of sequenced motor movements with the goal that they would be able to recall and enact the sequence. Abigail initially participated in the "Jedi training"; however, she became increasingly frustrated with the repetition of the choreographed moves because she was having difficulty recalling the specific sequence. Eventually, Abigail began verbalizing her displeasure. After she began screaming and crying, she was removed from the group. A unit staff member assisted in calming her down. However, she was not able to return to the group for 25 minutes. Once she returned, she was able to sit and wait her turn to spar with the OT, who was posing as another Star Wars character. While she waited, she was observed cheering for her peers when they completed their turn. Although she forgot the sequence of the routine, she remained calm and expressed that she enjoyed the activity when it was over.

Questions to Consider

Goal Areas and Treatment Focus

1. This week, what are Abigail's strengths?
2. Write short-term goals for Abigail for this week.
3. Design a group for Abigail and other children on the unit that will be supportive of her goals.
4. What are some ways OT can structure the group so Abigail can participate successfully?
5. What strategies could Abigail try in the group in order to manage the noise level and respond to her peers effectively?
6. How would an OT approach with Abigail differ from the approaches used by other staff members on the unit?
7. What are some evidence-based strategies that you can use with Abigail to lead to goal achievement?

Safety Precautions

1. Does Abigail pose any safety concerns?
2. What precautions should be put in place to address these concerns?

Plans for Discharging Home and Returning to School

1. What tools might you suggest Abigail use at home and at school to help her attend to classroom activities and attend physical education and music classes?
2. What resources would you put together for mom and Abigail so they could learn more about her sensory challenges?
3. What community resources might you suggest for Abigail and mom related to her current level of function, her interests, and her sensory needs?
4. Keeping in mind that Abigail will grow up, what community resources might you share with mom and Abigail to support her as she moves through her developmental stages (high school, work, independent living)?

Resources

Look at information related to adoption from Russia and other eastern European countries. Also familiarize yourself with adoption from orphanages and mental health issues that are associated with these children. Common issues include reactive attachment disorder, ADHD, and conduct disorders.

Davidson, D. (2010). Psychosocial issues affection social participation. In J. Case-Smith & J. O'Brien (Eds). *Occupational therapy in children* (6th ed., pp. 404-433). St. Louis: Elsevier.

Henry, D., Wheeler, T., & Sava, D. I. (2004). *Sensory integration tools for teens: Strategies to promote sensory integration*. Youngtown, AZ: Henry Occupational Therapy Services, Inc.

Murray-Slutsky, C., & Paris, B. A. (2005). *Is it sensory or is it behavior? Behavior problem identification and intervention*. San Antonio, TX: PsychCorp.

Tiffany: Pediatric Depression/Community-Based Mental Health

Brad E. Egan, OTD, MA, OTR/L and Eric Howard, COTA/L

History and Background Information

Tiffany, age 16 years, was diagnosed with depression 3 years ago. She was admitted to this shelter 3 days ago as a walk-in. Tiffany told intake staff members that she had run away from home nearly 4 weeks ago, was out of money and hungry, and had no safe place to go. She completed intake paperwork and reported the following information.

Mental Health History

Tiffany was diagnosed with depression at the age of 13. She reports that she felt a lot of anger and hostility toward friends and family during this time. In addition, she stopped doing homework, began to fail classes, stopped going out with friends, and lost interest in after school activities like choir and Spanish club. At her mother's request, she was evaluated by a psychiatrist, who diagnosed her with depression and prescribed Lexapro (escitalopram). Tiffany reports that she did not like taking Lexapro because it made her feel tired and restless. She also noted that she attempted suicide by taking a bottle of acetaminophen during her freshman year of high school. Following the suicide attempt, she was hospitalized for 2 weeks. Her psychiatrist discontinued her prescription for Lexapro and prescribed 20 mg of Prozac (fluoxetine) daily. Tiffany reports that she has not taken any medication in over 6 weeks. She also indicated that she is not sure if the medication even helps. She identified that she has used Vicodin (acetaminophen/hydrocodone) and ecstasy recreationally. At the time of intake, Tiffany was slightly disheveled; she denied any suicidal or homicidal thoughts, denied being under the influence of any illicit substances, and presented with a stable mood.

Medical History

Unremarkable.

Family History

Prior to running away, Tiffany lived with her mother, father, and older brother. Tiffany's father is a car salesman and her mother works as a bank teller. Her brother is a student at a local community college and spends most of his time at his girlfriend's house. Tiffany describes her parents as being "too conservative," "too controlling," and rarely affectionate with her. In addition, Tiffany reports that she has been fighting with her mother over dropping out of school during her junior year, shortly before running away. Tiffany was close with one male first cousin who is similar in age but reports that they have not really spoken in 2 years. She reports feeling like the "black sheep" of the family.

Educational History

Tiffany completed 10th grade and dropped out of high school the first semester of her junior year. Tiffany indicated that she "hates" school and is particularly upset with her ninth-grade math teacher, who spoke with her mother about changes she had observed in Tiffany's behavior. Tiffany also reported that she was an honor student in elementary school and during the first 2 years of junior high school. She does not regret dropping out of school and has no interest in returning. However, Tiffany is aware that she will likely need a GED in order to get a job.

Evaluation Information

Occupational Profile

An occupational profile was initiated by the occupational therapy assistant (OTA) on the 4th day after Tiffany arrived at the shelter.

Although Tiffany responded with "I don't know" for most of the questions asked during the interview, she did provide information about a typical day. Tiffany reports that she typically sleeps until noon or later and spends most of her time in her bedroom. When asked why she sleeps till noon, she noted that she "hates the mornings." She usually showers once every 3 days, which had become a point of contention between her and her parents. Unless her mother makes tacos or a favorite food for dinner, Tiffany often makes peanut butter and jelly sandwiches and eats them in her bedroom alone. When asked why she came to the shelter, Tiffany said that she was fearful of being physically harmed by some of the strangers with whom she had been "hanging out." She describes herself as "useless" and indicated that she did not think that anyone really cared about her except her grandmother, who lives more than 300 miles away. Tiffany initially said that she was not good at anything, but after rephrasing the question, Tiffany told the OTA that she is good at sketching. She did not elaborate on what she likes to sketch. She reports that she has not completed a sketch in a long time because she gets too distracted by all of the things on her mind. When asked about her current goals and priorities, Tiffany was unable to identify anything more specific than "finding a place to live." She was adamant that she did not want to return home or go back to school.

After the occupational profile interview, the OTA and OT collaborated to determine which assessments might be useful in identifying more information about Tiffany's interests (past, present, and future) and perceptions about her skills and abilities. In addition, both practitioners thought it would be necessary for Tiffany to identify more specific goals that could support her in successfully finding a place to live. The OT suggested that Tiffany complete the Occupational Self-Assessment (OSA) and the Adolescent Leisure Interest Profile (ALIP).

Assessment Results

The OTR met with Tiffany on day 5 of her stay at the shelter to complete the OSA and ALIP. Tiffany was initially guarded about completing the assessments. However, after the OTR explained the purpose of each one, she agreed. See Tiffany's report in Table 6-1.

Tiffany's evaluation data largely suggest that she is unable to identify many strengths, roles, interests or occupations she does well. The OT interpreted this information as evidence that Tiffany is presenting with volitional subsystem problems, namely personal causation, because she

TABLE 6-1

OSA: MYSELF AND MY ENVIRONMENT

	HOW WELL TIFFANY DOES IT				*HOW IMPORTANT IT IS TO TIFFANY*				
	Lot of problems	***Some difficulty***	***Well***	***Extremely well***	***Not so important***	***Important***	***More important***	***Most important***	***I would like to change***
Concentrating on my tasks	Lot of problems	**Some difficulty**	Well	Extremely well	Not so important	Important	**More important**	Most important	*Not having so much on my mind*
Getting where I need to go	Lot of problems	**Some difficulty**	Well	Extremely well	Not so important	**Important**	More important	Most important	*No car or transportation*
Managing my finances	**Lot of problems**	Some difficulty	Well	Extremely well	Not so important	Important	More important	**Most important**	*Need a job*
Expressing myself to others	**Lot of problems**	Some difficulty	Well	Extremely well	Not so important	**Important**	More important	Most important	*I don't have friends*
Having a satisfying routine	Lot of problems	**Some difficulty**	Well	Extremely well	Not so important	Important	More important	**Most important**	*Bored a lot*
Being involved as a student, worker, volunteer, and/or family member	**Lot of problems**	Some difficulty	Well	Extremely well	Not so important	Important	More important	**Most important**	*Need a job*
Doing activities I like	Lot of problems	Some difficulty	**Well**	Extremely well	Not so important	Important	**More important**	Most important	*I'm pretty good at sketching and video games*
A place to live and take care of myself	**Lot of problems**	Some difficulty	Well	Extremely well	Not so important	Important	More important	**Most important**	*That's why I'm here; need a place*

Adapted from Baron, K., Kielhofner, G., Iyenger, A., Goldhammer, V., & Wolenski, J. (2006). *Occupational Self Assessment (OSA) (Version 2.2)*. Chicago, IL: Model of Human Occupation Clearinghouse.

(continued)

Table 6-1 (continued)

ALIP

	HOW INTERESTED ARE YOU IN THIS ACTIVITY?	HOW OFTEN DO YOU DO THIS ACTIVITY?	HOW WELL DO YOU DO THIS ACTIVITY?	HOW MUCH DO YOU ENJOY THIS ACTIVITY?	WHO DO YOU DO THIS ACTIVITY WITH?
Sports Activities	NONE	NONE	NONE	NONE	NONE
Outdoor Activities	NONE	NONE	NONE	NONE	NONE
Exercise Activities					
Aerobics	Somewhat	Less than once a month	Well	Somewhat	By myself
Relaxation Activities					
Watching TV	Very	3 to 7 times a week	Very well	Very much	By myself
Listening to Music	Somewhat	3 to 7 times a week	Very well	Somewhat	By myself
Playing Video Games	Very	3 to 7 times a week	Very well	Somewhat	By myself
Sleeping Late	Very	3 to 7 times a week	Very well	Very much	By myself
Intellectual Activities	NONE	NONE	NONE	NONE	NONE
Creative Activities					
Drawing	Very	Once or twice a month	Well/very well	Very much	By myself
Socializing Activities	NONE	NONE	NONE	NONE	NONE
Club/Community Activities	NONE	NONE	NONE	NONE	NONE

Adapted from Henry, A. (2000). *Pediatric Interest Profiles*. Tucson, AZ: Therapy Skill Builders. Retrieved from: http://www.uic.edu/depts/moho/images/assessments/PIPs%20Manual.pdf

only identified one item on the entire OSA that she does well. Although Tiffany identified getting a job, managing her finances, and finding a place to live as priority areas to be addressed in OT, in a follow-up interview the OT collaborated with her to identify smaller action steps and goals that were still aligned with her priority areas yet appropriate given the maximum 30-day time limit of the setting. The OT and Tiffany also discussed how meeting the goals set in OT could potentially support a greater sense of both capacity and efficacy.

Findings from Tiffany's OSA and ALIP reinforce her current feelings about having some difficulty organizing a satisfying routine. Her reported routine appears to be mostly organized around solitary and relaxing activities, which she reports is not very satisfying. In the follow-up interview, the OT asked Tiffany to describe the skills she uses and practices when engaging in the four main activities that make up her routine (watching television, listening to music, playing video games, and sleeping late) and to compare those skills to the skills needed to get a job and an apartment. After a long pause, Tiffany reported that it would be a good idea for her to start getting up earlier and to have some responsibility. The OT and Tiffany also agreed that opportunities to interact and express herself to others may be helpful in future situations with coworkers or landlords.

Based on the interviews and self-assessment reports, the OT, OTA, and Tiffany collaborated to determine the following interventions based on the priority areas noted in the assessments:

1. The OTA intentionally assigned Tiffany the chore of setting up the morning continental breakfast with a team of three other clients Monday through Wednesday. The OTA felt that the breakfast group (rather than a daily cleaning chore) would be more beneficial in developing an early-morning routine, decreasing the amount of time spent sleeping late, and increasing the amount of time interacting with others, while gaining valuable skills that could be easily generalized to the workforce or to future home management occupations.
2. The OT suggested that the OTA have a conversation with Tiffany regarding the potential benefits of utilizing the GED tutorial services offered two times a week in the facility's computer lab.
3. To provide Tiffany with opportunities to continue to engage in an occupation she values (sketching/drawing) while also exploring social and communication skill development, the OTA suggested that Tiffany will organize a nightly Pictionary (Hasbro) game group with peers.
4. The OTA also enrolled Tiffany in the mandatory daily grooming group for teenage girls. Her daily ADL goals will be to shower or bathe, brush her teeth, brush her hair, apply deodorant, and wear clean clothes. In addition, she must wash her hair at least every other day and launder her clothes a minimum of two times per week. The OTA suggests providing Tiffany with the following choices so that she can exercise some autonomy in making decisions about her personal care: bathing in the morning or in the evening, choosing when to wash her hair, determining her own laundry schedule, and identifying a personal grooming goal.

Occupational Therapy Weekly Progress Note

Tiffany appears to be more comfortable interacting with staff and other peers during OT groups. In fact, she reported that she enjoyed the Pictionary group and brought a suggestion to staff to buy Cranium (Hasbro). Tiffany reported that she thinks she will need a GED to get a job she would like but feels that she has too much on her mind right now to think about an educational goal. She told the OTA that she is confident that she could get a dishwashing job at a restaurant without a GED. Her case manager reported that she expressed interest in applying for housing at the transitional living facility once her 30 days were up at the shelter (Table 6-2).

The OTA and OT agreed to continue with the current OT plan of care. The progress note was signed by both professionals.

Practice Setting

Safe Zone is an emergency shelter for teens between 14 to 18 years of age. Safe Zone serves a maximum of 12 male and 12 female clients each night and will hold beds for clients in good standing for up to 30 consecutive days. Safe Zone provides youths with food, shelter, and a lending closet for clothes, towels, and sheets. It is open from 6 PM to 10 AM daily, 365 days a year. Staff, which consists of two full-time case managers, a part-time OTA, an OT consultant, a nutrition consultant, a full-time spiritual care counselor, and a dance therapist who leads one group per week, provide assistance with vocational, educational, relationship, and spiritual skills for self-sufficiency and independent living. In addition, a nurse practitioner provides a broad range of medical services each Wednesday night, which include, but are not limited to, performing physical exams, coordinating referrals, ordering lab tests, and medication counseling. Safe Zone operates out of the annex of a Unitarian church. The building has six single-sex bedrooms, each housing two sets of bunk beds, three single-occupancy bathrooms, an open kitchen with a full stove and microwave, a computer lab equipped with high-speed Internet access and five computers, a conference room with seating for 12, and a lounge area with a television and pool table. A typical continental breakfast is set up

TABLE 6-2

TIFFANY'S OCCUPATIONAL THERAPY GOALS

SHORT-TERM GOALS	*CURRENT STATUS*	*MET/NOT MET*
Tiffany will organize and lead an evening Pictionary group at least 2x/wk with peers in the shelter.	Although Tiffany agreed to the goal, she needed assistance from OT staff to determine strategies for inviting peers to the first game night group. In addition, she had difficulty assuming the role of group leader and practiced leading the group during a one-on-one session with the OTA. During the first group, Tiffany needed help in explaining the rules of the game to peers who were unfamiliar with Pictionary and she was the last person to take a turn each round. She successfully led the second game night on Friday evening and utilized the strategies identified in her one-on-one session with the OTA. However, she still waited to be the last person to take a turn each round.	Not met. Continue with current goal.
Tiffany will perform bathing and grooming tasks daily using the ADL group to structure her routine.	She missed two ADL groups because she reported not feeling well. She wore the same clothes two days in row despite cueing from staff and encouragement to wash her clothes. Tiffany showered daily. However, she was unable to follow the morning shower schedule that she signed up for 3 of the 7 days and had to wait to shower until everyone else was done.	Not met. Continue with current goal.
LONG-TERM GOALS		
Tiffany will be out of bed by no later than 7 am each morning in order to independently make herself a simple breakfast and complete ADL routine by 8 am.	Tiffany overslept Monday and Tuesday and missed the 6 am start time for the breakfast prep group. She reported that her alarm did not go off. She completed all of the breakfast chores on Wednesday but did not socialize with any of her peers.	Not met. Continue with current goal.
Tiffany will independently bathe and groom every day.	Tiffany is currently utilizing the structure and support of the grooming group.	Deferred

by four clients each morning and served from 6:45 to 8 AM. Clients who do not help with breakfast setup are required to complete an assigned cleaning chore before leaving each morning. Clients are required to vacate the premises from 10 AM to 6 PM daily and must reserve their room in advance if they plan on returning that evening. Clients who are not returning must strip their beds and turn in dirty bedding to staff. Clients who reserve a room and do not show up and clients who do not complete their assigned chores lose sleeping privileges for at least 30 days. In addition, clients who are caught using alcohol or drugs on the premises or who present under the influence of any drugs or alcohol will be denied services for up to 6 months. Clients who successfully participate in services at the shelter are eligible to apply for residency at an affiliated transitional living facility for homeless teens and adults up to the age of 21.

Questions to Consider

1. What are the roles and responsibilities of the OT and the OTA in this case?
2. Describe ways that OTs and OTAs can collaborate in this setting as well as in others.
3. What additional interventions might be helpful in addressing Tiffany's desire to get a job?
4. What additional assessments or strategies may be helpful in identifying how Tiffany spends her time?
5. Based on Tiffany's occupational profile and goals, what group intervention(s) could the OTA design to address some of her current barriers to occupational performance?
6. How might the OT practitioners discuss the main concepts of the Model of Human Occupation with Tiffany in a way that makes sense to her?

7. In addition to interpreting the evaluation data, how might the OT provide support to the OTA in Tiffany's case?
8. What information would be important for the OT practitioners to provide to the referring nurse practitioner?
9. How might the OTA specifically support Tiffany in the community when the shelter is closed from 10 am to 6 pm?
10. What are some potential challenges that Tiffany could encounter at discharge?
11. What discharge recommendations might the OT and OTA consider as Tiffany transitions from the shelter to a transitional living facility?

References

Baron, K., Kielhofner, G., Iyenger, A., Goldhammer, V., & Wolenski, J. (2006). *Occupational Self-Assessment* (OSA) (Version 2.2). Chicago: Model of Human Occupation Clearinghouse.

Henry, A. (2000). *Pediatric Interest Profiles*. Tucson, AZ: Therapy Skill Builders. Retrieved from: http://www.uic.edu/depts/moho/images/assessments/PIPs%20Manual.pdf

Resource

Teen Living Programs. Retrieved from http://www.teenliving.org/3.0/home.html

Sophia: Early Intervention/ Infant Mental Health

Kris Pizur-Barnekow, PhD, OTR/L;
Jennifer Nash, PhD, OTR/L;
Susan Wendel, MS, OTR/L; and
Molly Chopper

History and Background Information

Molly is a single mother of twin girls, Sophia and Bella, who are now 20 months chronological age (adjusted age 16.5 months). The girls were born extremely premature at 25 weeks gestation and required a lengthy stay in the hospital. Bella was hospitalized in the Neonatal Intensive Care Unit (NICU) for 4 months and Sophia was hospitalized for 4.5 months. In addition to their prematurity, the girls were diagnosed with a rare genetic skin disorder, congenital erosive and vesicular dermatosis, affecting 90% of their bodies. As newborns, their skin would blister, causing it to rip and tear. Nurses and caregivers could only minimally touch and reposition the girls due to the fragility of their skin. As a result of this condition, Bella and Sophia have scarring and hypopigmentation of their skin throughout their extremities and torso.

Bella's current development is unremarkable and she is not receiving EI services. Sophia is diagnosed with global developmental delays and is enrolled in EI services. The girls are also enrolled in Early Head Start (EHS). The family receives a weekly visit from an EHS home visitor and they participate in some of the monthly socialization play groups. Sophia's past medical history is significant for three surgeries. When she was 2 weeks old, she had surgery to repair a patent ductus arteriosus defect. She had eye surgery for retinopathy of prematurity at 4 months and a bowel repair at 13 months. Sophia is susceptible to lung infections and frequent illness. She has had pneumonia requiring hospitalization on four separate occasions. In addition to care from her pediatrician, Sophia receives tertiary medical care from specialists, including a cardiologist for an enlarged aorta, a pulmonologist for lung disease, and a dermatologist for her congenital skin disorder.

Soon after the twins were born, Molly and the girls moved from Idaho to Seattle, Washington to be closer to a network of friends who could offer them support and companionship. Molly and the girls live in a two-bedroom apartment on the lower level of a rental home. Their living space is large enough for the girls to have room to play and explore. Their home is near a community playground, which Molly and the twins visit on a regular basis. They also enjoy daily walks around their neighborhood. Since the birth of the twins, Molly is enrolled in online classes toward a bachelor's degree in psychology. Her long-term goal is to become a clinical psychologist and to inspire her daughters. Molly is a parent representative on a board for the local EHS Program.

Bella and Sophia attend an EI program at a children's clinic serving children primarily from birth to 3 years who have neurodevelopmental disabilities. The clinic participates in Part C funding and is required to offer services within a natural environment. Children under 18 months of age are offered home-based services. At 18 months, children may be considered for placement in the clinic's toddler classroom program as appropriate to the needs of the child. Twenty-five percent of the toddler classrooms are integrated with typically developing children; in that case, the classroom is considered a natural environment. Bella is enrolled at the clinic as a typical peer model. Sophia is enrolled to receive EI services and has an Individual Family Service Plan (IFSP). The girls participate in a 2-hour toddler classroom twice a week. Sophia's OT and speech therapy services are conducted both as individual pull-out sessions and within the context of the classroom.

Evaluation Information

Parent Interview

OT: How would you describe Sophia?

Molly: Very tender, loving, little being. Sophia enjoys her own little world that she lives in. She has been through so much in her short life already, surgeries and hospital visits are a lot of what has contributed to her feeling like it's okay to take her time. She has been very slow in her development up until now. She has this little sparkle that melts my heart.

OT: Did you have support during those times?

Molly: When I first had them I didn't have much support (my mom and sister were good for a phone call). I lived in the Ronald McDonald House in Spokane while they were in the hospital. Even after discharging from the NICU to our place in Idaho, I was home most of the time. It was hard to find someone to come over for just a little bit, so I could run to the store for groceries. Most of my support was in Seattle (five to six friends). That's why we moved from Idaho to Seattle in June (very soon after the girls were born).

OT: How would you describe your relationship with your child?

Molly: Very nurturing and loving.

OT: Can you describe what a day might look like for you and your child, starting with when she gets up to when she goes to bed?

Molly: Sophia's a good sleeper. Sometimes she'll sleep until 9 AM. We do have a good morning routine. Change diapers. Go into the living room for play time and rub their little backs. Then it's time for breakfast. They sit in their high chairs. Breakfast is the meal where I try to introduce new things (spoon and fork), maybe introduce some new foods. Then it's cartoon time. They watch cartoons while I clean up the house. Then we go for a walk, color. Lunchtime. Back in the high chairs. Now that Sophia is starting to crawl, I try to get her to follow me into other rooms. I try to tempt her into following me around. Usually when they take a nap, I try to do my school work. Then they're up and they're playing. In the evening, after dinner and jammies are on we read books and I try to focus on getting her to do gross motor and read books. I sit and play with them for about an hour, hour and a half. Mornings and evenings are really our special time together.

OT: What worries, if any, do you have about your child right now?

Molly: My concern about Sophia, I worry about her social life down the line. I know how things go through her brain is a little bit slower than the average kid. I just worry that she will get picked on in life, maybe not be able to fully play with her sister and her peers. I don't want her to face that in her life, getting picked on.

OT: What do you feel you need most right now?

Molly: Time. More time. Energy. I wish I had a nanny. I don't feel that I need much more than that. Next year though, the girls will be going to Head Start or a developmental preschool a few hours each day, which will free up some time each day for me to do what I need to do. It's the same old more energy and time dance.

OT: When did you first have a worry about your child? When did you first realize your child might have a special need?

Molly: In the NICU, close to the time of discharge. The doctors, nurses, and OT, they all said that Sophia would have some hurdles. Her lungs were weak and she was susceptible to getting sick.

OT: What were your feelings at the time of this realization?

Molly: I just worried that the worst would happen. Along with that, knowing that hospital visits would be with two of them (one sick, one not). Scared. Scared about her health, scared that I wouldn't be able to do everything. Wondering if I would be capable of doing it on my own. At the same time, I have always felt that how I feel affects the girls. If I'm fearful and scared, that feeds into their atmosphere. So I try to stay loving and positive, even if deep down I'm scared. There were some times I was worried about Sophia's ability to function in the world and her development in all areas; a lot of that has lifted.

OT: Have your feelings changed over time?

Molly: Yes. Definitely. Over time, getting to know her and being with her and understanding her. She's going to be just fine. No matter what. However it looks. Whatever road blocks come up, she's going to be fine. She's a beautiful little being. I have grown to have more acceptance and those things don't matter so much to me anymore.

OT: What is it like to be the caregiver for your child with her specific needs?

Molly: Sometimes it's kind of frustrating. Just because she has a lot of intestinal issues. Anything around bowel movements, she can have a lot of pain. It's hard to constantly be carrying her everywhere. Trying to resolve her problem (not breathing right, painful bowel movement). On a great day, Sophia and her sister entertain each other, and Sophia engages in a lot of activities, but when she's having a bad day; it can be pretty brutal. It's more than just frustrating. There's a lot of joy in watching her little achievements. With Bella, she was crawling, then walking, things happened so quickly. With Sophia, her achievements are almost more exciting. In that anticipation, wondering if it would ever happen. Like when she started crawling, I called everyone and told everyone. Sue [her current OT] was the one I was most excited to tell. I couldn't wait for Sue to see it. I knew she would be so happy. She has worked just as hard as I have toward this.

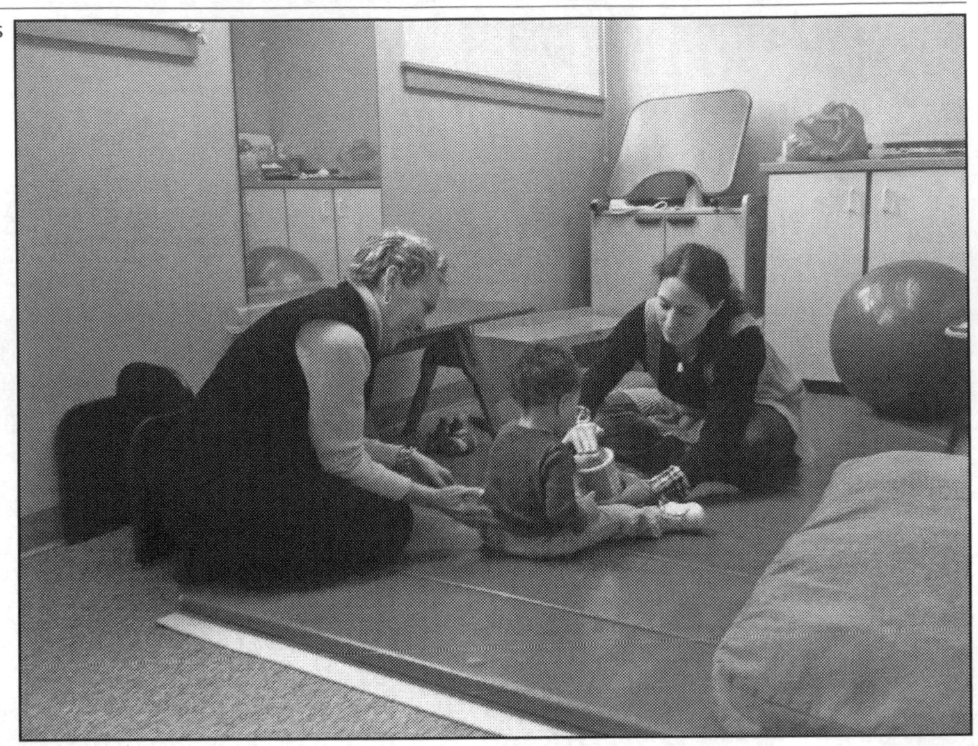

Figure 6-1. Sophia places objects into a container.

OT: What kinds of services have your child and family received to help with the special need?

Molly: We are in the EHS program. Early education, occupational therapy, and speech therapy services through the Children's Clinic. A lot of medical specialists at the Children's Hospital. Sophia sees a cardiologist for her enlarged aorta, a pulmonologist for her lung disease, a dermatologist for her rare skin disorder, and an ophthalmologist.

OT: What new skills are you working on with Sophia?

Molly: Walking and feeding herself. With speech, being able to communicate with me instead of throwing a fit and expecting me to be psychic. Moving more, feeding herself, and communicating.

OT: How do you imagine your future relationship with your child?

Molly: Having open communication with her. More of the same of what we're doing. I would like more interaction. I'm excited about when Sophia can talk to me. I look forward to playing more games.

Analysis of Occupational Performance

Play

Sophia is an adorable, curious toddler who has overcome many medical challenges. Sophia participates in reciprocal play with verbal and physical cues. She rolls a ball back and forth during play with mom. She prefers toys that make noise (e.g., balls with bells). Sophia spontaneously closes the doors of a pop-up toy and with moderate assist manipulates buttons to engage the doors to open. She inserts objects into a container with a large opening (Figure 6-1) and is working on placing a circular shape in a shape sorter. Sophia engages best in purposefully directed play when guided and supported by a caregiver. Sometimes Sophia's solitary play is repetitive and lacks a targeted intent, such as repeatedly tossing a toy to the floor to make noise.

Activities of Daily Living

Sophia removes socks when prompted, feeds herself yogurt with minimal assistance using a child-sized spoon, and finger feeds cereal using a raking grasp. Sophia's self-feeding takes a lot of time and does not fully meet her nutritional needs. She becomes distracted and loses her focus during feeding. Therefore, Sophia's mother continues to feed Sophia some amount of each meal (Figure 6-2). Per mother's report, sleeping, eating, and dressing routines are relatively predictable unless one of the girls is ill.

Mobility

Sophia creeps on all fours independently and transitions from supine to sitting and back to the floor. She stands with support when placed up against furniture.

Goal Areas and Treatment Focus

Through the interview process, the OT learns a lot about Molly's experience as a mother and caregiver. It is apparent

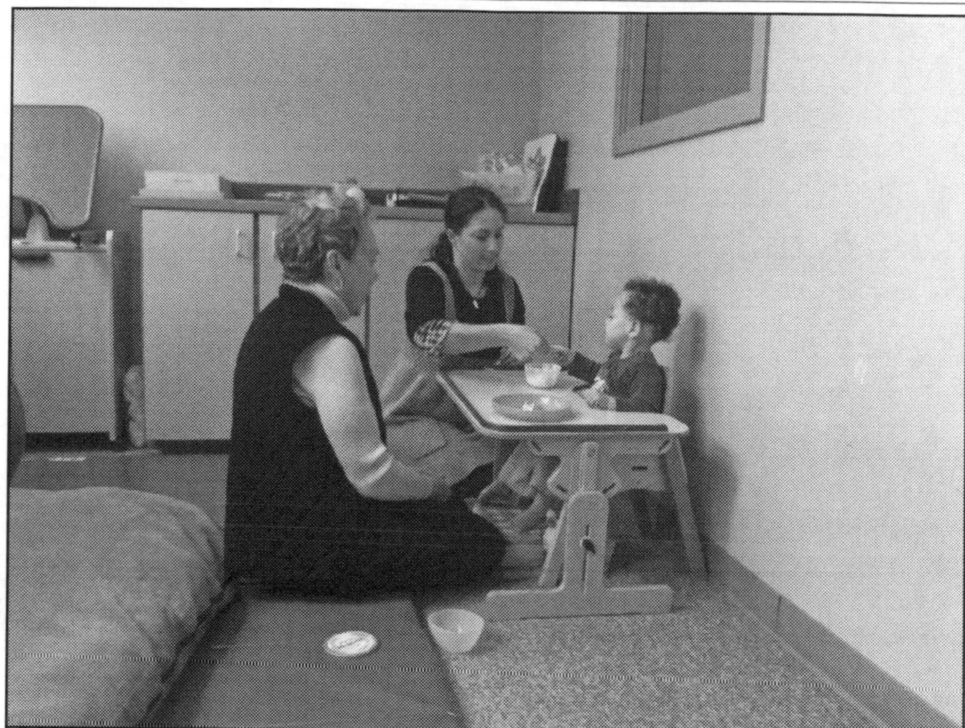

Figure 6-2. Sophia's mom assisting her with eating.

that Molly is a responsive and loving mother who wants the best for her daughters. In particular, Molly identifies that she would like to see Sophia walk and feed herself. Because walking and self-feeding are Molly's priorities, the OT's intervention plan includes treatment strategies and goals that address these priorities.

The OT approach uses parent coaching to promote caregiver-child interactions to foster a healthy relationship between caregiver and child, provide family education about developmental milestones, and promote play and activities to work toward achieving the caregiver's desired goals and priorities. The intervention sessions engage the parent/caregiver as an active participant and the focus of the intervention sessions is facilitating co-occupational participation between the caregiver and child. The desired outcome is to support the parent/caregiver in his or her relationship with the child and foster high-quality attachment and bonding.

Goals for Sophia

- Long-term goal: Sophia will independently self-feed a variety of soft textured foods using a spoon and fork in 6 months.
- Short-term goal: Sophia will independently self-feed yogurt or other soft, sticky foods using a spoon once per day, 5 days per week within 2 months.
- Long-term goal: Sophia will independently walk 10 steps in 6 months.
- Short-term goal: Sophia will cruise/walk five steps while holding onto furniture once per day, 7 days per week within 2 months.
- Long-term goal: Sophia will independently engage in a purposeful play scheme with two different toys in 6 months.
- Short-term goal: Sophia will place a circle shape into a shape sorter without assistance during three consecutive play opportunities within 2 months.

Safety Precautions

Sophia is medically fragile with an enlarged aorta, occasional intestinal distress, and a weakened respiratory system. Because of this, precaution and care must be taken to create a safe play environment that decreases the likelihood of exposure to infection.

In the parent interview, Molly described the feelings she had when she realized that Sophia had special needs. While Molly's feelings have changed over time and her feelings of anxiety and worry have decreased, the OT recognizes that Molly is at risk for developing symptoms of perinatal posttraumatic stress disorder given all that she has experienced during the postnatal period (Callahan & Hynan, 2002; Pizur-Barnekow & Erickson, 2011). The OT monitors Molly for signs of avoidance, reexperiencing, or hyperarousal, and provides support to Molly in the future if Sophia's health condition changes or declines.

Questions to Consider

1. Construct an occupational profile for Sophia.
2. What other questions might you ask to gain additional information from Molly? How would you use this information to inform therapy?
3. Generate a list of Sophia's needs.
4. Generate a list of Sophia's strengths and other factors that will support her development.
5. Develop an in-home treatment plan to address Sophia's goals.
6. Consider the other professionals that might be involved in providing therapy services to Sophia and how the OT might collaborate with each of them. Are any of Sophia's goals better addressed by another professional?
7. Develop a treatment plan for Sophia to take place in the toddler room at the children's clinic.
8. Describe how you would coach Molly and Sophia's teacher to provide more opportunities for Sophia to practice the functional skills outlined in her goals.
9. What are some specific examples of signs of avoidance, reexperiencing, or hyperarousal that the OT should look for when working with Molly?
10. Locate local resources that could be shared with Molly. What are the resources? How might they be supportive to Molly? Is there a fee involved in accessing the resources?
11. When should Molly begin to seek transition services for Sophia?
12. What might some of Sophia's needs be at the time of transition? How can treatment be designed now to reduce these needs in the future?

References

Callahan, J. L., & Hynan, M. T. (2002). Identifying mothers at risk for postnatal emotional distress: Further evidence for the validity of the perinatal posttraumatic stress disorder questionnaire. *Journal of Perinatology, 22*, 448–454.

Pizur-Barnekow, K., & Erickson, S. (2011). Perinatal post-traumatic stress disorder: Implications for occupational therapy in early intervention practice. *Occupational Therapy in Mental Health, 27*, 126-139.

Resource

Hanft, B., Rush, D., & Shelden, M. (2004). *Coaching families and colleagues in early childhood*. Baltimore, MD: Brookes Publishing.

William: Bipolar Disorder/School

Sally W. Schultz, PhD, OTR, LPC

History and Background

William, age 14 years, has returned to school after being discharged from a 3-week psychiatric hospitalization due to extreme disruptive and aggressive behaviors toward others. He was diagnosed with bipolar disorder at age 10. Various psychoactive medications have been trialed with minimal success. William's mood and affect can range from serious depression and disengagement to extreme excitability and agitation. Prior to the hospitalization, he was educated within a self-contained classroom and included for physical education (PE) class when his behavior was under control.

Evaluation Information

Occupational Profile

Although William scores above average on intelligence testing, he was retained in both kindergarten and fifth grade for failing to make adequate progress. His lack of progress was attributed to his emotional status and frequent behavioral outbursts. William's family has limited understanding of mental health problems. He is the fourth of five children. Both of his parents work full-time outside the home. The other children in the family are described as typically developing children. William is notably smaller in stature than his male siblings. His mother reported that William admires his father's ability to fix things around the house, but he has little patience to learn how to do things. She stated, "Whenever he and his dad try to do something together it ends up in a big fight, with William tearing it up and threatening his father." William's teachers reported that he displays similar outbursts of aggressive behavior whenever he is paired with another student on an activity and during team games in PE class.

An informal assessment of William's sensorimotor functioning was completed and it was determined that he did not have any significant impairments or developmental delays.

The educational diagnostician's evaluation revealed no presence of any identifiable learning disabilities. The school counselor and OT observed William within his classroom, during lunch in his classroom, on his way in and out of school, and during PE activities. They concluded that he has a significantly impaired adaptive repertoire of skills to use when facing social and/or educational difficulties. In other words, he uses negative behaviors rather than prosocial skills like negotiation and problem solving, when he becomes frustrated. This conclusion was based on their observations that when William encountered challenging situations, he would shut down and withdraw, make a joke out of it, or "begin hitting or throwing." He typically responded to such challenging situations with one of these three responses. They also noted that his aggressive responses appeared to be unpredictable (e.g., on some occasions when William was frustrated he would "laugh it off") and seem to occur with disproportionate relationship to what is going on around him.

Referral to Occupational Therapy Activity Group Therapy

Based on an overall assessment of William's evaluation data during an educational planning session, the team recommended that William be included in an OT group program designed to help students increase self-management skills through the use of self-directed in vivo occupation-based activities.

Overview of the Therapy Group Based on Occupational Adaptation

The counselor and the OT collaborated to develop and implement this group. The group is based on established principles of group interventions with children and adolescents (Slavson, 1947), the *Theory of Occupational Adaptation* (Schkade & McClung, 2001; Schultz, 1992, 2003, 2014; Schultz & Schkade, 1992), and client-centered methods of interaction (Rogers, 1951). It meets Monday, Wednesday, and Friday from 11 am until 1 pm, and at the time of William's addition to the program, it had been in place for about 6 months. The group is limited to 7 males from approximately age 13 to 16. The OT is the primary facilitator for the group. The OT is assisted by two Level II Fieldwork OT interns.

The program emphasizes development of a therapeutic alliance between the OT and the students within the context of occupation-based activities that are meaningful to the participants. The group therapy environment provides individual and parallel activities along with opportunities for students to work together on projects. The goal is to increase the students' sense of mastery, self-efficacy, and social skills through a therapeutic milieu environment.

An Exchange During Group Therapy With William

The group has begun and the OT notices that William is becoming agitated because the airplane he is putting together keeps falling over; he is beginning to become angry. The OT comes closer into his space and comments in a matter-of-fact way, "For some reason, the plane keeps falling over." She gingerly moves further into William's space and leans over to look at the plane and begins the process of "wondering out loud" what the problem may be. Through this method, she helps William extricate himself from the tension of the situation. William doesn't have to demonstrate his typical adaptive response. As the OT continues the process, she "grades" her words and comments to give William the opportunity to make his own discovery of a solution to the problem. When William doesn't begin to engage in wondering with her, the OT progressively becomes more concrete in her words while still attempting to activate him in identifying his own solution. The OT uses such comments as, "I wonder if the glue had enough time to dry?" A critical aspect of this therapeutic dialogue is that the OT is not looking at the student, thereby conveying that she is not placing blame on the student and reinforcing that she is "just thinking out loud." The OT continues to grade her comments until William begins to reengage with the activity himself. William says, "I think the wing wasn't lined up right. Maybe the glue wasn't dry either." At that point, the OT steps out of his space and engages with others as needed.

Questions to Consider

Goals/Treatment Plan

1. Identify a problem list for William that is consistent with the occupational adaptation-based activity group therapy.
2. What strengths does William have?
3. What long-term goals would be appropriate for William? (Be sure they are consistent with the theoretical approach.)
4. What short-term goals would you identify using the theoretical approach as presented here? How would you measure progress?
5. If William's teachers want you to incorporate goals that are inconsistent with the theoretical approach, how would you handle it?

Safety Precautions

1. What are the primary safety concerns that you will need address while William is in your treatment group?
2. How will you handle his using tools that are potentially dangerous?

Self-Care/Leisure/Work

1. What guidance might you give to William's parents?

Equipment/Adaptations

1. What equipment or environmental considerations or modifications might you want to implement in the therapy room?

Neuromusculoskeletal

1. Are there any neuromusculoskeletal issues that should be considered?

Psychosocial

1. How would you address psychosocial issues that arise between students during the group?

Teacher/Staff Education

1. How would you describe your intervention to William's special education teacher?
2. What guidance might you provide to her on the approach you are using the activity group?

Duration of Activity Therapy Group

1. What do you believe is the appropriate time frame to start seeing a positive effect on William in this group?
2. If you begin to observe William becoming more adaptive in the group sessions, how will you go about helping him to transition this into the remainder of his school experience?

References

Rogers, C. R. (1951). *Client-centered therapy: Its current practice, implications, and theory.* Boston: Houghton Mifflin.

Schkade, J., & McClung, M. (2001). *Occupational adaptation in practice: Concepts and cases.* Thorofare, NJ: SLACK Incorporated.

Schultz, S. (1992). School-based occupational therapy for students with behavioral disorders. *Occupational Therapy in Health Care,* 8(2-3), 173-196.

Schultz, S. (2003). Psychosocial occupational therapy in schools: Identify challenges and clarify the role of occupational therapy in promoting adaptive functioning. *OT Practice,* September, CE 1-8.

Schultz, S. (2014). Theory of occupational adaptation. In B. Schell, G. Gillen, M. Scaffa, E. Cohn (Eds.), *Willard and Spackman's occupational therapy* (12th ed., pp. 527-540). Philadelphia: J.B. Lippincott.

Schultz, S., & Bullock, L. (1991). Occupational therapy: An underutilized little-known related service for students with behavioral disorders. *Programming for adolescents with behavioral disorders.* Arlington: Council for Exceptional Children.

Schultz, S., & Schkade, J. (1992). Occupational adaptation: Toward a holistic approach to contemporary practice, Part 2. *American Journal of Occupational Therapy, 46,* 917-926.

Slavson, S. (1947). *The practice of group therapy.* New York: International Universities.

James: Posttraumatic Stress Disorder/ Inpatient Psychiatry

Ann Aviles de Bradley, PhD, OTR/L

History and Background Information

James, age 17 years, presents with an extensive history of early maltreatment and rapidly ensuing sexual behavior problems. His developmental history was remarkable for adoption by his paternal aunt after extensive early physical abuse by his biological parents. James and his siblings were removed and placed with a family member (aunt). His aunt had children of her own and soon realized that she could not care for three additional children. In less than 1 year, James and his siblings were moved to a nonrelative foster home. At this placement, his foster brother sexually abused James. He told his foster mother and she did not believe him. The abuse went on for months, until James began to run away from his foster home to escape the abuse. When James finally returned to the foster home, however, his foster mother felt he was unmanageable and requested that he no longer be placed there. After leaving this foster home, James was placed in three different group homes. Each time, he was moved because of his unruly behavior. He was referred to the child and adolescent psychiatric inpatient unit for multiple aggressive acts, with the most recent being assaulting staff at his current group home.

James was diagnosed as follows: PTSD (chronic); sex abuse of a child—victim and perpetrator issues; severe, primary support issues. James currently resides in a residential treatment program for adolescent males. He was clinically observed to be a bright and articulate adolescent with generally good social skills. However, he is often sarcastic and passive-aggressive in his interactions with staff. Because James will be turning 18 years old in the next 10 months, the staff is concerned about his transition out of the child welfare system. James demonstrates elevated scores on the Trauma Symptom Checklist for Children (TSCC) (Briere, 1996) in the areas of posttraumatic stress (PTS), sexual concerns (SC), and sexual distress (SC-D). As is true of many children who are sexually abused, James's responses reveal elevated scores in areas relevant to his history of sexual abuse. James also endorsed two critical items: "Wanting to hurt myself" and "Feeling scared of men."

Clinical staff have noted that although James demonstrates good social skills, once he begins to develop positive social relationships with adults, he begins to act aggressively toward staff (primarily through verbal "attacks"), in particular toward male staff.

The child and adolescent psychiatric unit provided several group treatment options, including art therapy, group psychotherapy, and OT. The art therapy group focused on self-expression through various mediums such as painting, drawing, and art projects. This facilitated and supported James in expressing feelings and thoughts through art to address and resolve his concerns, fears, and conflicts. Group psychotherapy emphasizes mutual sharing, support, and constructive feedback. Because all of James's peers were wards of the state, many had similar experiences with abuse and neglect. This group provided a safe space in which youths engaged in self-exploration and expressions, facilitating self-awareness of behaviors and patterns that either facilitated or limited healthy behaviors. The OT group focuses on acquiring and practicing skills needed for successful engagement in various occupational roles (e.g., student, friend, worker, etc.). The OT also implemented a system in which youth could practice money management. Youth would earn "Cooperative Cash" based on their behaviors throughout the week, and on Fridays this "cash" could be used to purchase items from the mobile store—a rolling cart that contained several items such as cologne and perfume, and more fun items such as candy and magazines.

Interdisciplinary Perspectives

Youth Perspective

James expresses the need for support with managing his feelings and engaging in school activities. He is aware that the support he is receiving will end soon and worries that he will not be successful once on his own. While he recognizes the inappropriateness of his behavior, he feels "out of control" as if he is outside of his body when these behaviors occur. He believes he has improved due to the services provided by his group home, but feels that he should be more self-sufficient in order to have a successful transition from the child welfare system.

Social Worker Perspective

James's social worker played a critical role in the facilitation of his goals and coordination of the various individuals involved in his care. The social worker had personal experiences with being a ward of the state, which facilitated their rapport and also provided the clinical team with insight and awareness regarding a concerted effort to address James's issues and concerns. The social worker expressed to the clinical team the importance of forming healthy relationship dynamics between James and the adults working with him. Further, the social worker recognized the significance of creating connections to the school community in which James was situated as well as the need to identify community agencies that would welcome and support James in his transition out of state care. As a result, each member of the clinical team was tasked with identifying a community agency that would build on the skills being developed on the adolescent psychiatric unit.

Psychiatrist Perspective

The child psychiatrist working with James on the adolescent unit has been able to improve his behavior by managing his medications. When James was first admitted, the psychiatrist completed a med "wash" in order to discern the physiological and behavioral components of James's PTSD. She has expressed to the clinical staff that James is responding well to the changes in medication and is in need of behavioral and ADL services.

James is able to identify "emotional numbness," "irritability/anger," "distrust," and "intrusive thoughts and feelings" as his primary PTSD symptoms and areas of greatest distress/dysfunction. He gave as an example of emotional numbness, feeling devastated but not being able to cry when a close friend was murdered 1 year or so before. He stated that although he felt physically sick (e.g., nauseated) upon learning of his friend's death, he was "emotionally blank" and "flat as a board." James expressed a strongly felt need for interpersonal control, stating that he rarely asked for help and instead preferred to "do it myself"; additionally, he identifies that because of his trust issues he sabotages relationships to prevent himself from being "hurt" and "let down." He states that the most terrifying feeling he had recurrently experienced in his life was "helplessness." In discussing this, he stated that as a child he always felt very small and that everyone and the world around him always seemed very big.

Treatment Principles

It is important for persons working with youths who are wards of the state to approach youths in a caring and respectful manner. Roth and Brooks-Gunn (2000) identify parental caring, connectedness, and involvement with adolescents as of fundamental importance, being associated with decreased likelihood of delinquency and substance abuse. Therefore, youths who are not developing in supportive environments require programs that will provide a safe, "family-like" environment, where caring adults will support and facilitate the development of life skills (Roth & Brooks-Gunn, 2000). Youths who are able to create strong relationships with adults (e.g., counselors, teachers, therapists) are less likely to engage in delinquent behaviors (Resnick, Bearman, Blum, et al, 1997). Furthermore, creating trusting, caring relationships is necessary for a youth to feel comfortable and confident in asking adults for assistance in obtaining life-skill training. Providers need to recognize and emphasize youths' strengths and personal resources when working with them on their transition into adulthood; this is especially significant for those who have experienced instability in their personal lives, such as children who are wards of the state. Providers must also understand the complexity of emotions that youth are experiencing. Although some youths have been removed from their homes because of neglect or abuse, many continue to

Figure 6-3. James and his OT.

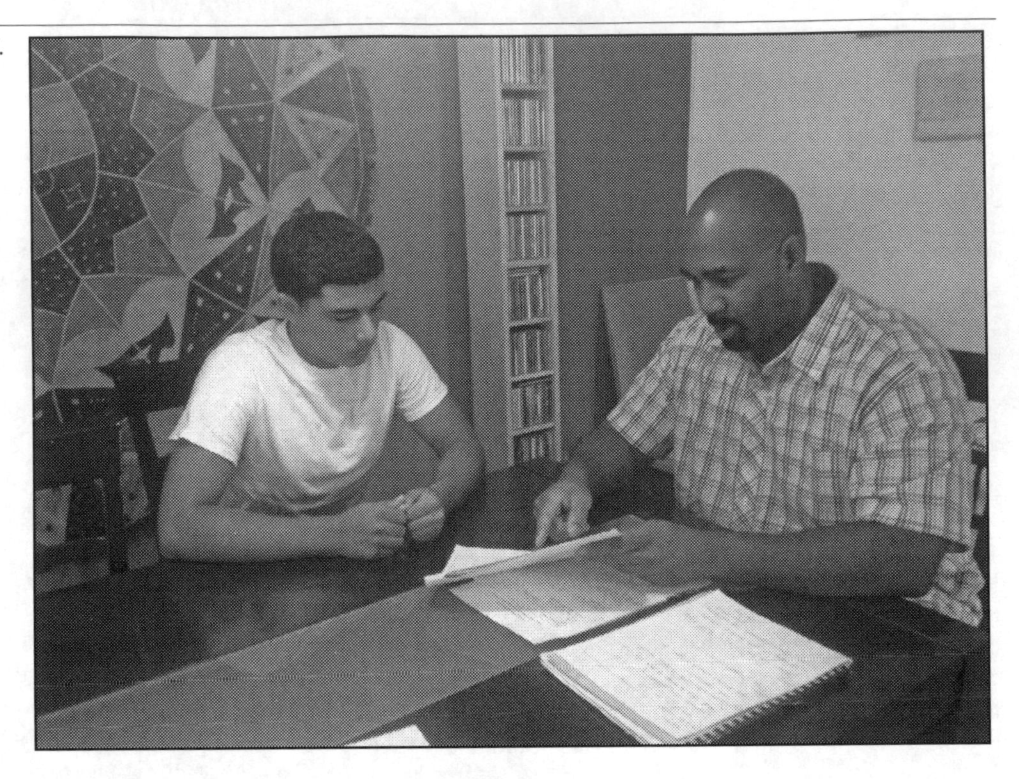

have contact with their families and often want to maintain these relationships despite the stress and strain it causes them.

Evaluation Information

Occupational Profile

James enjoys listening to music and playing basketball and video games. When he has been able to sustain appropriate behavior, he has participated in the open gym at his local park. James is on track to graduate from high school and expresses a desire to attend community college and work part-time. The plan for discharge is for James to return to the residential facility.

The OT and James completed the Occupational Self-Assessment (OSA) and The Ansell-Casey Life Skill Assessment (ACLSA) (Figure 6-3). The OSA allows youths to self-identify their areas of strength and weakness in regard to life skills, while simultaneously measuring how the environment(s) they function in support or inhibit their life-skill abilities. The ACLSA is an evaluation of youth independent living skills. It assesses daily living tasks, housing and community resources, money management, self-care, social development (communication, relationships, community values), work and study habits (career planning, decision-making, study skills). The short form assessment (for ages 11 to 18) provides a brief summary of youth abilities.

James was able to identify areas of strength as well as areas of weakness on the OSA. James's strengths include being involved as a student, worker, volunteer, and/or family member (has success as a student); working toward my goals (will graduate high school this year); and places where I can go and enjoy myself.

Areas James identified as problems include identifying and solving problems, getting along with others, and people who support and encourage me.

James identified the following as areas he would like to improve: (1) a place to live and take care of myself, (2) identifying and solving problems, (3) getting along with others, and (4) managing my finances. Information obtained from the ACLSA demonstrates James's lack of knowledge in daily living tasks and money management.

Occupational Therapy Goal Areas

- Increase positive coping skills (interpersonal) and problem solving
- Develop job readiness and home management skills
- Decrease anxiety when interacting with adults (specifically adult males)
- Develop money management skills

Questions to Consider

Occupational Performance Areas

1. How will you address James's aggression?

2. What coping skills are needed to facilitate positive and healthy relationships between James and adult males?
3. How will you address James's transition out of the child welfare system? Which life skills are most important in supporting a successful transition in his adult role?
4. What types of clinical and community contexts need to be considered for equipping James with the skills necessary for successful engagement in his current and future occupational roles?
5. Design a treatment group that will address one of James's goal areas.

Youth Education

1. What areas of individual and community education will you address with James?
2. What types of community organizations will be helpful in supporting James's transition out of the child welfare system?
3. What ongoing services will James need to achieve self-sufficiency?
4. Explain why it is important to include him in all steps of the process (problem solving decision making, resource gathering).
5. How would you collaborate with other professionals and James on his goals?

Other Considerations

1. Describe and justify the contributions an occupational therapist makes to the team in facilitating James' future success.

References

Baron, K., Kielhofner, G., Iyenger, A., Goldhammer, V., & Wolenski, J. (2006). *Occupational Self-Assessment* (OSA) (Version 2.2). Chicago: Model of Human Occupation Clearinghouse.

Breire, J. (1996). *Trauma Symptom Checklist for Children* (TSCC). Lutz, Florida: PAR.

Casey Family Programs & Ansell, D. (n.d.). Ansell-Casey Life Skill Assessment (ACLSA). Retrieved from: http://www.casey.org/cls/assessments/LifeSkills.pdf

Resources

Resnick, M. D., Bearman, P. S., Blum, R. W., Bauman, K. E., Harris, K. M., Jones, J., ...Udry, J. R. (1997). Protecting adolescents from harm: Findings from the National Longitudinal Study on Adolescent Health. *Journal of the American Medical Association, 278*(10), 823-832.

Roth, J., & Brooks-Gunn, J. (2000). What do adolescents need for healthy development? Implications for youth policy. *Social Policy Report, Giving Child and Youth Development Knowledge Away, 14*(1), 3-19.

Emma: Anxiety Disorder/Inpatient

Kristin Winston, PhD, OTR/L and Jamie Harmon, MS, OTR/L

History and Background

Emma, age 16 years, was admitted to a local psychiatric inpatient hospital earlier this month due to panic attacks that were becoming increasingly severe and interfering with occupations at home, work, and school.

Her mother reported that Emma has always struggled socially and emotionally compared to her similarly aged peers. Emma was diagnosed with an anxiety disorder at the age of 7, shortly after Hurricane Katrina, when her family was displaced for over 8 months. Since then, Emma's family has been accustomed to frequent calls from school, continuous therapies, and unpredictable behaviors. Most recently, Emma had been demonstrating increased anxiety and worry, which resulted in alienating friends, loss of a part-time job, decreased attention to self-care, and decreased ability to function in school.

Emma has been in a regular education program and her goals have always been oriented toward attending college and pursuing a career in biology. Up until this hospitalization, Emma had been receiving reasonable accommodations under Section 504 for issues related to anxiety at school. Emma's teachers describe her as having difficulties and anxiety over school work and social activities, difficulty attending to tasks, having low self-esteem, and being easily distracted. These behaviors are not always present, but have recently become problematic in terms of her success in daily occupations.

Evaluation Information

Occupational Profile

Emma's family consists of herself, an older brother who is 18 and away at college, and a younger sister who is 14. Emma's parents have been married for 20 years. Both of her parents work outside the home; her father is employed full-time as a high school teacher and her mother works part-time as a bank teller. Emma's family is very supportive and has been very involved in her programming.

Throughout Emma's first week in the hospital, she spent many hours with various members of the treatment team, including the psychiatrist, psychologist, behavioralist, social worker, OT, nurses, MD residents, and teachers. Each of the team members had his/her own assessments to complete and began formalizing a comprehensive intervention plan for Emma. Within the first 24 hours, Emma was placed on a positive support behavior plan that was followed by all staff (24 hours a day), and she was assessed by the occupational therapy department to focus on safety and ability to participate in daily occupations, including ADL, school work, and socialization. During the first week, she began attending the hospital's school-based program, where she received her educational services during her hospital stay.

Analysis of Occupational Performance

Emma's assessment with the OT went very well and Emma began asking to work with OT multiple times per day. The OT worked with Emma to determine strengths and barriers by completing the *Canadian Occupational Performance Measure* (Law et al, 2005), where Emma's occupational performance concerns were: taking care of her appearance (Performance Score 6, Importance 9, Satisfaction 4), getting her part-time job back (Performance 1, Importance, 10, Satisfaction 1), going to movies with friends (Performance 4, Importance, 5, Satisfaction, 5),and being successful in her classes at school (Performance 5, Importance 10, Satisfaction 4).

Emma also completed the Adolescent/Adult Sensory Profile (Brown & Dunn, 2002) and her scores indicated sensory sensitivity as her overall pattern of response. This was particularly evident in relationship to auditory, tactile, and vestibular information. Emma demonstrated difficulty managing and coping with various stimuli in her environment. At the time of admission, she appeared to spend much of her day working to stay in difficult situations and fighting the desire to leave difficult situations, and she had significant difficulty accessing coping skills and enjoying any of her leisure time. She had trouble with attention to task and was easily distracted by her environment. Emma appeared very worried about how she was doing and what would happen next.

Progress Information

Throughout week 2, Emma began to show some signs of improvement. Although she still expressed anxiety and worry, she was able to participate in group activities with her peers with support from the staff. Emma was able to work with the therapists and social workers to complete her assessments and begin therapy. She was able to make it through most of her school day and complete the majority of her schoolwork, though her attention was poor and her anxiety remained high.

Following her short stay on the inpatient unit, the plan for Emma is to return home with her family and back to attending her high school as she was prior to her hospitalization. She is to continue her medication, which will be followed by outpatient visits with the psychiatrist. Emma and her family will continue to receive outpatient counseling support as well.

As the OT who will be working with Emma upon returning to high school, you have met with the current inpatient OT to discuss programming and Emma's goals for returning home. Emma will now be receiving a formal transition plan under IDEA part B in the category of emotional disturbance.

Questions to Consider

Goals/Treatment

1. What will your goals for transitioning planning look like given the background information and assessment information you currently have?
2. What frame of reference will guide your further assessment and intervention?

Planning for Discharge

1. Identify three long-term transition goals and two short-term objectives for each goal.
2. Identify one appropriate intervention strategy for three of the short-term objectives. Include the rationale for your choice of strategy (developmental theory, frames of reference, support in the literature), identify what your role will be and what Emma's role will be in the activity.

References

Brown, C., & Dunn, W. (2002). *Adolescent/adult sensory profile.* San Antonio, TX: Pearson.

Law, M., Baptiste, S., Carswell, A., McColl, M., Polatajko, H., & Pollock, N. (2005). *Canadian occupational performance measure* (4th ed.). Ottawa, Ontario: Canadian Association of Occupational Therapists.

Chapter 7

Introduction to Community Settings

Occupational therapists (OTs) are increasingly providing services to children and youth in community-based settings. Sometimes the services are being provided to children directly, as they would in more traditional settings (i.e., schools and hospitals). Other times, the OTs act as consultants to organizations that serve children and youth.

Expanding our role to meet the occupational needs of children in the community is in keeping with the American Occupational Therapy Association's Centennial Vision (AOTA, 2007). OTs who work with community organizations may be involved in needs assessments, program development, and measuring program outcomes. In addition, they may be responsible for developing educational materials, training other staff, and day-to-day operations.

Community practice provides an opportunity for OTs to meet the occupational needs of society (AOTA, 2007) and develop innovative avenues for service delivery. As we are part of a global community, this type of practice extends beyond one's backyard and can mean traveling to meet the occupational needs of children and youth abroad.

Questions to Consider

1. What is a population of children and youth that you feel is underserved?
2. If you could create a community practice with these children or youths at the focus, what would it look like? What would you do? What resources would you need?

Reference

American Occupational Therapy Association. (2007). AOTA's centennial vision and executive summary. *American Journal of Occupational Therapy, 61*(6), 613-614.

Michael: Anoxic Brain Injury/Hippotherapy

Monica Griffin, OTD, OTR/L, C/NDT

History and Background Information

Michael, age 5 years, has a diagnosis of anoxic brain injury. At 3 years of age, Michael suffered from an asthma attack that led to an anoxic episode and the diagnosis of his brain injury. For 2.5 years, Michael has received 20+ hours of therapy a week, to which hippotherapy was added as a treatment strategy within the last 4 months.

Evaluation Information

Occupational Profile

Prior to his injury, Michael was a very active boy who loved to play with his three older brothers. He is very interested in sports such as baseball and enjoys going on vacations with his family. Michael is a very determined and energetic child who loves interacting and playing with peers. Currently, Michael attends preschool 3 days a week and has a very rigorous therapy schedule to aid in his recovery.

Michael's mother reports that he needs maximum assistance with many activities of daily living (ADL). These areas include dressing, bathing, bowel and bladder management, functional mobility, and personal hygiene

Cahill SM, Bowyer P, eds. *Cases in Pediatric Occupational Therapy: Assessment and Intervention (pp 155-173).*

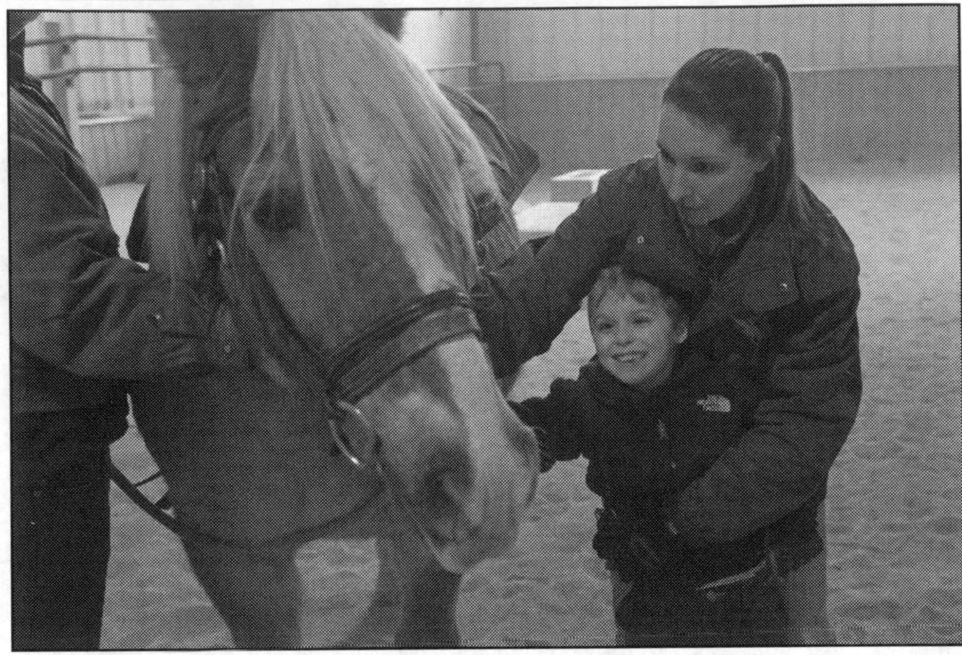

Figure 7-1. Michael getting used to the horse.

and grooming. Michael's mother reports that he is able to self-feed with increased time. He is currently finger-feeding and working toward using utensils. His mother reported that within the past couple of months, he started receiving his entire caloric intake orally. He continues to receive hydration through his g-tube, although he is working toward drinking thin liquids.

Michael is very motivated to participate in play activities, although occasionally this area of occupation is difficult for Michael due to limited communication. Michael's mother reported that he is able to vocalize various words/phrases but they can only be recognizable if said within a given context.

Analysis of Occupational Performance

Michael has active range of motion within normal limits for his upper extremities. He presents with left-hand dominance for activities but demonstrates a more efficient pincer grasp with his right hand. Michael's carpometacarpal (CMC) joint in his right thumb frequently subluxes during grasping activities. He is able to transfer objects between hands independently and is able to visually target and grasp a toy of interest inconsistently due to his fluctuating tone. Michael is participating in bilateral coordination activities with improved ease. He is able to stabilize an object with his right hand and manipulate with his left hand.

Michael rolls as his primary means of mobility throughout his environment, although he is able to assume a quadruped stance independently. Currently, Michael is working toward maintaining quadruped for an increased period of time with minimal assistance. Michael is able to weightbear through his lower extremities independently and needs moderate to maximum assistance for balance when standing and walking.

Cognitively, Michael can understand simple directions, such as, "Give me the red ball." He is able to engage in interactions and make his needs known through gestures and vocalizations. Michael is working on using an augmentative communication device for communication in speech therapy to increase his independence in all environments.

Upon incorporating hippotherapy, Michael needed maximum assistance for sitting balance. He was able to maintain upright sitting for a maximum of 30 to 45 seconds inconsistently while participating in a functional activity. His upper extremities frequently locked into extension for stabilization and he presented with head and neck hyperextension due to decreased strength and stability. Michael also had significant flexion in his thoracic spine as a result of weak abdominals and poor paraspinal muscule activity. Furthermore, Michael demonstrated difficulty vocalizing due to stabilizing with his jaw secondary to decreased strength. His primary goal areas for OT were to improve postural control, proximal stability, upper extremity strength, and trunk strength.

The first hippotherapy session focused primarily on evaluating Michael's response to the horse (Figure 7-1). Immediately, it was noted that Michael could not tolerate wearing a helmet on the horse. It was evident that he had severe head and neck instability, which could have caused more damage with the added weight of the helmet. After the helmet was removed, Michael was better able to control his head. The therapist then observed that Michael

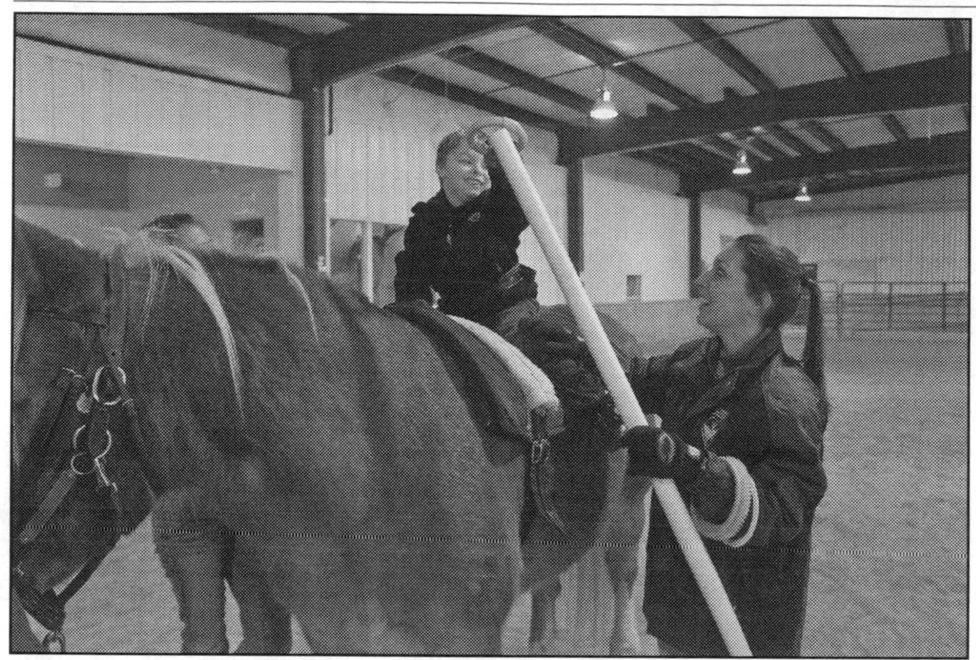

Figure 7-2. Michael reaching on horseback.

presented with significant flexion throughout his trunk, which corresponds with his posture while sitting on a bench or bolster. Michael also presents with tightness in his lower extremities, which makes it difficult to straddle the barrel of the horse.

While on the horse, Michael sits on a bareback pad in order to feel the warmth of the horse, facilitate stretching of his lower extremities, and provide him with a large base of support for improved postural control. Michael needs two side walkers to help him with his balance while riding, and a leader is used to control and guide the horse. During sessions, Michael typically participates in activities that challenge his postural system. For example, the therapist instructs the leader to guide the horse around cones or in circles in order to facilitate a righting reaction. The more twists and turns, the harder it is for Michael to maintain an upright posture. In addition to balance reactions, Michael also works on upper extremity weight bearing and reaching activities to promote strengthening and control. For these activities, Michael will work on reaching for rings or toys to improve the accuracy of his upper extremities (Figure 7-2). He is also positioned backwards or in quadruped to facilitate weight bearing on his arms to increase strength and stability.

Progress Information

Since beginning hippotherapy, Michael has dramatically improved his sitting balance and upper extremity strength and control. Currently, he is able to sit on a bolster with contact guard assistance while participating in a functional tabletop activity. Michael is able to more consistently reach for toys in his environment with improved accuracy in order to play. His head and neck stability is also improving, suggesting increased strength throughout his trunk and postural system. Michael's parents report that their primary goals for him are to increase independence with ADL and instrumental activities of daily living (IADL) such as feeding, dressing, bathing, functional mobility, and communication management.

In Michael's case, one of the main areas all three disciplines (OT, physical therapy, and speech and language pathology) were working toward was to increase his proximal stability and strength in order to make gains distally. These gains would positively impact his gross-motor skills, fine-motor skills, ADL, and communication skills. As a result, hippotherapy was suggested as a treatment strategy to meet these goal areas. Since Michael started OT sessions integrating hippotherapy, he has greatly enjoyed each and every week. The horse, volunteers, and therapists afford Michael the opportunity to interact with everyone in his environment in a purposeful manner. It is evident that Michael is greatly motivated by this meaningful task that promotes active participation.

Questions to Consider

1. Write out a problem list for Michael.
2. What strengths does Michael possess that can be used throughout hippotherapy treatment sessions in order to attain functional outcomes?

3. What short-term goals would you set for Michael in order to work toward increasing his independence in the following ADL?
   a. Feeding
   b. Bathing
   c. Dressing
   d. Functional mobility
4. Describe how traditional OT and hippotherapy will support Michael's development toward his goals. Discuss how the two different types of treatment complement one another.
5. Describe the type of adaptive equipment Michael may need to increase his independence in the following ADL:
   a. Feeding
   b. Bathing
   c. Dressing
6. How might the subluxation occurring at Michael's CMC joint be addressed?
7. What types of environmental adaptations or strategies need to be used to help Michael sequence multiple steps for ADL?
8. What are some ways to support Michael psychologically as he grows and matures into adolescence?
9. A common dilemma that arises when adding hippotherapy as a treatment strategy is that therapists, parents, and doctors are unaware that hippotherapy exists. Furthermore, many medical professionals are unaware of the purpose or benefit that a horse's movement can have on a child's function, therefore they overlook the possibilities hippotherapy can have on a child's prognosis. Even if a therapist does not know about this treatment strategy, it is the therapist's responsibility to inform the family about what options are available in order to provide the child with the best care possible. Locate two resources that could be shared with families, therapists, or doctors who are interested in learning more about hippotherapy.

Resources

American Occupational Therapy Association. (2008). Occupational therapy practice framework: Domain and process (2nd ed.). *American Journal of Occupational Therapy, 62*, 625-683.

Engel, B., & MacKinnon, J. (2007). *Enhancing human occupation through hippotherapy.* Bethesda, MD: American Occupational Therapy Association.

Snider, L., Korner-Bitensky, N., Kammann, C., Warner, S., & Saleh, M. (2007). Horseback riding as therapy for children with cerebral palsy: Is there evidence of its effectiveness? *Physical & Occupational Therapy in Pediatrics, 27*(2), 5-23.

Opening Doors/ Community Organization

Brittany Diasio, MOT, OTR/L;
Brooke Dudley, MOT, OTR/L;
Brianne N. Heiland, MOT, OTR/L;
Elizabeth Kohler-Rausch, OTR/L; and
Kiley Rich, MOT, OTR/L

History and Background Information

Organization

The mission of the organization is to provide programming, opportunities, and resources to individuals with developmental disabilities, 14 to 30 years old, so that they can pursue educational, social, and occupational interests. The organization's goal is to foster an environment where individuals with developmental disabilities can be active and experience self-enrichment and self-advocacy while being recognized for their unique and exceptional abilities within the larger community.

Programming at the organization ranges from artistic to sports-focused, with an emphasis on continually providing opportunities for participation across the diverse range of skills and abilities of the participants. New programming runs seasonally in 4- and 5-week sessions.

Client Population

The client population at the organization includes individuals with developmental disabilities ages 14 to 30 years old. The performance deficits of the clientele range from physical to cognitive. Specific diagnoses include Down syndrome, cerebral palsy, and autism spectrum diagnoses. Opening Doors would like to collaborate with an OT to expand their cooking program. The OT does a cursory task analysis related to cooking.

Benefits of Cooking (Moyer, 2009)

- Enjoyable for many
- Learning how to prepare healthy and nutritious meals
- Increases independence
- Opportunity for social interaction
- Saves money

Performance Skills for Cooking

- Cooking requires a variety of skills, ranging from cognitive to physical.

Cognitive Skills

- Comprehension of the recipe
- Sequencing
- Multitasking
- Problem solving
- Mathematical calculations
- Selecting appropriate tools and ingredients
- Organizing task objects and timing

Motor Skills

- Bending
- Reaching
- Lifting
- Carrying
- Manipulating task objects
- Cutting
- Chopping
- Stirring
- Gross grasp
- Pincer grasp

Sensory Perceptual Skills

- Positioning of one's body safely while interacting with objects, tools, and equipment
- Interpreting hot and cold temperatures
- Tasting the flavors of the food
- Tactile sensation of various food textures while preparing
- Interpreting different smells (burning while cooking)
- Auditory cues (timers, popping of food)

Evaluation Information

Occupational Profile

In addition to completing the task analysis, the OTs completed interviews with the staff, conducted a site visit, and received a brief description of the current cooking program. The next cooking program would have a Thanksgiving theme and allow every member of the class to participate in each session. The initial sessions would focus on learning cooking techniques and practice making recipes. During the last session, the entire class would cook a typical Thanksgiving meal to enjoy with the other members and staff at the organization.

Analysis of Occupational Performance

In order to prioritize concerns, the OTs needed to gain an understanding of the activity demands and the environment for the cooking program. From staff interviews, the consulting therapists discovered that past programs have utilized simple recipes with minimal use of adaptive strategies and equipment. An environmental analysis revealed the current kitchen resources and areas of need for standard and adaptive equipment. Currently, the organization has a kitchen available that is being used for both program participants and staff. The kitchen includes a larger countertop with many cabinets, a sink, a full-size refrigerator, a full-size gas stove, vinyl flooring, iridescent lighting, and a large work table with eight chairs. The kitchen is separated from the next room with a partial collapsible door. The kitchen is supplied with basic utensils and basic kitchen items. Adapted equipment includes a cutting board and rocker knife. Financial resources are limited due to the organization receiving mostly private funding minus 3% provided by government funding. The organization also relies on volunteers to assist in program implementation.

Client Factors: Body Functions

Due to the wide range of abilities and body functions of the client population, the OTs consider many possibilities in client ability levels and participation (Radomski & Trombly Latham, 2008). Clients were viewed on a continuum including lower functioning to higher functioning clients with developmental disabilities. The varying abilities of these individuals presented a challenge for equal participation within the weekly cooking tasks. The following are some of the client's concerns.

Neuromusculoskeletal and Movement-Related

- Spasticity
- Low tone
- Involuntary movement reactions
- Decreased strength and range of motion
- Decreased fine- and gross-motor control
- Impaired eye-hand coordination
- Difficulties with bilateral coordination
- Decreased standing and sitting balance

Sensory Functions

- Decreased ability to modulate sensory input
- Decreased ability to discriminate sensory input
- Vision deficits including low vision
- Diminished sensation including light touch, pain, and temperature
- Diminished sense of body in space
- Diminished hearing

Mental

- Decreased processing speed
- Difficulty with attention
- Decreased IQ
- Impaired safety awareness
- Impaired memory
- Diminished impulse control
- Difficulties regulating emotions
- Impaired executive functions
- Dyspraxia

Voice and Speech

- Impaired vocalizations
- Alternative vocalization functions and technology considerations
- Difficulties understanding spoken speech

Cardiovascular

- Decreased endurance
- Difficulties regulating blood pressure

Client Factors: Performance Skills

Similarly to body functions, client factors related to performance skills were analyzed on a continuum from low to high in order to meet the diverse needs of the client population (AOTA, 2008). Skill sets vary from clients new to cooking tasks to those familiar with simple meal prep activities. Consultation recommendations included the following.

Recipe Simplification

- Break down steps so each item is one short statement
- Use simple, consistent terminology

Picture System

- Use pictures of the items used in the recipe

Measurement Color-Coding System

- Implement a color-coding system for typically used measurements
- Use the symbol in the recipe and also place it on the appropriate measuring device

Repositioning Techniques

- Remove (or open) cabinet doors to allow someone in a wheelchair to slide his or her chair and legs under the counter to be positioned closer to the counter.
- Mount mirrors above the stove top to allow people in wheelchairs to see what they are cooking.
- Allow clients to sit or stand while working.
- Provide support to extremities.
- Allow clients to experiment with different adaptive equipment and select what works best for the individual (Table 7-1).

Environmental and Equipment Adaptations

Safety

- Always make sure clients are educated on the proper way to use equipment.
- Provide supervision during cooking tasks.
- Be aware of any precautions or concerns of clients.

Questions to Consider

Goal Areas and Treatment Focus

1. How can the OT ensure equal involvement for all participants in the cooking program?
2. How will the OT present the program to staff and participants?
3. How can the OT facilitate social interaction amongst participants?
4. How can the OT create opportunities to challenge and advance participant skills?

Safety Precautions

1. How will the OT and/or staff designate safe and appropriate tasks for each individual in the program?
2. Are enough staff members available to closely supervise individuals engaging in potentially dangerous cooking tasks?

Intervention Plan

1. How can the OT train staff regarding all consultation recommendations?
2. How will the OT monitor effectiveness throughout the intervention process?
3. How will the OT adapt if the recommendations do not fully meet the needs of the participants?

Planning for Discharge

1. How can the OT best prepare staff to carry out the cooking program in the future? (Or future sustainability?)
2. How can the OT ensure consistent application of the recipe simplification system?
3. How can the OT assess the effectiveness of the program following implementation?
4. Will the OT provide opportunity for retraining or additional consultation to address the organization's future needs?

Table 7-1

Environmental and Equipment Adaptations

EQUIPMENT	HOW IT CAN BE USED	WHO CAN BENEFIT FROM THIS
Dycem nonslip mats	Dycem may be placed underneath plates, bowls, and other kitchen containers in order to prevent these containers from sliding. Dycem provides a more stable surface to work on. Dycem may also be used to open a tight jar with a twist off lid. Dycem may be used in many recipes such as the green bean casserole when the ingredients need to be mixed in the bowl.	Students who exhibit poor motor capabilities, coordination, or bilateral integration may benefit from this product.
Single-hand cutting board	A large adapted cutting board can be used to help stabilize food. Vegetables, fruit, and meats can be stabilized by being placed onto the spikes while the other hand cuts. A cutting board with raised edges can help prevent bread from sliding when spreading topping. Some models include a vice, which can be used to hold not only food but also jars and mixing bowls. This cutting board can be used to slice cheese for the broccoli and cheese casserole and for cutting fruit and sweet potatoes.	Individuals with motor impairments, including unilateral weakness and spasticity, CP, attention deficits, autism, and general cognitive deficits.
Special pan holder	A pan holder can help to stabilize a pot or pan while stirring. It prevents the pan from turning and sliding, which can often cause spills. One that as suction cup feet will help to secure the pan holder to the stove. A pan holder can be beneficial for the sweet potatoes and stuffing.	Individuals with motor impairments, including unilateral weakness and spasticity, CP, Down syndrome, autism, and general cognitive deficits.
Rocker knife	A rocker knife allows the individual to use gentle pressure to cut. Pressure placed onto the knife using the whole hand, and rocking back and forth allows the knife to cut. This tool can facilitate one hand cutting. A rocker knife can be used to help prepare the stuffing and fruit turkey.	Individuals with decreased strength and dexterity, motor impairment including unilateral weakness and spasticity, Down syndrome, and general cognitive deficits.
Weighted utensils	Weighted utensils may assist students with poor dexterity and coordination. Weighted utensils also provide more sensory input. These utensils may be incorporated in the cream cheese fruit dip recipe when stirring the ingredients.	These utensils may benefit students with poor coordination, ataxia, or require more sensory input.
Color-coded measuring system	Color coding assists in the cognitive aspects involved with cooking. This becomes important when exact measurements are needed. Color coding measuring instruments eliminates the need for math skills. Color coding is especially useful when measuring many ingredients such as in traditional holiday stuffing recipe.	This technique will benefit any student with cognitive difficulties such as students with autism, Down syndrome, etc.
Colored foam tubing	Foam tubing may be incorporated to provide better ergonomics on utensil and pan handles. Foam tubing could be incorporated on a whisk for the corn pudding recipe.	Foam tubing may benefit any student with poor hand strength allowing for more ease of grip.
Can drainer	This allows for easier draining of canned items. This tool comes in varying sizes to fit different cans. This device helps ensure the contents for the recipe are held in the can while the liquid is only released. The corn pudding recipe could incorporate this tool for draining the can of corn.	This tool may be utilized for students with decreased hand function, unsteady grip, or decreased control of force in movements.

(continued)

Table 7-1 (continued)

Environmental and Equipment Adaptations

EQUIPMENT	*HOW IT CAN BE USED*	*WHO CAN BENEFIT FROM THIS*
Slap chopper	This device allows one to chop and dice without exposing fingers to a blade. Items must be small enough first to fit into the container. Items are diced with the push of a large button. This item may be used in the recipe traditional holiday stuffing to chop the celery.	The slap chopper may be used for students who have limited ability to use a knife due to poor hand function or decreased judgment and safety awareness.
Double-handled pots, pans, etc.	Double-handled kitchen items allow for better joint protection by evenly distributing the weight between the two upper limbs. Items such as these may be useful in the candied sweet potato recipe when carrying the pan to and from the stove.	Students with decreased coordination and strength may benefit from double handled kitchen items.
Plastic lettuce knives	These knives have no sharp blades and may be used to cut a variety of items such as fruits, vegetables, and bread. This tool requires more force with more firm items such as carrots. This knife may be incorporated into the fruit turkey recipe when cutting the fruit.	Students with decreased judgment and safety awareness will benefit from this tool. Students with poor hand coordination and dexterity may benefit as well.
Rope loops	Loops of rope may be incorporated on cabinet, door, and refrigerator handles to allow for easier access. This may be useful when collecting ingredients for the scalloped potatoes recipe such as the milk and butter.	Students with limited hand function may find using loops to open cabinets and doors easier.
Electric equipment (i.e., can opener, mixer, blender)	Electric equipment helps to conserve energy when cooking by reducing the physical demands and the time for meal preparation. When choosing electric equipment, make sure it is still easy to use and maneuver. For example, one handed cordless can openers may be made only in a right hand model. An electric can opener may be beneficial in the pumpkin pie recipe in order to open the can of pumpkin.	Students with CP, Down syndrome, autism, etc. may benefit from electric equipment.
Spring-loaded tongs	Spring-loaded tongs allow for a more gross grasp to be utilized when picking up objects while also working on the hand strength needed for fine motor coordination. Spring-loaded tongs may be used in the fruit turkey recipe when placing the fruit on the plate.	Students with poor bilateral coordination may benefit from this product.
Egg cracker	There are various different pieces of equipment that are made to facilitate egg cracking. Some models not only crack the egg, but also separate the yolk and prevent the egg shell from getting into the food. This tool may be used for the holiday stuffing, pumpkin pie, and corn pudding, which all require eggs.	Students with decreased hand strength and dexterity may benefit from this tool.
Hot/cold faucet indicator	This indicator changes the water color depending on it's temperature. Blue indicates that the water is cold or room temperature, and red indicates hot water. The indicator turns off when the water is shut off.	Individuals with sensory and cognitive deficits, Down syndrome, autism, etc. may benefit from this product.
Sponge mitt	A sponge mitt can be used to wash dishes for those with limited grasp who may have trouble holding onto a washcloth or regular sponge.	Individuals with limited grasp and other fine motor difficulties, general hand weakness, and spasticity may benefit from this product.

Adapted from Patterson Medical Holdings, Inc., (2013). Kitchen supplies. Retrieved from http://www.pattersonmedical.com/app.aspx?cmd=searchResults&sk=kitchen

References

American Occupational Therapy Association. (2008). Occupational therapy practice framework: Domain and process (2nd ed.). *American Journal of Occupational Therapy, 62*, 625-683.

Moyer, A. (2009). *Why teach cooking skills to children with special needs?* Retrieved from http://www.yourspecialchef.com/ysc_production/_design/app/_show/ static/Why Teach Cooking Skills

Patterson Medical Holdings, Inc., (2013). *Kitchen supplies.* Retrieved from http://www.pattersonmedical.com/app.aspx?cmd=searchResults&sk=kitchen

Radomski, M., & Trombly Latham, C. (2008). *Occupational therapy for physical dysfunction* (6th ed.). Philadelphia: Lippincott Williams & Wilkins.

Ivan: Status Post Burns and Left Lower Extremity Amputation/Village in Ecuador

Mark Kovic, OTD, OTR/L

History and Background Information

Ivan, age 5 years, sustained approximately one-third total body surface area (TBSA) burns as a result of a fire of unknown cause. He sustained burns to aspects of both of his legs, both arms, and his face. He has a left trans-tibial, trans-fibial lower extremity (LE) amputation (Figure 7-3).

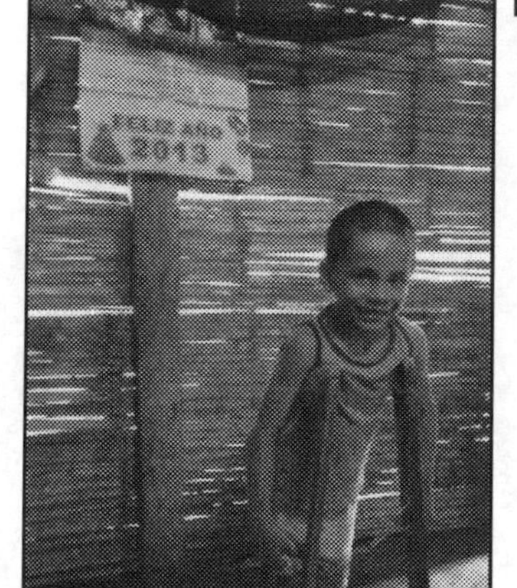

Figure 7-3. Ivan.

Ivan received physiotherapy twice per week for approximately 1 hour per session in the city of Guayaquil, Ecuador, from January through March. Health care, including therapy/ancillary services, is provided to Ecuadorans free of charge at state-run hospitals and clinics. Currently, he is waiting to be fit for a prosthesis (Handal, Lozoff, Breilh, & Harlow, 2007).

Ivan lives in rural coastal Balzar, Guayas, Ecuador. Balzar is a town of approximately 50,000 residents located in Guayas Province. This town is situated approximately 90 kilometers (approximately 55 miles) north of Guayaquil, which is the seat of the local provincial government.

Ivan's primary caregiver is his youngest aunt, Bermania. Bermania is a single parent of three children below the age of 7 who earns a living by planting and harvesting rice. Her sister is Ivan's mother. Prior to being taken care of by Bermania, Ivan, his mother, and his brother were being taken care of by Ivan's grandmother. However, Ivan's grandmother recently died as a result of being run over by a motorcycle. Currently, Bermania is the only caregiver for Ivan, her children, her sister, and Ivan's younger brother.

Ivan's mother has a history of mental health concerns. She has never been evaluated by a psychiatrist to determine her illness, yet she is currently unable to handle her basic self-care needs. Ivan's younger brother is 3 years old. Ivan's younger brother was reportedly conceived as a result of a sexual assault on Ivan's mother when she disappeared during a period of unmanaged mental illness.

The OT's connection to Ivan began when a project coordinator spoke to the Guayas Province Vice-Prefectura asking for specific support for Ivan and his family. The project coordinator organized key stakeholders to make sure that Ivan would be able to meet with a support team from an international non-governmental organization (NGO). This NGO is grounded in its mission to work with improving the quality of life of the citizens of Ecuador. Members of the NGO support team included the OT, a PT, the director of the NGO, members of the local Club de Liones (Lions Club) chapter, and representatives of the province/prefectura government. The team met Ivan in March in his current residence in order to observe and consult with the family as indicated regarding current or future needs.

Consultation Information

There are no community-based OT personnel within an approximate 100-mile radius of this family. Occupational therapy personnel are in limited supply in urban areas in coastal Ecuador and in even more limited supply in rural areas in this particular region. Thus, this consultation was made and plans were implemented given this knowledge and expectation of the likelihood of limited follow-up services.

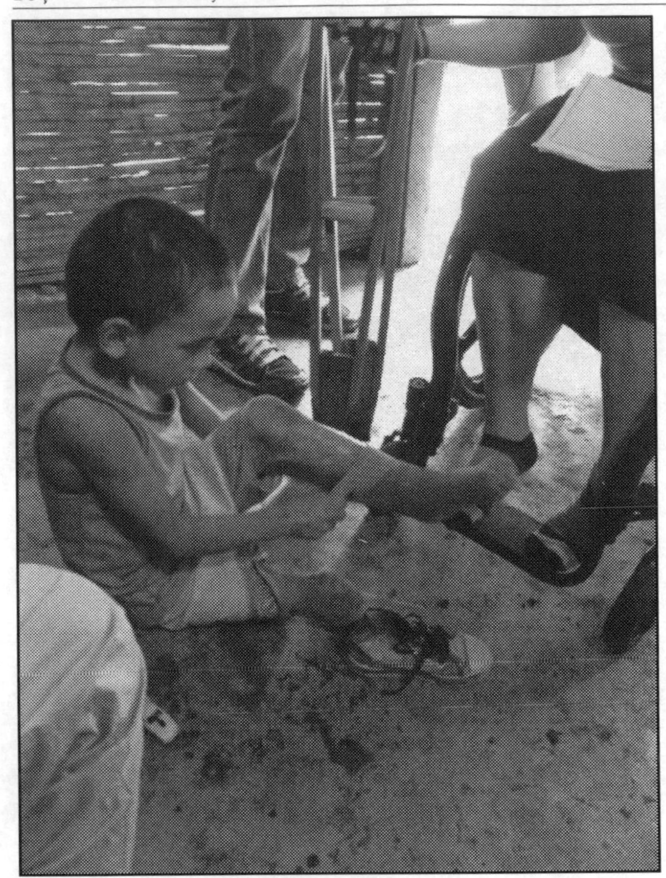

Figure 7-4. Ivan donning his sock.

Ivan was observed in a natural environment engaging in his usual daily activities. Ivan lives with his family is a four-room house without a front door and with limited running water. Ivan's family has limited access to electricity. His mother, aunt, grandfather, brother, and three cousins also live in the house. This house is approximately 1000 square feet. There is a dirt path that leads to a dirt road approximately 100 feet in length. In the rainy season, this entire area is often muddy and has limited accessibility.

It was necessary to observe Ivan engage in various age-appropriate activities to determine whether his burn scars were impeding his occupational performance. No formal assessments were completed. Rather, while Ivan engaged in play activities, his upper extremity range of motion and strength were assessed and determined to be within functional limits.

Lower extremity range of motion was also assessed in this fashion and appeared to be within functional limits.

Ivan was asked to doff and then don his sock and shoe (Figure 7-4). When he removed these items, the team observed that his great and second toes appeared to be dislocated toward the medial aspect of his body. The scars that run alongside the superior aspect of his foot appeared to be contributing to this deformity. Ivan did not report any pain or discomfort. His aunt stated that she had already made his medical treatment team, including his regular physiotherapist, aware of this deformity.

Ivan and his family speak Spanish. The following questions and responses are presented in translation and taken from conversations that occurred during the visit.

OT: How is Ivan doing with playing with his friends since the accident?

Ivan's aunt: Ivan always plays with his cousins. He is the leader of the group. He seems to have adjusted well after the fire.

OT: Does Ivan tell you anything about his burns, such as with pain or discomfort?

Ivan's aunt: No. He never complains. He is as happy as he has always been. He is always smiling. That makes me smile.

OT: Is he using his hands and moving around when he plays?

Ivan's aunt: Ivan jumps around. He sometimes sits on his legs by crossing them. He will kneel. He does not usually stand when he plays unless he needs to go get a toy.

OT: Can Ivan dress himself? Can he do his buttons and zippers?

Ivan's aunt: That was one of the first things he tried to do after the accident. He wants to do all of that for himself. He never asks for help. I think he wants to do it on his own. He can't always do buttons, snaps, or zippers. He can put his shirt and pants on.

OT: Does he use his hands to do what he needs to do?

Ivan's aunt: He sometimes will use his other [left] hand to move some things around in his right hand. I only see him do this when he is writing or coloring. He does not do this when he plays with his friends or when he eats or drinks.

Analysis of Occupational Performance

Per report from his aunt, Ivan independently completes all of his self-care. He bathes himself without difficulty using hot water and a washtub. He also feeds himself but needs assistance with cutting food. Ivan dons/doffs pullover short-sleeved shirts independently. Ivan is able to complete his lower body dressing with modified strategies. He completes donning/doffing his shorts and jeans, not including fasteners. He is able to don/doff his sock and shoe and tie the shoe with extra time. His strategy to sit on the ground (or any low to the ground surface) appears to be sufficient to complete this particular activity.

Ivan plays alongside his friends and family members at the floor/ground level. When he plays with toys or is drawing, he does so in a modified kneeling position. Because his knee is intact on his unaffected side, he is able to utilize this extremity for support in a variety of positions.

Ivan colors and writes in various positions (Figure 7-5). He was observed in a seated position while he worked on his lap. He is right hand dominant and he is able to

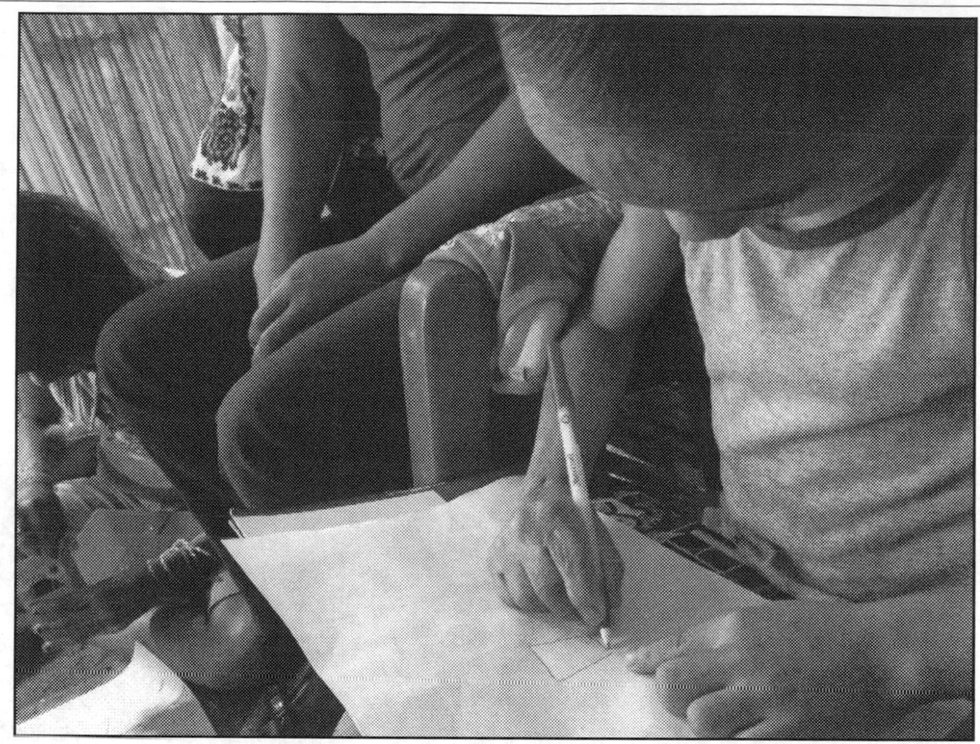

Figure 7-5. Ivan writing.

incorporate the right hand into these activities, except sometimes when he wants to manipulate a writing utensil in his right hand. manipulating writing utensils, such as turning a pencil around to access the eraser or adjust a crayon in his hand, is accomplished by Ivan bringing his left hand to complete these adjustments. It appeared that he compensated in this way approximately 50% of the time, yet he did so effectively.

Ivan ambulates using wooden crutches. However, he is unable to carry things when he is using his crutches. At this time, Ivan moves around in his home environment more quickly and efficiently on all four limbs.

Ivan's aunt completes most of the home management tasks; however, she sometimes requires Ivan's assistance with meal preparation and laundry. Because of Ivan's difficulty using his crutches, he is unable to transport laundry from the washtub to the clothes line without it getting dirty. Ivan is also unable to peel potatoes or other vegetables or chop vegetables into small pieces. Although Ivan is only 5 years old, it is not uncommon for other children this age in Ivan's village to complete these tasks.

Ivan will begin to attend school this fall. Ivan's school is located 2 miles from his home and children in the village are expected to walk to and from school in all types of weather. Ivan will need to bring his lunch to school and carry his books back and forth.

The NGO team will have an opportunity to visit Ivan one more time before they leave the village later this week.

Questions to Consider

1. Locate the village of Balzar on a map, as well as socioeconomic information about this village.
2. What are some typical obstacles that are generally encountered by children in Ecuador?
3. What are some additional questions that you might ask Ivan's aunt to get a better sense of his occupational performance?
4. What are some other occupations in which you would like to observe Ivan engaging?
5. Discuss the psychosocial aspects associated with Ivan's case. How do you think such factors have influenced his development? Do you anticipate any additional challenges related to these issues in the future?
6. Based on the information from the consultation, what are Ivan's strengths and needs? Prioritize his needs.
7. Discuss how you anticipate Ivan's needs will change in the future.
8. What sort of obstacles do you imagine he will encounter when he starts going to school? What are some possible solutions to these obstacles?
9. Describe specific ways that OT could be used to address Ivan's occupational performance difficulties when the NGO team returns to Ivan's house later this week. Consider any equipment that the OT would bring or fabricate to support Ivan. Also, describe how information will be provided to Ivan's aunt.

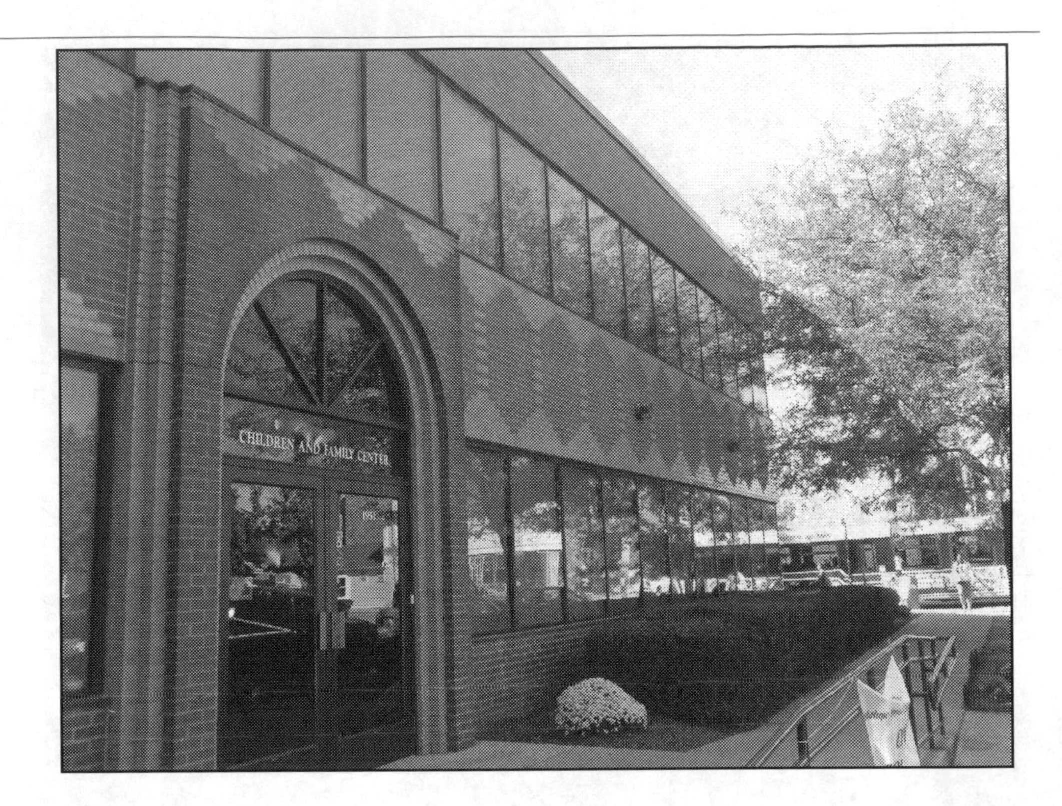

Figure 7-6. La Fuente.

10. Ivan currently sees a physiotherapist. What information would you like to communicate to the physiotherapist? How do you think the physiotherapist could help to support Ivan's occupational performance after the OT leaves Ecuador?
11. What are the challenges and opportunities associated with providing OT services in underserved communities abroad?
12. What are the knowledge, skills, and attitudes that OT practitioners must possess to be able to effectively provide services to underserved communities abroad?

Reference

Handal, A. J., Lozoff, B., Breilh, J., & Harlow, S.D. (2007). Sociodemographic and nutritional correlates of neurobehavioral development: A study of young children in a rural region of Ecuador. *Public Health, 21,*292-300.

Resources

Issues facing children In Ecuador. Retrieved May 1, 2013 from www.unicef.org/onfobycountry/ecuador.html

Parkes, M. W., Spiegel, J., Breilh, J., Cabarcas, F., Huish, R., & Yassi, A. (2009). Promoting the health of marginalized populations through international collaboration and educational innovations. *Bulletin World Health Organization, 87,* 312-319.

La Fuente: Community-Based Parent Education and Advocacy Training in Special Education

Cindy DeRuiter, OTD, OTR/L

History and Background Information

Community Organization History

La Fuente is a small, nonprofit, community-based organization serving people with disabilities and their families in a large metropolitan area (Figure 7-6). La Fuente serves people from birth to older adulthood through a variety of programs and services, including youth programming, vocational training, community-based housing options, and family support groups. Many of La Fuente's services focus on strengthening families and equipping parents and caregivers to meet the needs of their child with a disability. This takes the form of providing respite care, parent education and training courses, self-advocacy training, and family support groups.

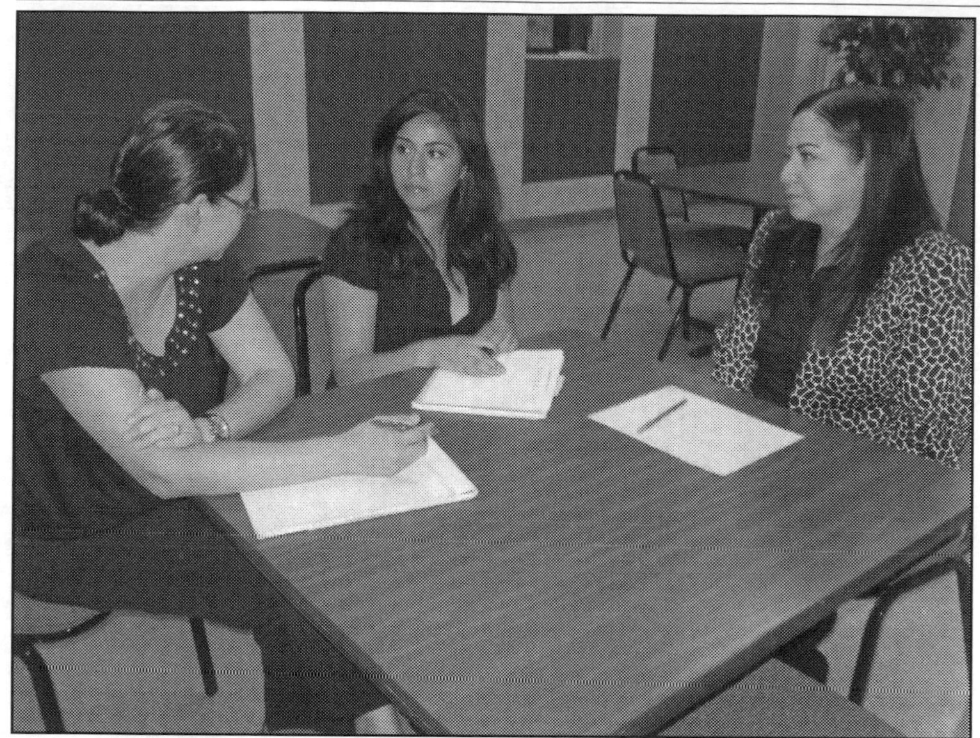

Figure 7-7. Parents expressing a desire to receive education and training in special education policy.

La Fuente is rooted in the Hispanic community and primarily serves Spanish-speaking clients, though people of all backgrounds are welcomed. La Fuente is located in a predominantly Hispanic neighborhood of a large metropolitan area, where the majority of residents live at or below the poverty level. Most parents living in this neighborhood have not earned their high school diploma or GED, and many speak limited English. In recent years, this neighborhood has been plagued by increasing gang violence and crime. As a whole, this neighborhood is well-organized, with a large network of community and social service organizations, churches, and schools. This neighborhood is built on the rich cultural traditions of its Mexican immigrant population as well as resident-led community rebuilding efforts. La Fuente is a major contributor to strengthening this vibrant neighborhood and providing much needed disability and social services to its residents.

As a community-based nonprofit organization, La Fuente relies on fundraising, donations, and grants to supports its programming. La Fuente often partners with local corporations and universities for research and funding opportunities. Because they do not currently employ an OT on staff, La Fuente frequently draws upon its connections to the local university's OT program for consultative OT services.

Description of Need

Parents involved in La Fuente's youth programs have frequently expressed frustration with the quality of their interactions with professionals in the special education system. They report that they feel misunderstood by school professionals and are often confused and intimidated by the special education process. Parents have shared that they lack knowledge about their rights and the rights of their child under special education policy, and that they know little about how the special education system works. Educational and language barriers present a persistent problem for these parents as well; often, legal documents such as the student's Individualized Education Plan (IEP) and information on Procedural Safeguards (that is, a description of parents' rights and the process of making or challenging educational decisions within the special education system) are not translated into parents' native language, or are written at too high a reading level. Furthermore, these parents tend to feel ill-equipped to express their desires and goals for their child's education and are afraid to ask questions in meetings, largely due to limited English proficiency and a view of themselves as passive participants in the educational decision-making process. Overall, this lack of information, intimidation, and language and educational barriers contribute to a sense of disempowerment and frustration for the families La Fuente serves.

Recently, a group of parents currently participating in La Fuente's respite program have expressed a desire to receive education and training in special education policy so that they can better advocate for their child's right to a free, appropriate public education (Figure 7-7). La Fuente does not currently offer a special education advocacy training program. Administrative staff at La Fuente reached out to the local university's OT program, asking them to design and implement a programmatic intervention that

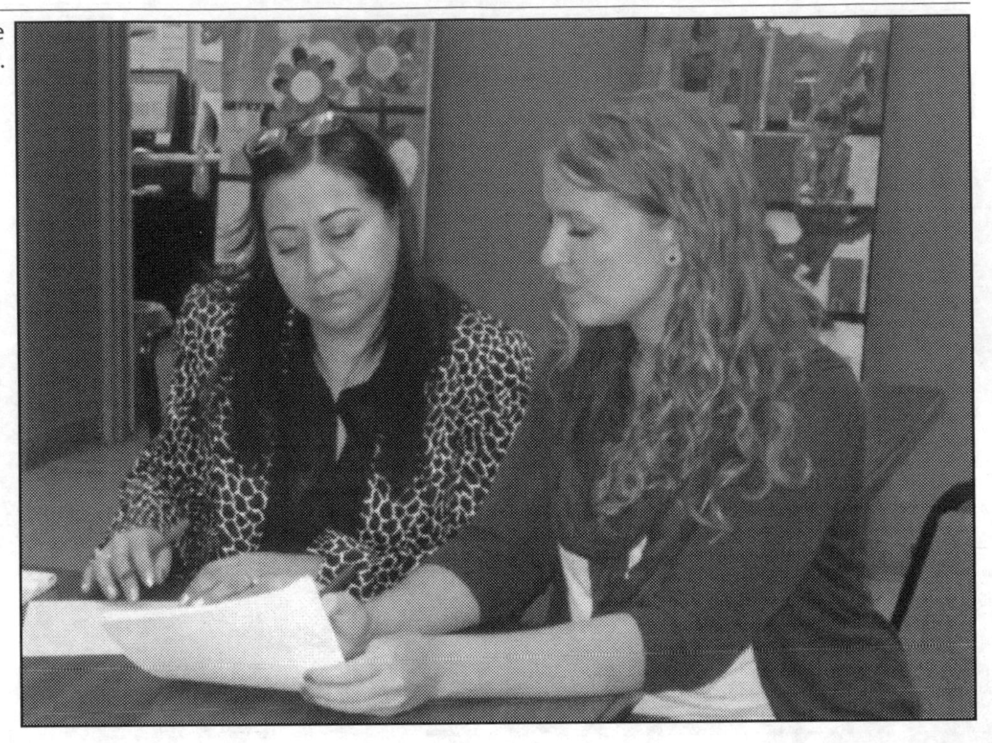

Figure 7-8. Staff at La Fuente want the OT to design a program.

would educate parents and empower them to advocate for their child's educational needs. Staff at La Fuente want the OT to design a programmatic intervention that combines parent education, advocacy training, developing support networks, and knowledge of available disability resources in the community (Figure 7-8).

La Fuente's goals for this intervention are that participating parents will demonstrate the following:

- Improved knowledge of disability and special education policy
- Increased self-efficacy in advocating for the child with a disability in the special education context
- Increased awareness of advocacy networks and disability resources in the community and online

In the long run, staff at La Fuente hope that participants in the program will have improved access to quality education for their child with a disability, and that they will feel they are empowered, capable, and knowledgeable advocates.

Evaluation Information

Literature Review

The OT assigned to the case conducted a brief review of literature on common special education issues faced by families like the ones served by La Fuente. She found that families from diverse backgrounds, like the ones La Fuente serves, are often marginalized and underprepared to interact with professionals in the special education system. These parents are often confused, overwhelmed, and underinformed about how the special education system is structured and what their rights are within that system (Cheatham, Hart, Malian, & McDonald, 2012; Reiman, Beck, Coppola, & Engiles, 2010). Language and cultural barriers pose a significant problem to parent-school interactions; parents often feel misunderstood, intimidated, or ill-equipped to ask questions and give input about their desires for their child's education (Burke, 2013; Lo, 2008). In addition, many teachers do not receive cultural competency training to help them deal with families who come from diverse backgrounds (Murray, Handyside, Straka, & Arton-Titus, 2013). Finally, both parents and school professionals have great demands placed on their time and resources that prevent them from being able to fully engage with one another in the educational decision-making process (Gershwin Mueller, Milian, & Lopez, 2009).

Program Review

The OT also conducted a review of existing family advocacy training and special education programs available in the area, as well as available disability and family support resources. She found that several programs exist that partially meet the requirements La Fuente has set forth for this intervention. Some local organizations offer classes to help parents understand special education policy. Some advocacy groups provide training to help parents develop communication skills. Other organizations provide parents with links to legal aid and dispute resolution services specific to special education cases. The OT found that, while each of these programs serves its purpose well, there is

Table 7-2

Results From a Demographic Survey

Participant's Age		*Education*		*Language Spoken/Read*		*Child's Age*		*Child's Diagnosis*	
18 to 24	2	Less than high school	4	Spanish only	7	3 to 5	3	Autism/developmental delay	4
25 to 34	2	High school diploma/GED	3	English only	0	6 to 8	4	Intellectual disability	2
35 to 44	5	Some college/vocational training	1	Bilingual	3	8 to 10	2	Physical/orthopedic impairment (e.g., muscular dystrophy)	2
45 to 54	1	Bachelor's degree	2	Other	0	11 to 13	1	Learning disability/ADHD	2

Note: This survey was conducted by the occupational therapist. Data reflect results from 10 parents of children with disabilities who will participate in the intervention.

currently no program in place that combines all three elements (education, advocacy training, and resource finding and networking) that La Fuente requires. The OT plans to meet with potential participants to conduct an informal survey of their needs and desires in order to guide her in developing this programmatic intervention.

Demographic Survey

To familiarize herself with the 10 parents who would be involved in this program, the OT conducted a brief demographic survey prior to creating the program. Results of this demographic survey are found in Table 7-2.

Concerns Report Method

To evaluate the needs of La Fuente's families, the OT used a concerns report method (Fawcett, 1993). A concerns report method is a tool for involving participants in a community or program in identifying, prioritizing, and addressing concerns. After discussing their experiences and frustrations with the special education system, parents listed and prioritized their top areas of concern related to the special education advocacy process. Families' top concerns are as follows:

- Difficulty communicating with school personnel
- Lack of information about programming and services the school offers
- Lack of options for special recreation in the community
- Professionals' negative attitudes toward the child and/or family
- Lack of follow-through on implementing the IEP

Parent Goal Setting

Before participating in the program, families were asked to reflect on their experiences in special education and set education and advocacy goals for themselves. After discussing their experiences, issues, and frustrations with one another, each parent set a goal for him- or herself regarding special education advocacy. Examples of goals parents set include the following:

- Learning how the special education system is structured and which professionals provide which services
- Understanding how special education teachers are trained
- Improving written and verbal communication skills in order to discuss issues with school professionals
- Becoming familiar with the legal process for handling educational conflicts

Program Design

Based on the above information, the OT will design an interactive four-session intervention with the following 3 components covered:

1. Parent education. The OT will educate parents on special education policy, their rights under the Individuals with Disabilities Education Act (IDEA), and how the special education system is structured.
2. Advocacy training. Parents engaged in hands-on advocacy training, practicing their skills using case studies and role-playing activities.
3. Networking and resource finding. The OT introduced parents to disability and advocacy resources in their

community and provided opportunities for parents to network with representatives from other community disability organizations.

The OT plans to incorporate interactive activities throughout the program. In addition, the OT plans to build in ample time for self-reflection to help parents track their progress and understand the new role they will take on as advocates. She will provide opportunities for parents to "check in" on their goals and progress during each session.

Questions to Consider

1. Why is it appropriate for an OT to develop this program?
2. What considerations must the OT take into account when working with this population?
3. What resources and supports are needed for this program?
4. What considerations must the OT take into account when working with a nonprofit community organization?
5. Why is it important to review background literature and information on existing programs?
6. What factors should the OT consider when developing content for this program?
7. Are there any resources the OT can draw from to help her develop program content?
8. What information do parents need to know about the special education system?
9. What component skills are necessary for parents to develop in order to advocate for their child's education?
10. What resources might be helpful to parents interacting with the special education system?
11. What theories should the OT draw upon to help her develop this intervention?
12. How can the OT measure participants' progress?
13. How might the OT be able to support parents on this journey after the intervention concludes?
14. What are some potential challenges participants may encounter when participating in this program? What are some challenges the OT may encounter?

References

Burke, M. M. (2013). Improving parental involvement: Training special education advocates. *Journal of Disability Policy Studies, 23*, 225-235.

Cheatham, G. A., Hart, J. E., Malian, I., & McDonald, J. (2012). Six things to never say or hear during an IEP meeting: Educators as advocates for families. *Teaching Exceptional Children, 44*(3), 50-57.

Fawcett, S. B. (1993). *Concerns report handbook: Planning for community health.* Lawrence, KS: University of Kansas.

Gershwin Mueller, T., Milian, M.M., & Lopez, M. I. (2009). Latina mothers' views of a parent-to-parent support group in the special education system. *Research & Practice for Persons with Severe Disabilities, 34*(3-4), 112-122.

Lo, L. (2008). Chinese families' level of participation and experiences in IEP meetings. *Preventing School Failure, 53*(1), 21-27.

Murray, M. M., Handyside, L. M., Straka, L. A., & Arton-Titus, T. V. (2013). Parent empowerment: Connecting with preservice special education teachers. *School Community Journal, 23*(1), 145-168.

Reiman, J. W., Beck, L., Coppola, T., & Engiles, A. (2010). *Parents' experiences with the IEP process: Considerations for improving practice.* Eugene, OR: Center for Appropriate Dispute Resolution in Special Education (CADRE).

Resource

Jackson, L. (Ed.). *Occupational therapy services for children and youth under IDEA* (3rd ed.). Bethesda, MD: AOTA Press.

Carlos: Duchenne Muscular Dystrophy/Hospice

Wanda Mahoney, PhD, OTR/L

History and Background Information

Carlos, age 16 years, has a diagnosis of Duchenne muscular dystrophy (DMD), mild intellectual disability, scoliosis (spinal fusion surgery with metal rods 4 years ago), heart arrhythmia (managed well with digoxin medication), and pneumonia with recent tracheostomy and oxygen.

Carlos lives with his mother, father, and 12-year-old sister, Ana, in a one-story, 1200-square-foot house with three bedrooms and one bathroom in a large metropolitan area in the Midwest. The family speaks Spanish and English fluently. Carlos's mother and father are originally from Guatemala, although they have lived in the United States for over 20 years. His father works in an office and has increased the number of hours he works to try to cover increased health care costs. His mother is his primary caregiver; she has rheumatoid arthritis and reports that caring for Carlos has been increasingly difficult with her pain and his decreasing abilities. She reports that using the Hoyer lift has become very difficult. She also reports being increasingly anxious and upset about her son's declining health and impending death, her own struggles with her physical health, her daughter becoming increasingly withdrawn, her husband being away from home longer, and concerns about the family's finances.

The family made modifications to their home 5 years ago to accommodate Carlos's wheelchair (ramp into home, widened doorways). The bathroom is rather small, so Carlos transfers to the Hoyer lift prior to entering the bathroom. They have an older wheelchair-accessible van that they use to transport Carlos in the community.

Medical History

Carlos was admitted to the hospital 1 month ago for pneumonia. While there, he had tracheostomy surgery and was discharged from hospital to home with hospice services due to DMD with pneumonia complications. His hospice services include an aide three times per week, nursing once a week, and social work twice a month. OT frequency is to be determined.

In order to qualify for hospice services, an individual's physician has to certify that the patient is expected to have less than 6 months to live and no curative treatment will be provided (AOTA, 2011).

Carlos has private insurance through his father's employer. The hospice benefit follows Medicare regulations, but cost is associated with amount of services (not a flat rate), and the family is responsible for 20% of the cost of services.

Carlos currently has a power wheelchair with specialized seating system and joystick controls, Hoyer lift with manual controls, and a specialized bathing/toileting chair. He has an oxygen tank in a bag on the back of his wheelchair with tubing connected to a mask on his track with an elastic band around the neck.

The hospital team recommended a Hoyer lift with electronic controls, although it may take up to a month for insurance approval and to receive the equipment.

Educational History

Carlos attended a local high school until his hospitalization for pneumonia 1 month ago. He participated in general education courses with modifications to reading material, a computer activated with a specialized switch (joystick similar to wheelchair control), and an aide to assist with transfers for toileting. He reads at approximately a fifth-grade level. Once he is discharged home, he will have a teacher providing educational services at home for 2 hours per day.

Referral Process

When preparing for discharge from the hospital, Carlos and his family met with the hospice care intake coordinator to discuss hospice services and what Carlos's doctor had recommended. The family was concerned about finances, and although they wanted to make sure that Carlos was comfortable and his mother had help with caregiving, they were also concerned about the costs of multiple services. They determined that they wanted to start with the aide three times a week and consider increasing the frequency in the future. They wanted the nurse to only come once a week to monitor Carlos's respiratory status and health. Because of the family stress, the coordinator recommended social work services, and the family agreed to twice a month. Carlos expressed concern about what he was going to do at home all day and how he didn't want to be babied by all these people coming to the house. The coordinator said that this may be something that OT could address, and if the family agreed, she would bring it up with Carlos's doctor. Carlos's doctor provided an OT referral to "evaluate and treat" with hospice services.

During a team discussion prior to the first home visits, the nurse told the OT that the aide assigned to Carlos has only worked with older adults. The nurse planned to talk to the aide prior to her first visit about what may be different working with an adolescent and asked for assistance training the aide on specific concerns related to Carlos.

Occupational Therapy Evaluation

The OT visited the home on the day after Carlos was discharged from the hospital. The OT planned to determine Carlos's and the family's priorities, safety with transfers and other physically demanding aspects of care, key areas of occupational performance that Carlos would like to address, and possible adaptations to enable ongoing participation in desired occupations. The OT did not plan to administer any formal assessments, rather the OT planned to interview Carlos and his mother and observe performance in identified areas of concern. Because the mother had previously indicated concerns with using the Hoyer lift, the OT explicitly planned to assess safety with transfers.

When the OT arrived, Carlos was sitting in his wheelchair watching television. He reported that he has not seen any of his friends since being admitted to the hospital. He reported that he has not been able to keep in contact with them because he does not have a switch to use the computer at home and he feels weird that he hasn't been on Facebook in over a month. He reports that he likes watching sports, especially basketball and soccer. He reports that he played wheelchair soccer through last summer, and he played wheelchair basketball until about 2 years ago.

He reports that he is angry that it looks like he's going to die at 16. He said, "I always knew I would die young. That's part of my condition. But I should have made it to my 20s. They say that people live until their 20s with Duchenne's or even longer. I've never even had a girlfriend." He reports being worried about his mom also. He said that he knows this is so hard on her and her health is getting worse too. He said that he tries to do what he can, but it is a struggle. "Me going to the bathroom is really hard for her. I try to hold it as long as I can. It's hard because if I hold it too long, I could have an accident, which means she has to clean me up, which is even more work than taking me to the bathroom."

Carlos needs full assistance for all ADLs, which his mother provides. He reports that he could brush his teeth and feed himself (making a mess) up until about 1 year ago, but then he got too weak to lift his hand to his mouth. He explained, "I still choose my clothes and want to do what I can. My mom tries to baby me too much, and it doesn't help that she has to feed me and stuff like I was a baby. I want to do my own thing, but I can't. I can't even drive my wheelchair if my hand falls off the controls. I can only listen to music or watch TV if someone else turns it on for me. I want headphones when I listen to music so that I have at least some privacy. Privacy—that's really hard to come by. And any kind of control, too. I want a little control and say about what's going on with me."

Carlos eats soft foods safely, at a slow pace, with someone (usually his mother) feeding him. He drives his wheelchair throughout the house, except for the bathroom, independently. However, he does not have sufficient strength to lift his forearm against gravity, so he needs full assistance to place his hand on the joystick of his wheelchair. He has full head movement and some shoulder/scapular elevation, but little additional voluntary movement against gravity. He has some movement of his arms in gravity-eliminated planes. He has no voluntary movement of his lower extremities. He has full, intact sensation in upper and lower extremities and in his face. He talks slowly and stops every few minutes for what he calls a "breathing break."

Carlos' mother reported that she's having trouble figuring out how to keep the new oxygen tubing out of the way during transfers. The OT requested that Carlos and his mother demonstrate a transfer using the Hoyer lift. Carlos' mother breathed heavily and groaned while pumping the Hoyer lift up from a standing/leaning position. The oxygen tubing was positioned behind and around her so she had to crawl under the tubing once Carlos was out of his chair. She lifted the oxygen off the wheelchair and carried it by placing the strap on her shoulder and pushing the Hoyer lift toward the bathroom. She said, "as long as he is up, let's go to the bathroom." Carlos' mother groaned when she worked to pull down Carlos's sweatpants and boxer shorts. Carlos did not speak during the transfer. He said he was ok when positioned on the specialized toilet seat with a chest strap, and his mother stayed in the bathroom until Carlos said that he was done. Carlos' mother was sweating and her face was red when they came out of the bathroom. The OT transferred Carlos back to his wheelchair. Carlos was unable to state the steps to direct the OT to place him back in his wheelchair, although he did let the OT know when he was not properly lined up when seated in his wheelchair. He talked and used his eyes to point to the way he needed to go and did not correctly identify "right" and "left."

Questions to Consider

Personal Reflection

1. What are your own feelings about dying and end of life services? What is your idea of a "good death"? Are your feelings about dying and death different when considering children and adolescents dying? How would you address your own feelings so they did not interfere with the services you provided?
2. Consider that this case presents an unusual situation for the OT. If OTs typically provide services through hospice, they do not often work with children or adolescents. If OTs typically work with children and/or adolescents, they are not usually providing hospice services. Consider what difficulties an OT who typically works in hospice may experience with this case. Consider what difficulties an OT who typically works with adolescents may experience with this case.
3. As the OT in this case, what would you do if Carlos died before being discharged from OT services? Consider both the practical and psychological implications.

Priorities and Treatment Focus

1. What would be the most important things for the OT to address with Carlos? How does the setting of hospice impact what the OT would address?
2. How could the OT address Carlos's self-determination and desire for any privacy and control in his life? Explain why this would be important to address and how the OT could bring up these concerns with the family in a respectful manner.
3. Should the OT address Carlos's mother's difficulty using the Hoyer lift even though a new one has been ordered? Explain why or why not.
4. What assistive technology would help Carlos participate more fully in the activities that he is interested in? What funding sources or equipment loan programs may be available to obtain this equipment? Keep in mind how long the funding approval process usually takes.
5. What would you expect to be the duration of OT services? Explain your rationale. How would the OT determine the appropriate time to discharge Carlos from services?

Clinical Rationale

1. Would it be appropriate for the OT to attempt to remediate Carlos's issue with right/left discrimination? Explain why or why not.

2. How should the OT collaborate with the teacher who will be providing home-based education services?
3. How would you expect Carlos's mild intellectual disability to impact OT services at home?
4. How could an OT address Carlos's lack of interaction with his friends? Consider his barriers to electronic communication and how the OT could most easily address them.

Safety Precautions

1. What safety precautions would the OT need to take related to Carlos's spinal fusion surgery? Who would the OT need to train about these precautions?
2. What other precautions does the OT need to consider?

Reference

American Occupational Therapy Association. (2011). The role of occupational therapy in end-of-life care. *American Journal of Occupational Therapy, 65*(Suppl.), S66-S75. doi: 10.5014/ajot.2011.65

Resources

Bendixen, R., Senesac, C., Lott, D., & Vandenborne, K. (2012). Participation and quality of life in children with Duchenne muscular dystrophy using the International Classification of Functioning, Disability, and Health. *Health and Quality of Life Outcomes, 10*, 43-52. doi:10.1186/1477-7525-10-43

Centers for Disease Control and Prevention Muscular Dystrophy information: http://www.cdc.gov/ncbddd/musculardystrophy/index.html

Muscular Dystrophy Association information: http://mda.org/

Penner, L., Cantor, R., & Siegel, L. (2010). Joseph's wishes: Ethical decision-making in Duchenne muscular dystrophy. *The Mount Sinai Journal of Medicine, New York, 77*(4), 394-397. doi:10.1002/msj.20196

Simonds, A. (2004). Living and dying with respiratory failure: Facilitating decision making. *Chronic Respiratory Disease, 1*(1), 56-59. doi: 10.1191/1479972304cd014

Financial Disclosures

Deborah K. Anderson has no financial or proprietary interest in the materials presented herein.

Erin Anderson has no financial or proprietary interest in the materials presented herein.

Michelle Bednarek has no financial or proprietary interest in the materials presented herein.

Dr. Ann Aviles de Bradley has no financial or proprietary interest in the materials presented herein.

Jennifer Bobo has no financial or proprietary interest in the materials presented herein.

Dr. Patricia Bowyer has no financial or proprietary interest in the materials presented herein.

Dr. Kimberly Bryze has no financial or proprietary interest in the materials presented herein.

Dr. Susan M. Cahill has no financial or proprietary interest in the materials presented herein.

Kendall Carithers has no financial or proprietary interest in the materials presented herein.

Molly Chopper has no financial or proprietary interest in the materials presented herein.

Sara Clark has no financial or proprietary interest in the materials presented herein.

Jennifer Clone has no financial or proprietary interest in the materials presented herein.

Dr. Cindy DeRuiter has no financial or proprietary interest in the materials presented herein.

Brittany Diasio has no financial or proprietary interest in the materials presented herein.

Brooke Nicole Dudley has no financial or proprietary interest in the materials presented herein.

Dr. Brad E. Egan has no financial or proprietary interest in the materials presented herein.

Dr. Robin Elaine Fogerty has no financial or proprietary interest in the materials presented herein.

Rachel Galant has no financial or proprietary interest in the materials presented herein.

Marvieann Garcia-Rodriguez has no financial or proprietary interest in the materials presented herein.

Mary J. Greer has no financial or proprietary interest in the materials presented herein.

Dr. Monica Griffin has no financial or proprietary interest in the materials presented herein.

Jamie Harmon has no financial or proprietary interest in the materials presented herein.

Brianne N. Heiland has no financial or proprietary interest in the materials presented herein.

Susanne Higgins has no financial or proprietary interest in the materials presented herein.

Jennifer J. Hofherr has no financial or proprietary interest in the materials presented herein.

Eric Howard has no financial or proprietary interest in the materials presented herein.

Patricia W. Ideran has no financial or proprietary interest in the materials presented herein.

Dr. Sonia F. Kay has no financial or proprietary interest in the materials presented herein.

Elizabeth Kohler-Rausch has no financial or proprietary interest in the materials presented herein.

Dr. Mark Kovic has no financial or proprietary interest in the materials presented herein.

Maureen Connors Lenke has no financial or proprietary interest in the materials presented herein.

M. Veronica Llerena has no financial or proprietary interest in the materials presented herein.

Lisa Mahaffey has no financial or proprietary interest in the materials presented herein.

Dr. Wanda Mahoney has no financial or proprietary interest in the materials presented herein.

Thelma Haydee Montemayor has no financial or proprietary interest in the materials presented herein.

Agnieszka Moroni has no financial or proprietary interest in the materials presented herein.

Lauro A. Munoz has no financial or proprietary interest in the materials presented herein.

Dr. Jennifer Nash has no financial or proprietary interest in the materials presented herein.

Dr. Roberta K. O'Shea has no financial or proprietary interest in the materials presented herein.

Dr. Dana Pais has no financial or proprietary interest in the materials presented herein.

Dr. Kris Pizur-Barnekow has no financial or proprietary interest in the materials presented herein.

Dr. Gail A. Poskey has no financial or proprietary interest in the materials presented herein.

Kiley Rich has no financial or proprietary interest in the materials presented herein.

Heather Roberts has no financial or proprietary interest in the materials presented herein.

Lisa Robken has no financial or proprietary interest in the materials presented herein.

Jennifer Schmidt has no financial or proprietary interest in the materials presented herein.

Dr. Sally W. Schultz has no financial or proprietary interest in the materials presented herein.

Dr. Angela R. Shierk has no financial or proprietary interest in the materials presented herein.

Dr. Ashley Stoffel has no financial or proprietary interest in the materials presented herein.

Meghan Suman has no financial or proprietary interest in the materials presented herein.

Joanna Swanton has no financial or proprietary interest in the materials presented herein.

Carly Thom has no financial or proprietary interest in the materials presented herein.

Dr. Minetta Wallingford has no financial or proprietary interest in the materials presented herein.

Dr. Leon Washington has no financial or proprietary interest in the materials presented herein.

Susan Wendel has no financial or proprietary interest in the materials presented herein.

Melissa Williamson has no financial or proprietary interest in the materials presented herein.

Mickenzie Wilson has no financial or proprietary interest in the materials presented herein.

Dr. Kristin Winston has no financial or proprietary interest in the materials presented herein.

Meagan E. Wisniewski has no financial or proprietary interest in the materials presented herein.

Jennifer L. Ziemann has no financial or proprietary interest in the materials presented herein.

Index

activity therapy group, for bipolar disorder, 148-150
acute myeloid leukemia, with complications, 123-126
ADHD (attention deficit hyperactivity disorder), autism with, 48-54
adjustment disorder, anxiety with, 89-92
Adolescent Leisure Interest Profile, for depression, 138-144
Adolescent/Adult Sensory Profile, for anxiety, 153-154
aggressive behavior
  in adopted child, 136-138
  in school, 54-56
Alberta Infant Motor Scale, 11-12
amputation, left lower, 163-166
amyoplasia multiplex congenita, 128-131
ankle foot orthosis
  for cerebral palsy, 59-66
  for spina bifida, 120-123
Ansell-Casey Life Skill Assessment, for posttraumatic stress disorder, 150-153
anxiety and anxiety disorder, 153-154
  adjustment disorder with, 89-92
art projects, for cerebral palsy, 69-72
asthma, anoxic brain injury from, 155-158
attention deficit hyperactivity disorder, autism with, 48-54
auditory hypersensitivity, 93-98
autism
  ADHD with, 48-54
  feeding disorder with, 106-108, 127-128
  in private school setting, 72-76

balance
  in anoxic brain injury, 155-158
  in CHARGE syndrome, 103-106
  in traumatic brain injury, 110-114
Beery VIM test, 54-56
behavioral disorders, after child abuse, 84-88
bipolar disorder, in middle school, 54-56, 148-150
brain injury
  anoxic, 155-158
  traumatic, 110-114
brain tumor surgery sequelae, 98-101
bronchopulmonary dysplasia, 9-12, 13-16
burn rehabilitation, 163-166

Canadian Occupational Performance Measure
  for amyoplasia multiplex congenita, 128-131
  for autism, 106-108
Canadian Occupational Performance Measure, for anxiety, 153-154
cardiac myopathy, after leukemia treatment, 123-126
caregiver education, for caring of disabled family members, 166-170
cerebral palsy
  consultative services in, 79-81
  hand difficulties in, 59-66
  hemiplegia in, 69-72
cervical spinal cord injury
  in four year old, 117-119
  in teenager, 131-134
CHARGE syndrome, 28, 103-106
chemotherapy, for leukemia, 123-126
child abuse
  neuromotor sequelae of, 84-88
  posttraumatic stress disorder after, 150-153
Child Occupational Self-Assessment (COSA)
  for cerebral palsy, 59-66
  for Down syndrome, 76-79

Children's Orientation and Amnesia Test, in traumatic brain injury, 110-114
cognitive impairment, in private school setting, 72-76
cognitive skills, in autism, 72-76
communication
  in cerebral palsy, 59-66
  in CHARGE syndrome, 103-106
  in sensory processing disorder, 40-45
community settings, 155-173
  anoxic brain injury, 155-158
  burn rehabilitation, 163-166
  depression, 138-144
  Duchenne muscular dystrophy hospice care, 170-173
  hippotherapy, 155-158
  La Fuente organization for parent education, 166-170
  left lower amputation, 163-166
  Opening Doors organization, 158-163
complex regional pain syndrome, 114-117
computer skills
  in autism, 72-76
  in complex regional pain syndrome, 114-117
  in emotional disturbance, 54-56
concerns report method, in La Fuente program, 166-170
conduct disorder, after child abuse, 84-88
congenital erosive and vesicular dermatosis, 144-148
consultative services, for cerebral palsy, 79-81
contusions, of brain, 110-114
cooking classes, for developmentally disabled people, 158-163
coordination, in CHARGE syndrome, 103-106
corpus callosum, agenesis of, 31-33

dating skills training program, Jefferson Union High School, 82-84
depression, 138-144
developmental delay
  in congenital erosive and vesicular dermatosis, 144-148
  in corpus callosum agenesis, 31-33
  educational organization for, 158-163
  hip dysplasia with, 38-40
  sensory processing disorder with, 40-45
Developmental Test of Visual-Motor Integration, for child abuse sequelae, 84-88
Disruptive Mood Dysregulation Disorder, 136-138
Down syndrome, 76-79
dressing
  in autism, 72-76
  in CHARGE syndrome, 103-106
  in spina bifida, 114-117
  in spinal cord injury, 117-119
Duchenne muscular dystrophy, hospice care for, 170-173
dyspraxia, 33-37

early intervention, 25-45
  congenital erosive and vesicular dermatosis, 144-148
  corpus callosum agenesis, 31-33
  description of, 25-26
  developmental delay
    hip dysplasia with, 26-30, 38-40
    sensory processing disorder with, 40-45
  dyspraxia, 33-37
  goals of, 25
  mental health, 144-148
  natural environment concept in, 25
  occupational therapy role in, 26
  sensory dysmodulation, 33-37
Ecuador, burn patient rehabilitation in, 163-166
emotional control
  in CHARGE syndrome, 103-106
  in premature infant, 16-21
emotional disturbance
  after child abuse, 84-88
  in middle school, 54-56
environment, for cerebral palsy, 59-66
equipment
  for CHARGE syndrome, 103-106
  for complex regional pain syndrome, 114-117
  for cooking, 158-163

failure to thrive, in sensory processing disorder, 40-45
feeding problems
  in amyoplasia multiplex congenita, 128-131
  in autism, 72-76, 106-108, 127-128
  in CHARGE syndrome, 103-106
  in congenital erosive and vesicular dermatosis, 144-148
  in corpus callosum agenesis, 31-33
  in developmental delay, 26-30
  in Duchenne muscular dystrophy, 170-173
  in motor disorder, 101-103
  in premature infant, 9-12, 13-16, 16-21, 21-24
  sensory dysmodulation with, 33-37
  in sensory processing disorder, 40-45
foster care, of former child abuse victim, 84-88
Full Individual Evaluation, for autism, 72-76
Functional Independence Measure for Children (WeeFIM), after traumatic brain injury, 110-114

gastroesophageal reflux, in premature infant, 9-12
Gilliam Autism Rating Scale, 48-54
glioblastoma multiforme, sequelae of, 98-101
global mental functions/, in traumatic brain injury, 110-114
group therapy, for bipolar disorder, 148-150

habituation
  in cerebral palsy, 59-66
  problems with, in sensory processing disorder, 40-45
hand
  amyoplasia multiplex congenita impact on, 128-131
  complex regional pain syndrome in, 114-117
handwashing habits, in autism, 72-76
Hawaii Early Learning Profile
  for autism and ADHD, 48-54
  for developmental delay, 38-40
hearing impairment, in CHARGE syndrome, 103-106
heart, congenital defects of
  corpus callosum agenesis with, 31-33
  in Down syndrome, 76-79
  in premature infant, 9-12, 13-16
hemiparesis/hemiplegia
  after brain tumor surgery, 98-101
  in cerebral palsy, 59-66, 69-72
  after traumatic brain injury, 110-114
hemorrhagic contusions, of brain, 110-114
hip dysplasia, developmental delay with, 26-30, 38-40
hippotherapy, for brain injury, 155-158
HIV/AIDS prevention program, 82-84
horses, therapeutic use of, for brain injury, 155-158
hospice care, for Duchenne muscular dystrophy, 170-173
hospital-based settings, 109-134
  amyoplasia multiplex congenita, 128-131
  anxiety disorder, 153-154
  autism, 127-128
  complex regional pain syndrome, 114-117
  description of, 109
  leukemia with complications, 123-126
  posttraumatic stress disorder, 150-153
  spina bifida, 120-123
  spinal cord injury
    in four year old, 117-119
    in teenager, 131-134
  traumatic brain injury, 110-114
Hoyer lift, for wheelchair, 170-173
hypersensitivity, sensory processing disorder with, 93-98

IDEA. *See* Individuals with Disabilities Education Act (IDEA)
IEP. *See* Individualized Education Program (IEP)
IFSP. *See* Individualized Family Service Plan (IFSP)
impulsivity, in adjustment disorder, 89-92
Individualized Education Program (IEP)
  for autism, 48-54
  description of, 47
  for Down syndrome, 76-79
  in La Fuente program, 166-170
  team for, 47-48
Individualized Family Service Plan (IFSP), 25-26
  for autism, 48-54
  for CHARGE syndrome, 103-106
  for congenital erosive and vesicular dermatosis, 144-148
Individuals with Disabilities Education Act (IDEA), 25-26
  corpus callosum agenesis, 32
  description of, 47
  least restrictive environment in, 47
  occupational therapy role in, 48
Infant and Toddler Sensory Profile, for autism, 106-108
Infant-Toddler Sensory Profile, 33-37
inpatient settings. *See* hospital-based settings
intellectual disabilities, after child abuse, 84-88

Jefferson Union High School District, sexuality and dating skills training program of, 82-84

knee-ankle-foot orthosis, for amyoplasia multiplex congenita, 128-131

La Fuente organization, for parent education, 166-170
leaf printing, for cerebral palsy, 69-72
learning disability, 67-69
least restrictive environment, in IDEA, 47
leukemia, with complications, 123-126

mental health settings, 135-154
  aggression, 136-138
  anxiety disorder, 153-154
  bipolar disorder, 148-150
  depression, 138-144
  Disruptive Mood Dysregulation Disorder, 136-138
  early intervention for infant, 144-148
  occupational therapy role in, 135
  posttraumatic stress disorder, 150-153
mitochondrial disorder, motor disorder from, 101-103
Model of Human Occupation
  for cerebral palsy, 59-66
  for leukemia patient, 123-126
Modified Ashworth Scale, in traumatic brain injury, 110-114
motor delay, with sensory processing disorder, 89-92
motor disorder, 101-103
motor skills
  in autism, 72-76
  in cerebral palsy, 59-66
  in CHARGE syndrome, 103-106
  in motor delay, 89-92
  in sensory processing disorder, 40-45
movement disorders, in premature infant, 16-21
muscular dystrophy, hospice care for, 170-173
myelomeningocele, 120-123

natural environment concept, in IDEA, 25
neonatal intensive care unit, 1-24
  occupational therapy role in, 1-2
  prematurity
    25 weeks gestation, 9-12, 13-16, 21-24
    29 weeks gestation, 2-9
    32 weeks gestation, 16-21
Neonatal Neurobehavioral Examination, 21-24
Neurodevelopmental and Behavioral Assessment form, for premature infant, 2-9
neuromotor sequelae, of child abuse, 84-88
neuromuscular coordination, in CHARGE syndrome, 103-106
neuromusculoskeletal dysfunction
  after leukemia treatment, 123-126
  in amyoplasia multiplex congenita, 128-131
  in anoxic brain injury, 155-158
  in complex regional pain syndrome, 114-117
  in developmental delay, 158-163
  in mitochondrial disorder, 101-103
  in premature infant, 16-21
  in traumatic brain injury, 110-114

Occupational Self-Assessment
  for depression, 138-144
  for posttraumatic stress disorder, 150-153
Opening Doors organization, for developmental disability education, 158-163
oppositional defiant disorder, in middle school, 54-56
orthosis
  ankle foot
    for cerebral palsy, 59-66
    for spina bifida, 120-123
  hand and forearm, for complex regional pain syndrome, 114-117
  knee-ankle-foot, for amyoplasia multiplex congenita, 128-131
outpatient services, 89-108
  autism, with feeding concerns, 106-108
  brain tumor surgery sequelae, 98-101
  CHARGE syndrome, 103-106
  description of, 89
  motor disorder, 101-103
  sensory processing disorder
    fine motor delay with, 89-92
    hypersensitivity with, 93-98
owl painting, for cerebral palsy, 69-72

pain, complex regional, 114-117
panic attacks, 155-156
parapodium, for spina bifida, 114-117
parent education, for caring of disabled family members, 166-170
Patient Rated Wrist/Hand Evaluation, for complex regional pain, 114-117
Peabody Developmental Motor Scale, 38-40
Peabody Developmental Motor Skills, for sensory processing disorder, 93-98
Peabody Developmental Scales, 33-37
performance skills, in emotional disturbance, 54-56
play, observation of, in sensory dysmodulation, 33-37
play dates, for developmental delay, 26-30
posttraumatic stress disorder, 150-153
prematurity
  25 weeks gestation
    maternal diabetes, 9-12
    neurodevelopmental problems, 21-24
    twin birth, 13-16
  32 weeks gestation, sensory overload, 16-21
  29 weeks gestation, Neurodevelopmental and Behavioral Assessment form for, 2-9
prevocational skills, in autism, 72-76
problem-solving team, for social emotional disabilities, 56-59
process skills
  in cerebral palsy, 59-66
  in sensory processing disorder, 40-45
psychosocial problems, in complex regional pain syndrome, 114-117

radiation therapy, for brain tumor, 98-101
range of motion, of arm and hand, in complex regional pain syndrome, 114-117
Response to Challenge item, in cerebral palsy, 59-66
retinopathy of prematurity, 9-12, 13-16

sand painting, for cerebral palsy, 69-72
school, transition to, in corpus callosum agenesis, 31-33
School Function Assessment, 48-54
  for cerebral palsy, 69-72
  for Down syndrome, 76-79
school systems practice, 47-88. *See also* Individualized Education Act (IDEA)
  autism
    with ADHD, 48-54
    private school setting, 72-76
  bipolar disorder, 148-150
  cerebral palsy
    consultative services in, 79-81
    hand difficulties in, 59-66
    hemiplegia in, 69-72
  child abuse sequelae, 84-88
  Down syndrome, 76-79

emotional disturbance, 54-56
learning disability, 67-69
sexuality training program, 82-84
social emotional disabilities with learning problems, 56-59

SCOPE (Short Child Occupational Profile)
for cerebral palsy, 59-66
for sensory processing disorder, 40-45

sensory dysmodulation, 33-37, 103-106

sensory processing disorder
in CHARGE syndrome, 103-106
developmental delay with, 40-45
fine motor delay with, 89-92
hypersensitivity with, 93-98

Sensory Processing Measure, for motor delay, 89-92

sensory processing skills, in autism, 72-76

Sensory Profile, for sensory processing disorder, 93-98

Sensory Profile Caregiver Questionnaire, for child abuse sequelae, 84-88

Sensory Profile-School Companion, 48-54

septic shock, 123-126

sexuality and dating skills training program, Jefferson Union High School, 82-84

Short Child Occupational Profile (SCOPE)
for cerebral palsy, 59-66
for sensory processing disorder, 40-45

sitting, after leukemia treatment, 123-126

social emotional disabilities, learning problems with, 56-59

social interactions, in sensory processing disorder, 89-92

social skills, in autism, 72-76

spastic hemiparesis, in cerebral palsy, 59-66, 69-72

speech disorders, 33-37
in sensory dysregulation, 33-37
in traumatic brain injury, 110-114

spina bifida, 120-123

spinal cord injury
in four year old, 117-119
in teenager, 131-134

strabismus, developmental delay with, 26-30

Synactive Theory of Behavioral Development, premature infant, 21-24

tactile hypersensitivity, 93-98

Test of Infant Motor Performance, 9-12

Test of Infant Motor Performance Screening Items, 9-12

toileting problems, in autism, 72-76

tracheostomy, for spinal cord injury, 131-134

Transdisciplinary Play-Based Assessment, 33-37

Trauma Symptom Checklist for Children, 150-153

traumatic brain injury, 110-114

Tuck Rehabilitation Hospital, outcome measures of, 110-114

twin, 25 weeks gestation, 13-16

Verbal Behavior Milestone Assessment and Placement Program, 48-54

Vineland Adaptive Behavior Scales, 48-54

visual impairment
in CHARGE syndrome, 103-106
in premature infant, 16-21
in traumatic brain injury, 110-114

volition
in cerebral palsy, 59-66
in sensory processing disorder, 40-45

wheelchair, for spinal cord injury, 117-119

Printed in the United States
by Baker & Taylor Publisher Services